Resilient Relationships

Designed to be used as a companion to couple therapy, this book is based on a trailblazing study of over 1400 individuals. It presents over 75 techniques to help relationships thrive in the long-term and provides insights into the challenges faced by contemporary couples.

Through in-depth interviews, this book takes pertinent questions from young couples and puts them to couples who have been together for decades. The time-tested secrets of thriving couples are presented in a new guise for a new generation. Capturing the effects of the COVID-19 pandemic, the study includes people from 52 countries and is the largest cross-sectional, multinational study on long-term relationships to date. It highlights the dynamic and protective factors that lead to relationship longevity, as well as societal pressures, to guide therapists on how to manage these with their clients. The authors uncover how long-term relationships promote resilience, emotional, mental, and physical health, and protect against loneliness and harmful behaviours.

Therapists and couples need to know what goes right in long-lasting relationships. Providing essential data and practical skills for psychologists, counsellors, and other professionals, this book is a must-read for anyone working with couples to explore and understand what leads to resilient relationships in a harsh, complex world.

Christian Heim, FRANZCP, PhD, is Clinical Director of Tasmania North Mental Health Services, a senior lecturer at the University of Queensland, and a Churchill Fellow who gives keynotes internationally on preventative mental health. In private psychiatry, he subspecialized in war-related and severe childhood sexual trauma, and couple therapy where mental illness is prominent.

Caroline Heim, PhD, is an associate professor at Queensland University of Technology. She has published two books in theatre studies. Caroline gives keynotes internationally, and her numerous articles cover various topics from global audiences to the mental health of her university students. Caroline is a certified Lifeline crisis counsellor and facilitator.

Resilient Relationships

Techniques for Surviving Hyper-individualism, Social Isolation, and a Mental Health Crisis

Christian Heim and Caroline Heim

Routledge
Taylor & Francis Group
LONDON AND NEW YORK

Designed cover image: Kimberly Hollingsworth

First published 2023
by Routledge
4 Park Square, Milton Park, Abingdon, Oxon OX14 4RN

and by Routledge
605 Third Avenue, New York, NY 10158

Routledge is an imprint of the Taylor & Francis Group, an informa business

British Library Cataloguing-in-Publication Data
A catalogue record for this book is available from the British Library

Library of Congress Cataloging-in-Publication Data
Names: Heim, Christian, 1960- author. | Heim, Caroline, author.
Title: Resilient relationships : techniques for surviving hyper-individualism, social isolation, and a mental health crisis / Christian Heim, PhD, Caroline Heim, PhD.
Description: Abingdon, Oxon ; New York, NY : Routledge, 2023. | Includes bibliographical references and index.
Identifiers: LCCN 2022051060 (print) | LCCN 2022051061 (ebook) | ISBN 9781032203928 (hardback) | ISBN 9781032203911 (paperback) | ISBN 9781003263395 (ebook)
Subjects: LCSH: Couples therapy. | Couples therapy—Case studies. | Mentally ill—Family relationships. | Mentally ill—Family relationships—Case studies. | Marital conflict.
Classification: LCC RC488.5 .H43 2023 (print) | LCC RC488.5 (ebook) | DDC 616.89/1562—dc23/eng/20230125
LC record available at https://lccn.loc.gov/2022051060
LC ebook record available at https://lccn.loc.gov/2022051061

ISBN: 9781032203928 (hbk)
ISBN: 9781032203911 (pbk)
ISBN: 9781003263395 (ebk)

DOI: 10.4324/9781003263395

Typeset in Sabon
by Apex CoVantage, LLC

Contents

About the authors

Christian Heim, FRANZCP, PhD is currently Clinical Director of Tasmania North Mental Health Services. He is a consultant psychiatrist in general adult psychiatry who has been in long-term private inpatient and outpatient practice. Christian subspecialized in war-related and severe childhood sexual trauma, and in couple therapy where mental illness is prominent. He is a Senior Lecturer at the University of Queensland and lectures to trainee psychiatrists. He has given keynote addresses internationally. A composer and pianist, previously Christian was a lecturer at several universities in classical music composition. He is a Churchill Fellow having researched the use of music in hospital environments, and is a recipient of the Newton-John Award for creativity in professional practice. His research area is preventative mental health, and in this he publishes and lectures to lawyers, doctors and therapists, university students, and the general public to help avoid burnout, compassion fatigue, mental illness, and to help couples keep their relationships together. Christian and Caroline have worked in theatre, counselling, and performing situations together and are developing an online presence.

Caroline Heim, PhD is an Associate Professor in Theatre at Queensland University of Technology and a global authority on theatre audiences and the psychology of relationships in the theatre. Her first book, Audience as Performer: the changing role of theatre audiences in the twenty-first century (Routledge 2016) is regarded as a leading authority on theatre audiences. Her second book, Actors and Audiences: conversations in the electric air (Routledge 2020) received an Honourable Mention in the Rob Jordan book prize. Caroline gives keynotes internationally, and her numerous articles cover various topics from global audiences to the mental health of her university students. Specializing in empirical research, she has interviewed over 200 actors and audience members internationally. Caroline's PhD (The University of Queensland) explored and trialled a new model for post-performance discussions. In the Creative industries, Education and Social Justice Faculty at QUT she lectures, coordinates courses, and has implemented a mental health program for her students using humour and clowning. Caroline is a certified Lifeline crisis counsellor and facilitator. Caroline and Christian have published and given conference papers together.

www.drchristianheim.com

Acknowledgements

Our sincere thanks go to the wonderfully brave couples who shared so much of their life stories and personal relationship experiences. We are deeply grateful for the generosity of each of the 90 couples we had the privilege of interviewing from many parts of the globe. Thank you for opening up your homes and stories to us.

The interviews would not have been possible to secure without the assistance of the following people who went out of their way to assist in the difficult task of recruiting willing couples or provide research resources: Rob Dunn, Laurel Gray, Michelle Fezza, Donna Burness and Paul Burness, Joy Lawn, Mark Grenning, Robin McKenzie, Marina Tuskan, Phil Mathers, Anne Mills, and Sue Brown. Special thanks goes to Merv Richens, who went above and beyond in helping us find interviewees through his many lifetime Probus connections. Several organizations were pivotal in facilitating the interviews and survey respondents, and we are very thankful for their assistance: Springwood Probus, Hobart Men's Probus, Exeter Probus, Bankstown Probus, Princess Cruises, Association Napolitana, Sydney Bulgarian Cultural and Social Association, the Estonian Society of Sydney and Curious Things.

We would also like to acknowledge our universities: Queensland University of Technology and The University of Queensland. QUT recognized the importance of this research in granting much needed research leave over these past five years. Our editor, Vilija Stephens at Routledge, has provided much enthusiasm and direction from the start and given much appreciated advice. Several readers offered valued critical comments: Dr Peter Devadason, Dr Cynthia Gray, Emma Felton, Peter Driessen, Shardé Heim, and Reuben Heim. The latter two's salty comments and savvy insights often shared over steaming hot chocolates, helped us bridge some generational gaps. A special thank you is due to Shardé for her help with all things technical and to Kimberly Hollingsworth for the metaphorical cover photograph.

Our own relationship would not have the resilience if it were not for enjoying and enduring the pleasures and trials of parenting our two wonderful sons: Benjamin and Reuben. They and supportive family and friends help us bridge the cultural divides in our relationship. Writing this book has been a challenging but deeply gratifying journey that has brought much long-term fulfilment.

Introduction

"How do you overcome the powerful influence of external world issues and their effects on the 'internal world' of your relationship?" This question, from our Surviving COVID-19 Survey, was asked by a person in a committed relationship of 3–5 years. It reveals the struggles of many young couples: needing to negotiate societal pressures which are at odds with their "internal world" and together life-story to build a resilient relationship. This book aims to answer this question and others like it for couples wanting to stay together and thrive amidst today's complexities. It is also for therapists working to help couples through insights gained from couples thriving 40+ years together.

Drawing from the primary evidence of over 1400 coupled individuals, and with consideration of current best evidence and informed by clinical practice, we present techniques and insights for twenty-first century couples wanting to reach relationship longevity amidst the pressures of hyper-individualism, social isolation, and the mental health crisis. Dynamic risk factors become the focus.[1] Static risk factors for divorce and break-up – marrying younger,[2] pre-engagement co-habitation,[3] previous divorce,[4] lower education level,[5] and parental divorce[6] – are unmodifiable for a couple already in relationship. Individual outcomes cannot be predicted,[7] risk factors are not stable over time,[8] and any couple can choose to stay together, as couples we interviewed did, in spite of apparent risks.[9] How did they do it?

Resilient relationships

Resilient couples help each other "adapt and maintain high well-being during stressful life situations"[10] to enhance "we-ness"[11] connection and relationship stability.[12] Resilience is, as we emphasize, steeped in attachment. How attachment underpins relationship resilience to help negotiate adversity is a theoretical focus of this book. Resilience is not random. We argue that choosing to adopt specific values helps strengthen attachment to build resilience. Divorce and separation occur due to one or both partners feeling

DOI: 10.4324/9781003263395-1

that they receive less than they need, or due to poor commitment.[13] Both of these can be mitigated against for those choosing relationship longevity.

Couples need resilience to bounce back from adversity. Hyper-individualism, social isolation, and the mental health crisis are major societal adversities impacting twenty-first century couples. Hyper-individualism appears to pit an individual against a relationship; social isolation is increased through social media and physical distancing to affect people within a household. Mental illness often impedes the effort needed by two to sustain a relationship. Based on clinical experience, these three are the most clinically relevant adversities ubiquitously affecting individuals and couples. Domestic abuse self-evidently harms relationships, and we acknowledge that climate change, political instability, economic hardship, uncertainty, justice inequities, changing gender identities, corruption, and overpopulation also impact relationships.

Literature review

The very wide umbrella of couple research includes couple therapy, couple counselling, relationship education programs, and independent researchers. Psychologists, counsellors, social workers, psychiatrists, academics, and more contribute to and move through several of these and other overlapping strands. Multiple perspectives are valued. Recent advances in neuroscience also impact relationship research, as do theoretical advances in sociology, anthropology, cultural studies, gender studies, evolutionary psychology, and more.

As coupling is a life experience affecting most people and as too many relationships fail,[14] people are desirous of information on this topic. In a haste to bring fresh, vital evidence to the public quickly, however, many complex concepts are over-simplified for social media. Scientific rigour, conceptual intricacies, and subtle problems of real-life applicability of insights can be lost. Best-seller advice may lack sufficient scientific basis and conversely, valid scientific material may not be accepted by the public even if packaged palatably. This is a side-effect of ultra-fast knowledge dissemination. Relationship complexities abound, exceptions abound, and too much remains unknown while new research vistas constantly present themselves.

Couple therapy is situated within family therapy; Lebow et al.'s *Couples Therapy Handbook* (2022) is the most recent authoritative text in this area. Noting the numerous independent researchers, counselling frameworks, and contributors to relationship education programs would be a major study in itself. Science still does not fully understand couple relationships,[15] and complexity in this area is only growing. Gender and sexual diversity, diverse relationships, the impact of religious contexts, and more detailed cultural perspectives, for instance, are yet to be adequately articulated. Varied contributions from myriad researchers aid our understanding. A vast number of studies articulate what contributes to relationship quality and through this assist couples reaching for relationship longevity. Far fewer studies directly consider thriving long-term relationships; our research adds to and serves as an adjunct to these, while adding much-needed context and couples' personal perspectives. This present study asks long-term couples "what keeps your relationship together?" Over the last century, surprisingly few studies have looked at this question with adequate sample sizes.

The first study we found to ask this question was Terman et al.'s study of 1938. Since then, a small number of cross-sectional studies have surveyed long-term couples on marital satisfaction and longevity, some using mixed methodology. Studies in this area are detailed in Chapter 5. Notable among them are Alford-Cooper's 1994 study assessing the marriage longevity of 1152 people married 50+ years and Sharlin et al.'s 1998 rigorous, multinational study assessing the satisfaction of 1220 people married 20+ years; both possibly motivated by the high divorce rates of that decade. Neither, however, contextualized the research within its social climate. Terman's study, for example, is more enlightening when read in conjunction with *Domestic Revolutions*[16] or *Marriage, a History*.[17] Historical contextualizing is relevant in longitudinal studies as societal changes can fast render a rigorous 20-year study obsolete.[18] Finkel's 2017 *The All or Nothing Marriage*, although not founded on an empirical relationship study, gives insightful historical context to its central thesis.

The study on which our book is based adds to the body of knowledge as the largest cross-sectional multi-national study of thriving long-term couples to date. It adds context and theoretical considerations and brings together empirical research, clinical experience, couples' values, consideration of the literature, and relevant aspects of the twenty-first century societal context. We present clinical techniques based on couples' comments and insights.

Study methodology

Background

Our book contains the findings of a cross-sectional study aiming to identify the main contributors to relationship longevity. Interviews of 90 resilient couples, defined as being married for 40+ years, form the core of three study arms. The other two arms are online surveys: one of couples thriving 40+ years, and an online survey of couples together more than three years who experienced COVID-19 lockdown. Qualitative methods were employed to reach deeper insights about participant experiences drawing from the research experience of Dr Caroline Heim:

> I have been conducting qualitative research since 2007: focus groups, semi-structured interviews and participant observation. My PhD developed a new form of focus groups for post-performance discussions in

the theatre[19] largely informed by Carl Rogers's model for group psychotherapy and education. My approach is used in theatres globally[20] and for group facilitation of university tutorials.[21] Its methodology emphasizes audience-centred rather than expert-driven facilitation: a moderator, rather than being an expert, becomes a facilitator privileging the audience voice and their meaning-making over expert-driven ideas.

Through my experience interviewing over 200 actors and audience members in six countries for my last two books,[22] I devised an innovative empirical research methodology for my field. This was of semi-structured interviews and participant observation[23] which was adapted as an over-arching qualitative research approach for this present study. In qualitative research, researcher bias remains problematic; yet, in an effort to remain scientific, studies remain relatively expert-driven in research questions, choice of language, and aims. To help ameliorate this and to ensure reflexivity, I aim to invert the natural expert-participant hierarchy by employing more of a phenomenological approach, emphasizing simple language, and generating questions from couples themselves to reach for more participant-centred research.

Dr Christian Heim and I have previously worked together in theatre and counselling situations. During a COVID-19 lockdown, when my university students were isolating and experiencing escalating mental health issues, we created a mental health program eliciting self-reported questions from university students.[24] Being cognisant of students' needs and approaches, we asked "if you could ask a psychiatrist a question, what would it be?" 241 student questions were answered in Q&A style using online lecture meetings, YouTube videos, Instagram and through podcasts to cater for student preferences in information accessing.

Our qualitative approach here is informed by the above: participant-generated questions, privileging the couple voice, interviews and questions on participants' terms (as far as possible), use of non-technical language, all aiming to understand couples' experiences and meaning-making. These ideals are inherent in qualitative research but we aimed to penetrate further. Our methodology follows best evidence-based practice for family therapy by integrating research evidence, clinical expertize and couple values.[25] Cited studies provide evidence, the study is informed by decades of clinical expertize, and my participant-led approach developed over 15 years of experience aims to faithfully represent couples' values.

Studies on couples most usually take a pathogenic approach by studying risk factors contributing to break-up such as poor communication, conflict, financial distress, behavioural problems, and intimacy issues.[26] Recent evidence, however, shows that improved behaviour and communication, for instance, do not always lead to relationship success,[27] and real-world therapy failure rates remain unacceptably high.[28] Therapists mostly intervene according to evidence on troubled relationships[29] as studies on flourishing relationships are few, dated, are based on relatively small numbers, and have not been contextualized.

To help ameliorate this, our research takes a salutogenic approach[30] to explore what contributes to healthy relationships in couples together 40+ years. Finkel asked, "Can spouses in mediocre marriages learn from those in flourishing marriages?"[31] Having been privy to the enlightening insights of thriving relationships, our answer is an enthusiastic "yes."

Study aim

Our study aimed to capture what thriving couples told us contributed to their relationship longevity. We initially sought to capture this by documenting the lived experiences of thriving couples in in-depth interviews only, supplemented by an online survey of this demographic. The pandemic, however, placed relationships centre-stage for the general population and created an opportunity for us to survey the relationship health of younger couples and their concerns. We were then able to devise a form of intergenerational discourse by asking younger couples (in relationships of 3+ years) what questions they may have for couples thriving 40+ years. These questions provided insight into pressures on younger couples and their relationship aspirations, and were asked in the thriving couples' interviews and survey. Our in-depth interviews prior to the pandemic covered what we thought was pertinent to younger couples, but we made minor adjustments to more fully focus on their questions. Our interview and survey questions[32] were initially based on clinical experience and extant evidence. Through progressive focussing towards "what really matters,"[33] however, questions from younger couples informed our thriving couples' interview and survey significantly.

Study design

Three study arms helped achieve our aim:

1. The Thriving Couples Interviews
2. The Surviving COVID-19 Survey
3. The Married 40+ Years Survey

Consistent with best practice, our study used mixed methodology.[34] In-depth semi-structured interviews, surveys, and participant observation were employed. Semi-structured interviews were chosen for their facility to drill down to what is actually going on in a relationship through open-ended questions and probing. Most studies on long-term couples rely on surveys which cannot probe or identify subtle tone of voice or the "shuffle and fidget"[35] signifying that deeper truths are present or being obfuscated.[36] Surveys cannot prize and validate couple responses to build further trust to facilitate sharing richer, more profound insights. Participant observation, therefore, became important. During each interview, the couple's behaviour towards the interviewer and towards each other was observed: tension, non-verbal signifiers, degrees of felt embarrassment, levels of humour, and more. Following each interview, the interviewer engaged in a de-brief session to recognize and capture the objective observations and subjective impressions.

Recruitment

90 couples married for 40–73 years (average 50 years) were interviewed between 2017 and 2022, representing 24 countries for the Thriving Couples Interviews. Following ethical approval,[37] recruitment commenced in 2017. The inclusion criterion was couples married 40+ years to each other. 'Married' rather than 'co-habitating' was chosen for its precise, measurable definition. Exclusion criteria included significant cognitive impairment in either spouse and an inability to converse in English.[38] Since same-sex marriage laws were in a state of flux, two same-sex couples together 30+ years were included as they had recently married. Recruitment was undertaken as follows:

> Following best practice recommendations of quota sampling,[39] I recruited couples from Probus clubs,[40] retirement villages, cruise ships, and multicultural organizations. To avoid bias, couples were not recruited from religious organizations. A few couples were recommended to me by already interviewed couples or by associates; anyone we personally knew was ineligible. Using approaches from my previous research,[41] we gave talks and seminars on relationships and, to assist recruitment, we asked for volunteers after these. Establishing a presenter-audience pre-relationship built trust to overcome inhibitions and resulted in healthy numbers of volunteers. Contrary to our aims, however, this placed Dr Christian Heim in an expert role, therefore I conducted all interviews. Email, telephone or in-person announcements at organizations yielded little as pre-interview trust had not been established. To ensure a range of ethnicities, I recruited couples from multi-cultural organisations in Sydney, Hobart and Brisbane, Australia. International cruises had an extensive range of countries represented, and diverse ethnicities were actively sought. To ensure diverse socio-economic representation, I contacted Probus clubs from low socio-economic areas and travelled regionally in the Australian states of New South Wales, Queensland and Tasmania to interview couples.

The anonymous online Surviving COVID-19 Survey took place in 2020. The primary inclusion criterion was couples living together in relationship for 3+ years. Couples were recruited through quota and snowball sampling:[42] online Prime Panels and word-of-mouth. Of the 303 completions of the anonymous survey, 13 were excluded due to poor response quality[43] leaving 290 included participants. These represented individuals in relationships of 3+ years from 21 countries representing 37 ethnicities. 63% were female, 36% male, and 1% non-binary.

The anonymous online Married 40+ Years Survey was undertaken in 2022 with the same inclusion and exclusion criteria as the couple interviews. Couples were recruited through quota sampling: Prime Panels and an email list of 250 retirees from cruise ships. There were 1087 completions of the anonymous survey with 155 excluded due to poor response quality leaving 932 included participants. These represented individuals married 40+ years from 47 countries and 81 ethnicities. 56% were female and 44% male. Household income for these participants before retiring was:

Less than $25,000	13.58%
$25,000 - $50,000	31.07%
$50,000 - $100,000	34.41%
$100,000 - $200,000	12.54%
More than $200,000	1.73%
I prefer not to say	6.67%

Cumulatively, 1402 individuals in long-term relationships from 52 countries were interviewed or surveyed making this the largest cross-sectional, multi-national study of long-term relationships to date.

Data collection: interviews and surveys

The 90 face-to-face[44] interviews took between 45 and 120 minutes and (with informed consent) were audio-recorded. Only first names were used in the book. Although much sensitive material was shared, only 5 couples choose to use pseudonyms. Interviews were conducted in private homes, coffee shops, or in privately hired or arranged rooms in retirement villages or on cruise ships. Interviews, transcribed verbatim, generated 450,147 words. Following an iterative approach, questions were adjusted to reach for an optimum insight yield. Saturation of content was apparent by the last half-dozen interviews.[45] A single interviewer was used:

> To help preserve a more couples-led approach, I interviewed all the couples as a facilitator rather than expert. I identified myself as a "researcher" and mentioned that I was not a trained psychiatrist,

> psychologist, or health professional, in an effort to lessen "white-coat" clinician-induced stress.[46] Rogers's climate setting, positive regard and prizing were integral to the interview technique.[47] Many theorists argue for the use of multiple interviewers but evidence suggests that a single interviewer working across participants is more adept at eliciting deeper responses and creating a safer climate for authentic disclosure.[48] It also ensured consistency in documentation, accountability, and progressive focussing.[49] Given our phenomenological approach, using one interviewer provided consistency in interviewer-comfort when probing sensitive issues.[50]

The Surviving COVID-19 Survey was conducted using Key Survey. The 32 questions took 15–20 minutes to complete. The Couples Thriving 40+ Years Survey was initially conducted on Key Survey, then transferred to Qualtrics due to licencing changes made at Queensland University of Technology. The 21 questions took 20–30 minutes to complete. Twelve hard copies of this survey were mailed to respondents unable to use computers; these were kept anonymous and added to the online data. Both surveys included Likert scale, multiple choice, and open-ended questions.

Data analysis

Transcriptions of couple interviews were analysed using Interpretive Phenomenological Analysis,[51] which identifies themes, patterns, and motif systems through an iterative process.[52] It does not pick up emotional subtext or word inferences. Replaying recordings and analyzing participant observation notes helped identify deeper meanings.

Single interviewer memory of couples' non-verbal exchanges became important. As Greenhalgh argues, "In most qualitative research, one person knows the data far better than anyone else, so the idea that two heads are better than one simply isn't true."[53] Analysis included dyadic data analysis from interviews and individual data analysis from the two surveys. To preserve differentiation, results from interviews and surveys were not cross-tabulated. Throughout the book, however, quantitative data from the Married 40+ Years Survey (932 respondents) was used to help validate qualitative data from the couple interviews. Tabled results and the survey questions can be found in the Appendices. All interview questions are included in Chapter 5.

Limitations

There were numerous limitations to our approach. Firstly, across the Thriving Couple Interviews and the Married 40+ Years Surveys, participants self-selected, and we believe couples self-selected if they were happier. This would have favoured our approach looking for factors that helped thriving. We noted that some participants used the interviews as a quasi-therapy tool to articulate their own relationship issues. This was prevalent in surveys as well and suggested to us that thriving couples take every opportunity to improve their relationship.

Secondly, our study suffers from recall bias. All past adversity, for example, would have been seen to add to couple thriving when earlier interviewing could have revealed something different. Thirdly, interviews could have suffered from positive 'face-saving' constructs adopted by couples, at times culturally inscribed. There was even, perhaps, a 'saving of face' between spouses themselves resulting in an overly-positive construction by the couple of their relationship. Interviewing couples separately may have rectified this, but participant observation of the warmth, tension, body language, and interactions of the couples would have been lost.

Cross-sectional research naturally suffers from a cohort effect.[54] This particularly affected our study as couples' attitudes were evidently shaped by the zeitgeist in which their individual and relationship attitudes were formed. Answering the central question – 'what makes relationships last?' – must, however, include generational and zeitgeist considerations to be relevant. Attitudes towards long-term relationships, divorce, communication styles, and gendered roles were also culturally inscribed, and our exploration of this is very limited. Finally, in this twenty-first century, concepts of marriage, relationships, and 'long-term' are being dis-articulated and re-articulated; our study does not address this, neither does it address the experiences of many diverse groups.

Our interviewed couples

Consent forms, data collection methods, and statistical outcomes fall short of depicting the life experience of people, particularly the 90 couples interviewed. Rapport is formed, and trust grows. Unique and appealing personal, behavioural, and cultural subtleties were witnessed through participant observation:

> I had the privilege of interviewing many of the couples in their homes. The decor, the cosy warmth, and photographs told the story of their relationship journey: cabinets overflowing with hundreds of souvenirs from around the world, shoe boxes filled with 'x-rated' love letters, a handmade bookshelf from a time of poverty, a priceless antique shipped from a couple's hometown in Italy. When I asked one couple what helped them through their many years of adversity, the husband pointed to a mantle-piece filled with family photographs and broke down sobbing. Many set the table for me with their finest dinnerware and served baked muffins or biscuits, or invited me to a home-cooked lunch. I had

glimpses into their cultural heritages as I sampled Estonian *Pasha*, marvelled at Russian hand-painted icons or toured an artist's studio hung with vibrant paintings from a Grecian homeland. I was once greeted by dozens of garden gnomes and another time by a boisterous Labrador, one of many guide dogs a couple had fostered. This was hospitality as I entered into private worlds created over 40+ years of "just ordinary run-of-the-mill, married couple stuff: nothing exceptional" (Malcolm and Jeanette, 64 yrs). Yet, there was something exceptional in each encountered couple for me to savour.

I interviewed chicken farmers, hairdressers, lawyers, shoe sales-representatives, tradespersons, nurses, cleaners, army colonels, homemakers, foresters, translators, school teachers and principals, boilermakers, prison wardens, pilots, secretaries, retail workers, builders, artists, ministers, bookkeepers, sailors, chemists, businesspeople, professional bikers, security officers, IT managers, carpenters, journalists, bankers, counsellors, accountants, bakers, engineers, real estate agents, professors, mechanics and more. Two couples were professional ballroom dancers, and one couple were singers. Couples' stories and insights have resulted in 1178 pages of transcription. Due to limited space, we were unable to include all their rich insights and experiences. We are indebted to these courageous couples who shared their sometimes painful but always rewarding journeys with us.

Language

In our theoretical discussions, terms such as 'core' and 'broader' attachment have precise meanings, but words such as 'marriage,' 'relationship,' 'couple dyad,' or 'love-partnership' are used more or less interchangeably. A writing style more acceptable to scientific consideration is employed for theoretical discussions, whereas a more personable tone captures more of couples' real-life experience and insights, including use of the first-person voice, as employed thus far.

Book structure

The book is divided into three parts. Part I (Chapters 1–3) discusses the societal context, Part II (Chapters 4–5) presents our findings, and Part III (Chapters 6–7) presents techniques based on findings and clinical experience.

Part I presents the twenty-first century social environment impacting relationships. Chapter 1 centres on hyper-individualism which appears to fundamentally work against relationship longevity. The chapter argues that the two can be reconciled after considering selfish genes, altruism, attachment theory, and Maslow's insights. Chapter 2, centring on mental health, argues that attachment underlies the reciprocal link between relationships and mental health more than is emphasized even in the literature. Protecting one protects them both. Chapter 3 considers the under-appreciated impact of social isolation, particularly atomization, screen technology, estrangement, and social distancing on long-term relationships.

Part II presents our findings. Chapter 4 presents findings from the Surviving COVID-19 Survey of 290 people cohabiting or married for 3+ years during the pandemic. Questions from younger people became questions for couples together 40+ years. Chapter 5 presents findings of couples thriving 40+ years. As the core chapter, it presents the findings of the 90 Thriving Couple Interviews supported by the results of 932 surveyed respondents in the Married 40+ Years Survey. It looks to answer the book's central question – 'what makes relationships last?' – through considering couples' 'glue-secrets' to relationship longevity.

Part III presents techniques drawn from the study's findings, clinical experience, and underpinning literature. Chapter 6 presents techniques for enhancing pro-relational values for building resilient relationships. Chapter 7 looks at techniques and insights directly concerned with resilience, and the book concludes with consideration of a term we introduce: 'together-actualization.' Three appendices cover couple-specific quotes and tabulated results.

Future research

Even before presenting our material, it is evident that our study opens up vistas for new research as our limitations need to be overcome. Our study represents 52 countries, but our work leaves over 140 countries and many more ethnicities unrepresented. Future research could address this and cross-language divides to include a much-needed culture-informed and more representative global approach. Future research could address couples living with varying degrees of physical or mental ability, with mental illness, in diverse gender and sexual expression, and with diverse religious identifications. This book may be useful for developing nations as they face hyper-individual pitfalls in their socio-economic progress; with growing social isolation (even in populous nations) and mental illness. Much research in this burgeoning area will be needed.

In line with existing evidence, our book emphasizes the importance of commitment and pro-relational values to strengthen underlying attachment for relationship longevity. It aims to help couples thrive in today's societal context. Through mixed methodology and a salutogenic approach, it links younger couples wanting to achieve relationship longevity with thriving couples who have achieved it. We warmly invite you to consider the twenty-first century external factors that threaten couples wanting to relationally survive, and glimpse into the internal worlds of couples who have learnt to thrive.

Notes

1 Markman, Howard J., Scott M. Stanley, and Susan L. Blumberg. *Fighting for your marriage: A deluxe revised edition of the classic best-seller for enhancing marriage and preventing divorce*. John Wiley & Sons, 2010, 33, 34.
2 Clements, Mari L., Scott M. Stanley, and Howard J. Markman. "Before they said "I do": Discriminating among marital outcomes over 13 years." *Journal of Marriage and Family* 66, no. 3 (2004): 613–626.
3 Stanley, Scott M., Galena K. Rhoades, Paul R. Amato, Howard J. Markman, and Christine A. Johnson. "The timing of cohabitation and engagement: Impact on first and second marriages." *Journal of Marriage and Family* 72, no. 4 (2010): 906–918.
4 Bramlett, Matthew D., and William D. Mosher. "Cohabitation, marriage, divorce, and remarriage in the United States." *Vital and Health Statistics* 23, no. 22 (2002): 1–93.
5 Lyngstad, Torkild Hovde. "The impact of parents' and spouses' education on divorce rates in Norway." *Demographic Research* 10 (2004): 121–142.
6 Wolfinger, Nicholas H., and Nicholas H. Wolfinger. *Understanding the divorce cycle: The children of divorce in their own marriages*. Cambridge University Press, 2005, 11. Karney, Benjamin R., and Thomas N. Bradbury. "Research on marital satisfaction and stability in the 2010s: Challenging conventional wisdom." *Journal of Marriage and Family* 82, no. 1 (2020): 100–116.
7 Heyman, Richard E., and Amy M. Smith Slep. "The hazards of predicting divorce without crossvalidation." *Journal of Marriage and Family* 63, no. 2 (2001): 473–479.
8 Teachman, Jay D. "Stability across cohorts in divorce risk factors." *Demography* 39, no. 2 (2002): 331–351.
9 http://edition.cnn.com/2010/LIVING/09/22/divorced.parents.children.marriage/index.html Retrieved 17 November 2021.
10 Sanford, Keith, Lindsey M. Backer-Fulghum, and Chelsea Carson. "Couple Resilience Inventory: Two dimensions of naturally occurring relationship behavior during stressful life events." *Psychological Assessment* 28, no. 10 (2016): 1243.
11 Gildersleeve, Sara, Jefferson A. Singer, Karen Skerrett, and Shelter Wein. "Coding 'we-ness' in couple's relationship stories: A method for assessing mutuality in couple therapy." *Psychotherapy Research* 27, no. 3 (2017): 313–325.
12 Often achieved through both embodied and intangible aspects of couple's experience. See Skerrett, Karen, and Karen Fergus, eds. *Couple resilience: Emerging perspectives*. Springer, 2015.
13 Amato, Paul R., and Bryndl Hohmann-Marriott. "A comparison of high-and low-distress marriages that end in divorce." *Journal of Marriage and Family* 69, no. 3 (2007): 621–638.
14 Sperry, Len, and Paul R. Peluso. *Couple therapy: Theory and effective practice*. Routledge, 2018, 3. Skerrett and Fergus, eds. *Couple resilience: Emerging perspectives*. Springer, 2015, ix.
15 Baucom, Donald H., Varda Shoham, Kim T. Mueser, Anthony D. Daiuto, and Timothy R. Stickle. "Empirically supported couple and family interventions for marital distress and adult mental health problems." *Journal of Consulting and Clinical Psychology* 66, no. 1 (1998): 53.
16 Mintz, Steven, and Susan Kellogg. *Domestic revolutions: A social history of American family life*. Simon and Schuster, 1989.
17 Coontz, Stephanie. *Marriage, a history: How love conquered marriage*. Penguin, 2006.

18 See Williams, Lee, JoEllen Patterson, and Todd M. Edwards. *Clinician's guide to research methods in family therapy: Foundations of evidence-based practice.* Guilford Publications, 2014.
19 Heim, Caroline. "Theatre audience contribution through the post-performance discussion." PhD Thesis, School of English, Media Studies and Art History, The University of Queensland (2009).
20 Heim, Caroline. "'Argue with us!': Audience co-creation through post-performance discussions." *New Theatre Quarterly* 28, no. 2 (2012): 189–197.
21 Heim, Caroline. "Tutorial facilitation in the humanities based on the tenets of Carl Rogers." *Higher Education* 63, no. 3 (2012): 289–298.
22 Heim, Caroline. *Actors and audiences: Conversations in the electric air.* Routledge, 2020. Heim, Caroline. *Audience as performer: The changing role of theatre audiences in the twenty-first century.* Routledge, 2015.
23 Heim, Caroline. "Participant observation in practice and techniques for overcoming researcher insecurity." Snyder-Young, Dani and Matt Omasta, eds. *Impacting theatre audiences: Methods for studying change.* Routledge, 2022.
24 Heim, Caroline, and Christian Heim. "Facilitating a supportive learning experience: The lecturer's role in addressing mental health issues of university students during COVID-19." *Journal of University Teaching and Learning Practice* 18, no. 6 (2021): 69–79.
25 Williams, Lee, JoEllen Patterson, and Todd M. Edwards. *Clinician's guide to research methods in family therapy: Foundations of evidence-based practice.* Guilford Publications, 2014, 146.
26 See for example: Lebow, Jay L., and Douglas K. Snyder. "Couple therapy in the 21st century." *Clinical Handbook of Couple Therapy* (2022): 635.
27 Karney, Benjamin R., and Thomas N. Bradbury. "Research on marital satisfaction and stability in the 2010s: Challenging conventional wisdom." *Journal of Marriage and Family* 82, no. 1 (2020): 100–116.
28 Bradbury, Thomas N., and Guy Bodenmann. "Interventions for couples." *Annual Review of Clinical Psychology* 16, no. 1 (2020): 99–123.
29 Wallerstein, Judith. *The good marriage: How and why love lasts.* Plunkett Lake Press, Revised 2019.
30 Antonovsky, Aaron. "Health, stress, and coping." *New Perspectives on Mental and Physical Well-being* (1979): 12–37.
31 Finkel, Eli J. *The all-or-nothing marriage: How the best marriages work.* Penguin, 2019, 27.
32 Many studies on couples use the MAT or DAT satisfaction scales. These, however, are not conducive to reaching for a more couples-led approach.
33 Sinkovics, Rudolf R., and Eva A. Alfoldi. "Progressive focusing and trustworthiness in qualitative research." *Management International Review* 52, no. 6 (2012): 817–845.
34 Howitt, Dennis. *Introduction to qualitative research methods in psychology: Putting theory into practice.* Pearson, 2019, 394.
35 Heim, *Audience as performer.*
36 Wallerstein, *The good marriage*, 16.
37 University of Queensland Ethics Approval Number: 2017001628.
38 As a single exception, we used a translator for our longest married couple.
39 See Greenhalgh, Trisha M., John Bidewell, Elaine Crisp, Amanda Lambros, and Jane Warland. *Understanding research methods for evidence-based practice in health.* John Wiley & Sons, 2020.
40 Australian and New Zealand clubs of active retirees.
41 Heim, "Theatre Audience Contribution." And Heim, "Argue with Us!"

42 Greenhalgh, Trisha M., John Bidewell, Elaine Crisp, Amanda Lambros, and Jane Warland. *Understanding research methods for evidence-based practice in health.* John Wiley & Sons, 2020, 101.
43 Dewitt, Barry, Baruch Fischhoff, Alexander L. Davis, Stephen B. Broomell, Mark S. Roberts, and Janel Hanmer. "Exclusion criteria as measurements I: Identifying invalid responses." *Medical Decision Making* 39, no. 6 (2019): 693–703.
44 Due to COVID-19 restrictions, three interviews were not done in person.
45 Guest, Greg, Emily Namey, and Mario Chen. "A simple method to assess and report thematic saturation in qualitative research." *PLoS One* 15, no. 5 (2020).
46 Pickering, Thomas G., William Gerin, and Amy R. Schwartz. "What is the white-coat effect and how should it be measured?." *Blood Pressure Monitoring* 7, no. 6 (2002): 293–300.
47 Heim, "Tutorial facilitation in the humanities."
48 Rosenblatt, Paul C. "One interviewer versus several: Modernist and postmodernist perspectives in qualitative family interviewing." *Journal of Family Theory & Review* 4, no. 2 (2012): 96–104.
49 Ibid.
50 Ibid.
51 Smith, Jonathan A., and Megumi Fieldsend. *Interpretative phenomenological analysis.* American Psychological Association, 2021.
52 IPA falls under the rubric of Thematic Analysis. See Greenhalgh, Trisha M., John Bidewell, Elaine Crisp, Amanda Lambros, and Jane Warland. *Understanding research methods for evidence-based practice in health.* John Wiley & Sons, 2020, 39.
53 Ibid, 34.
54 Williams, Lee, JoEllen Patterson, and Todd M. Edwards. *Clinician's guide to research methods in family therapy: Foundations of evidence-based practice.* Guilford Publications, 2014, 92.

Part I

The context

Chapter 1

Resilient relationships versus hyper-individualism: Selfish genes, altruism, and attachment

Hyper-individual ideals and long-term relationships are seemingly antithetical. Resilience becomes a valued attribute, for relationship longevity in particular. Leading up to and into the twenty-first century, our world was growing enormously in socio-economic prosperity, although in some countries more than others. These same decades, however, saw the highest global divorce rates, the lowest marriage rates, and the highest levels of social isolation and mental illness. These phenomena are linked. They are driven, at least in part, by hyper-individual ideals adversely impacting relationships in a lonely, screen-centred world. Resilient relationships, however, bounce back. They are highly prized.[1] Yet many bewildered young couples metaphorically gaze up at grandparents to ask, "how did you stay together forty years when we're struggling after forty days?"

What has changed for relationships in less than two generations? Is a lifelong love-relationship still a viable option in our changing world? Can it offer authentic encounter amidst society's complexities? Can it be "presence and 'being-with' in the face of harsh existential facts of life"?[2] A relationship needs to withstand hyper-individualism, social isolation, and the mental health crisis for partners to find lasting contentment both individually and together.

Our evidence in Chapter 4 shows that people want their relationships to last. Couples who have weathered many storms of adversity and thrive after 40+ years possess insights to help younger couples achieve their goal. To have relevance, however, their insights need to be understood in the light of twenty-first century problems affecting relationships. This book distils insights from our empirical study of more than 1400 coupled individuals across 52 nations representing more than 81 ethnicities, including in-depth interviews of 90 couples married 40 to 73 years.

In the spirit of Maslow,[3] we studied thriving couples rather than those presenting with problems. Insights from these couples are presented in their own words and form the basis of techniques to help contemporary couples and couple therapists. Our book presents time-tested insights in a new guise for a new generation.

Having crossed the threshold into a new millennium, couples thriving 40+ years experienced emergent hyper-individualism: relaxed divorce laws,

DOI: 10.4324/9781003263395-3

feminism, affluence, changed gender roles, diverse identities, individual empowerment, broadened life opportunity, the internet, social media, and more. Divorce rates in this couple cohort were higher than for more-recently married couples. Thriving couples in our study are still together after 40–73 years, whereas 50% of US couples and 44% of UK couples divorce after an average of 8 years (12 in the UK), and separation rates in non-married couples are significantly higher.[4]

Still, these couples' insights need to be presented within a contemporary context. What do 'compromise' and 'commitment' mean today? Where's the 'fun' and 'novelty'? Do 'sacrifice' and 'perseverance' have relevance in our present age? Insights are presented with the major societal pressures of hyper-individualism, social isolation, and mental illness in mind.

This chapter centres on hyper-individualism. To help understand couple relationships within the hyper-individual ideal, it explores the biological basis of relationships, surviving and thriving, selfish genes and altruism, attachment theory, and Maslow's hierarchy of needs. It also explores changing attitudes towards sexual expression and relationships, and aims to reconcile hyper-individual ideals with long-lasting relationships. Firstly, however, we consider hyper-individualism itself.

The current zeitgeist: hyper-individualism

Hyper-individualism is more than, extreme, or beyond individualism. At the time of publication, "hyper-individualism" was not in the Oxford English Dictionary online, yet something of a body of research has grown around the term. Broadly, hyper-individualism is "a tendency for people to act in a highly individual way without regard to society."[5] More astutely, it is "a cultural shift whereby everyone is expected to demonstrate a capacity of judgment and choice, and to shape their life in a conscious, intentional manner, as a self-centred project."[6] Crossing all diverse identifications, most all of us in humanity have a personal vested interest in understanding couple relationships. To keep the focus on relationships, our discussion by-passes the term's political implications.

Is relationship longevity compatible with two lives shaped as self-centred projects? The clash is between self-centredness and altruism, or in relationships, give and take. Cynically, hyper-individualism lifts narcissism and instant self-gratification to a sociological ideal (hardly endearing towards couple relationships). More optimistically, it values hard-won autonomy to reach for self-actualization and thriving, and this perspective can include thriving in couple relationships. To facilitate an optimistic view, we offer the following definition:

> Hyper-individualism is extreme individualism valuing self-expression, judgment and choice to shape a self-made life-story reaching for self-actualization.

Steeped in socio-economic prosperity,[7] our hyper-individual age holds many benefits to facilitate thriving relationships:

More equal opportunities
A higher standard of living
Increased career opportunities
Higher education and understanding
Information access to aid problem-solving
Increased access to therapy and skills building
More opportunity to choose a together-focussed lifestyle

Hyper-individualism has many unintended side-effects: less close relationships, less well-being,[8] narcissism,[9] identity problems and loneliness,[10] and disillusionment through a focus on life's negatives.[11] Values clashes often occur in hyper-individualism[12] as seen through culture wars.[13] Relationships are more likely to fail as they need to serve two sets of high expectations.[14] To stay together at all, two people let go of enough individual selfishness to engage in relational give and take. Hyper-individual ideals, however, drive against this. For individual and mutual satisfaction, we need to reconcile hyper-individualism and reaching for long-term relationship.

Self-centredness pulls against relationship togetherness.[15] As Maslow points out, however, reaching for self-actualization, an essentially self-centred pursuit, means nurturing rather than neglecting relationships.[16] Careful judgment and conscious choice are needed. As a background to help understand and reconcile this tension, we explore couple relationship surviving and thriving, Maslow's hierarchy, selfish genes and altruism, attachment and love, and changing sexual expression.

Couple relationships: surviving and thriving

Our twenty-first century aim is to thrive, but our ancestors needed to survive. Biologically, being a couple holds many survival advantages and helps solve problems of mating competition, reproducing, parenting, and resource provision.[17] Humans are socially co-operative, and the couple framework helps express this in parenting, socializing, and sexual expression.[18] Being a couple serves the sexual and social functions; the infant-caregiver dyad is for parenting needs.

Humans are highly dependent on parenting. Domestic cats stay with mothers for only three percent of their lives, pandas spend six percent of their lives dependent, orang-utans 22%. Even with our modern conveniences, humans are dependent on parents for about 25% of their lives. Only two hundred years ago it was over 50%. Our great potential requires great nurturing. Children continue to need dedicated caregivers and stable social structures just to survive, let alone thrive.

Why do we want fulfilling relationships? Why do we want our children to 'do well'? Beyond biological survival, we have "an inherent drive for self-improvement and growth"[19] to thrive and self-actualize.[20] "Thriving"[21] provides added psychological insight into our motivation and behaviour. To thrive is to grow, succeed, be effective, and experience well-being.[22] Few people aim to survive, most of us aim to thrive:

> My mission in life is not merely to survive, but to thrive; and to do so with some passion, some compassion, some humour and some style. (Maya Angelou)[23]

About five percent of UK infants medically fail to thrive.[24] This can be life-threatening. Adults too can fail to thrive, as can businesses, economies, elite athletes, and long-term relationships. Our human relationships and individual thriving are deeply connected: individual thriving[25] is promoted through thriving families,[26] thriving friendships,[27] thriving couple relationships,[28] and more.

That social connection contributes to individual thriving, health, and well-being is beyond question, but *how* it contributes is not fully understood. Evidence shows that, through oxytocin release, close social connection promotes biological and neurological changes to facilitate individual resilience for increased physical and mental well-being.[29] This is explored in coming chapters.

In this twenty-first century, we individually thrive far beyond our reproductive years and beyond 'survival of our species'. Couple relationships too have moved beyond biological survival needs. They now aim for mutual self-fulfilment: self- and together-expression in ever-growing diversity. Our diversity – like our extended life-expectancy, art, spirituality, self-expression, technological innovation, and mutual relationship fulfilment – is a consequence of thriving. Biological and psychosocial perspectives underpin our growing diversity[30] and accepting diversity is underpinned by the science of the mere exposure effect.[31] The couple framework has evolved to serve us beyond survival and reach for self-actualization.[32]

Increased self-focus in Maslow's hierarchy

Self-actualization, closely related to thriving, is "the need to become all that one is capable of being to develop one's fullest potential."[33] Aspirational and rewarding, it is, perhaps, the core desire underpinning human motivation. In 1943, Maslow presented his theory on human motivation, his hierarchy of needs:[34]

1 Biological (food and shelter to survival an environment)
2 Safety (home, family, employment and stability in society)

3 Love and belonging (family, friends and relationship)
4 Self-esteem (confidence and achievement)
5 Self-actualization (creative self-expression and thriving)

It is often seen as a pyramid to reflect its aspirational ascent:

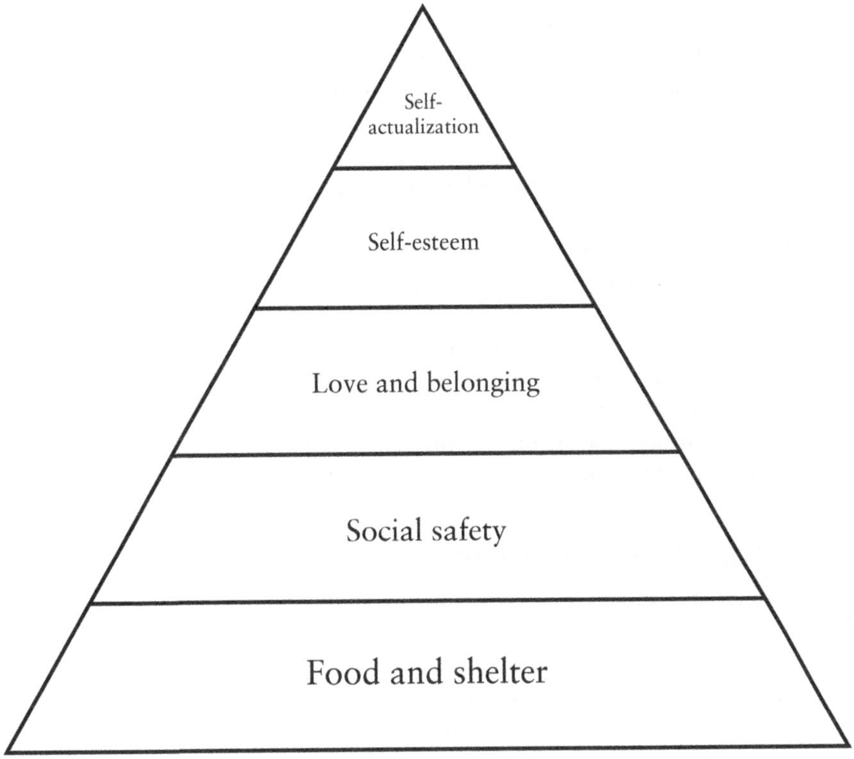

Figure 1.1

Socio-economic progress facilitates an upward ascent. On the ascent, however, the focus becomes increasingly self-centred: from an environment needing to be negotiated for food and shelter, to safety in society, to loving close people, and upwards towards esteem and actualization for the self alone. Economic progress allows more societies to fulfil more biological and safety needs, allowing more individuals to reach for self-actualization. In this way, socio-economic progress and individualism are linked.

Self-actualization, arguably, is the goal of hyper-individualism: 'I want to be me and do it my way.' This, however, creates relationship tension: 'do

I do it my way or my partner's way? Do I win or give in? What do I feel like doing? I don't want to be held back.'[35] This me versus you tension in a relationship mirrors the apparent tension between gene selfishness and altruism: 'hyper-individualism is just being true to my selfish genes, isn't it? Why give in to someone else's needs?'

"The selfish gene,"[36] as a 1976 book title and much-discussed scientific concept, has arguably entered social consciousness enough to embolden hyper-individual ideals, legitimize selfish behaviour for some, and influence our approach to life goals and values.[37] Yet we know that unbridled selfishness is at the root of relationship problems. As a neuroscientist plainly points out:

> Psychologists, couple researchers and neuroscientists have identified the individual and relationship qualities that make for satisfying and intimate couple connections. The bottom line? You need to be a *mensch* to do well relationally . . . a good, decent human being.[38]

After this revelation, Mona DeKoven Fishbane goes on to discuss the importance of values and virtues before moving on to her broader discussion on couple therapy and brain processes. Aren't good, decent human beings also driven by their selfish genes? Exploring selfish genes and altruism helps us understand this tension.

Selfish genes versus altruism

As Richard Dawkins points out:

> Let us try to *teach* generosity and altruism, because we are born selfish. Let us understand what our own selfish genes are up to, because we may then at least have the chance to upset their designs.[39]

Our selfish genes are the trouble-makers; altruism upsets their designs. Altruism – promoting another's welfare at cost to our own – increases another's chances of survival, selfishness increases our own; but both are needed for survival of our species.[40] Natural selection is understood to be driven at the gene level to motivate both individual selfishness and group altruism.[41] Asking whether humans are naturally selfish or altruistic becomes something of a false dichotomy as we need both, and they co-exist. We experience the two in apparent conflict but like night and day or Summer and Winter, they are part of a bigger picture. Parenting illustrates this.

> "I thought *I* was selfish!" says Sasha, "But holy hell, toddlers are the worst!" Four years into fatherhood, Sasha has a renewed appreciation for his parents as he adjusts to being one. The amphetamine use that

once dominated his life is a thing of the past. He found enough altruism to be a *mensch* and a father.[42]

Infants are totally selfish in their dependence on an altruistic care-giver. Selfishness is checked in toddlers as siblings arrive and parents must be shared; rivalries often ensue. Altruistic give-and-take is learnt in socializing with peers who increasingly shape our lives. When choosing a love partner, selfishness and altruism come into a balance as we begin to consider another's needs as almost equalling our own. Unsurprisingly, toddler-level selfishness tends to fail in adult love-relationships. In parenting, increased altruism is needed to fulfil children's needs; and most parents, like Sasha, become "good enough" as they rise to the immense challenge. Grandparents may often care for their children's children so continued altruism is needed. Fostering or adopting children requires more altruism as couples draw from their generosity and self-expression to provide a sense of family for biologically-unrelated children.

At each step in the human life-cycle, altruism balances selfishness. Furthermore, we learn more altruism as we age. Adults are expected to contribute to society if they can, and be rewarded for this. This too balances selfishness and altruism. "Upsetting" our selfish genes by finding this balance integrates selfishness and altruism in a bigger picture so we humans can individually and collectively survive and thrive.

Valuing altruism

We are each born with a potential to be anything from extremely selfish to extremely altruistic[43] depending on parental[44] and societal values,[45] cultural inheritance, learnt behaviour,[46] and choice.[47] We can choose to be altruistic[48] (or not) in response to experiencing empathy, just as we choose to eat a biscuit (or not) after experiencing its mouth-watering aroma.[49]

Medals are given to heroes because, as humans, we collectively value extreme, life-saving altruism. Reaching this takes growing up in a family and culture valuing altruism,[50] internalizing the ideal, and choosing it.[51] Relationship altruism likewise takes growing up in a family and culture valuing it, internalizing the ideal, and choosing it.[52] Individual choice is important: 'to live like my parents or to rebel?' is but one example. Societies valuing individualism breed less altruism,[53] but as a social contagion, altruism can produce more altruism.[54] Choosing altruism is difficult as it costs money, time, stress, and self-sacrifice.[55] Is relationship altruism worth it? Thriving couples share insight on this in future chapters.

In a relationship, selfishness preserves individuality while altruism preserves the relationship. Like night and day or Summer and Winter, as stated, the two are experienced as opposites but are complimentary and integrated in a bigger reality. Without selfishness individuality is lost, without altruism there would be no relationship. Altruism, being more challenging, merits more exploration.

Three types of altruism have been articulated:

Kin-based altruism
Reciprocity-based altruism
Empathy-altruism.[56]

Kin-based altruism, good done for family, is seen in male emperor penguins incubating eggs through a harsh winter, lionesses hunting for cubs' food, wolf-pairs adopting orphaned wolves, kangaroos carrying heavy joeys, gorillas protecting their troop, and more. It is ubiquitous, biological, and makes use of memory networks. In humans, it is seen in child-rearing, family ties, and people risking their lives to save their child or "two brothers . . . [or] eight cousins."[57] Kin-altruism grows and flourishes as a couple's sense of belonging and family grows.

Reciprocity-based altruism – doing good and expecting good in return – is the basis of free-market economies.[58] It involves limbic system trust, oxytocin, and dopamine. In nature, it exists in the pollination system, symbiotic interactions between sea anemone and clown fish, humans and beneficial microbes living in our intestines (microbiota), monkeys scratching each other's backs, and more. In relationships, it is give and take: mutual satisfaction and shared strengths and resources. One person may be giving in one aspect of the relationship while expecting return in another. This can be mutually satisfying and individually highly rewarding.

Empathy-altruism is being moved to do good without expected return. It involves anterior cingulate cortex empathy, amygdala empathic pain, pre-frontal cortex[59] valuing, and orbito-frontal cortex values-based decision-making. Empathy-altruism is compassion; initiated by empathy, feeling with someone, compassion feels for someone and consciously does something useful for them.[60] It involves frontal lobe thinking to render useful service based on empathy's limbic system emotional pain. Empathy-altruism is found in dogs' devotion to their owners[61] and in humpback whales saving other whale-species calves from orcas. It is found in abundance in humans; in soldiers, first responders, and heroes like the unsung couples in our research staying together against odds and reason to care for profoundly disabled children, deal with one person's severe mental illness, or forgive affairs.

We are all capable of altruism: of being good, decent, and *mensch*-like. It somehow shares life itself: "giving is more joyous than receiving . . . because in the act of giving lies the expression of my aliveness."[62] Any seemingly trivial deed which puts another's needs ahead of my own is altruism. In a relationship, altruism is expressed in small day-to-day interactions, going above-and-beyond, or working together to aid humanity. Deep intimacy in a relationship requires altruism, as you give of yourself to another person. It also involves selfishness, however, as you take what another person gives. This is mutual give and take: mutual altruism and selfishness together.

Altruism is a response to attachment:[63] core attachment in kin-based altruism, broader attachment in reciprocity and empathy-altruism. This is played out in our life-cycle: children are selfish, grow in independence, and learn reciprocity and empathy-altruism to take their place as adults in the group. Without altruism, collectively we would not survive. Neither would a relationship: selfishness preserves individuality, altruism preserves attachment.

Attachment theory: more influential than ever

"A baby cannot exist alone"[64] because an altruistic carer is always needed to pour love and care on the infant. Since Bowlby found that early separation left children at higher risk of criminality[65] and Spitz found that without affection even well-fed WWII infant orphans were at greater risk of illness and death,[66] attachment theory has become more influential than ever.[67] It holds eminence in the sciences[68] as the biology of attachment becomes clearer.[69] Attachment evolves[70] characteristic brain circuitry[71] to underpin both infant-carer and couple[72] relationships. Attachment is being "safe, secure and protected."[73] It is "confidence in protection."[74] We define it simply:

> Attachment is relational safety.

Relational safety is deeper than love; it is the underlying confidence that, as an infant, you can pee and poo all over your carer at night and, though sleep-deprived, they will still take care of you the next day. With such confidence, infants learn Eriksson's basic trust,[75] without it they cannot. Likewise, a couple need similar confidence to know that their relationship will continue in spite of hardship. This paves the way for intimacy rather than isolation[76] and is achieved by tempering selfishness and displaying altruism.

An adult-adult couple is the "prototypical"[77] adult attachment. It shares features with the carer-infant dyad[78] including common neural pathways.[79] The loss of a carer is life-threatening for an infant. Likewise, losing a long-term adult love-relationship can be life-threatening for an adult, as evidenced by heightened suicide risk in break-ups[80] and chronically in those separated[81] and divorced.[82] The loss of a friend, sibling, or work colleague tends not to threaten life. A couple dyad protects individual health[83] just as the infant-carer dyad protects against failure to thrive.[84] Adults thrive better when in relationship.[85]

Attachment involves strong forces of attraction and energy. It is essential to life: life-enhancing and life-preserving. Bowlby used the behaviour of hydrogen atoms as a metaphor for human bonding to show that much energy is involved in the making and breaking of human emotional bonds.[86]

Making an adult attachment bond takes energy: dating, becoming familiar, negotiating cultural, family and individual values, and endless nights discussing 'are we are right for each other?' Cementing the attachment takes energy: moving in, celebrating, adjusting social networks, and forsaking individual freedoms. Sustaining attachment takes energy: understanding, accepting, arguing, negotiating, dividing up chores, dove-tailing strengths, making plans, and forging shared values. Breaking an attachment bond, separating or divorcing, takes even more energy: negotiating heightened conflict, trial separation, preserving children's futures, separating from family and friends, legal and financial issues, and endless nights agonizing over 'were we ever right for each other?' If achievable, staying attached like a di-hydrogen molecule (two hydrogen atoms with a single bond) takes less energy.

Still, carer-infant and couple attachments require much effort. Such intense effort and energy are not needed for friendships, siblings, or work acquaintances. In the torrid challenges of a long-term relationship, solitude appears as a tantalizing option, but it is seldom chosen as we are biologically driven to find not only sex but to bond in relational safety.[87]

Theorists differentiate terms such as love, affect, romance, lust, couple, relationship, and attachment.[88] Defining these for research purposes is ongoing[89] and beyond our scope here. In this book, "core attachment" refers to the carer-infant or couple dyad, and "broader attachment" refers to feelings of closeness in human relationships.

Attachment principles hold throughout life: that, for safety and survival, we form close bonds with close people and these help us regulate our emotions, explore the world, grow independent, and become resilient.[90] Couple attachment (relational safety) is the foundation of love. It is expressed through intimacy,[91] commitment,[92] forgiveness,[93] communication, conflict resolution,[94] and more. Ideally, it provides safe-haven security to allow a couple to explore new vistas individually or together.

Couple therapists can help those struggling to balance self and other-needs in a relationship. They can help others appreciate and more fully understand the importance of attachment. Attachment is a biological necessity. In trying to thrive and in neglecting attachment needs, too many don't survive. How attachment relates to the mental health crisis is explored next chapter.

Attachment is important "from the cradle to the grave."[95] In our lifecycle, we grow from one core attachment, infant-carer, towards another, the couple dyad.[96] Like night and day and selfishness and altruism, attachment and independence are two sides of the same integrated coin: couple relationships in all their exhilaration and frustration.

Lifetime couple attachment is an ideal; a Jungian archetype.[97] Novels, movies, fairy-tales, and popular songs glorify romantic love leading to 'ever-after' relationship. Young adults expect to find a love-partner[98] and people thrive if their relationship thrives and are distressed if it falters.[99] Separated and divorced individuals seek new relationships,[100] and adults are deeply grieved by relationship loss through death. Attachment experiences somehow define us[101] and perhaps help unlock more potential in ourselves than we could individually realize. We humans need attachment to survive, let alone thrive,[102] but realizing this takes effort in a hyper-individual socio-cultural context.

Attachment and love in the brain

Ancient Greek helps us distinguish between attachment and love as it has multiple words for 'love.' Friendship-love, for example, is *philia*. Family love and love for children is *storge*. What science calls love, is closest to *eros:* erotic love connected to sex and survival. These love-types are distinct.[103]

Attachment is closer to *agape*.[104] It is altruistic love, at times unconditional, leading to relational safety, unity, and emotional health.[105] The altruistic nature of attachment is seen in the carer-infant dyad and in selfless cherishing in a couple. Initial and ongoing erotic attraction in the couple dyad is *eros*, but the growing sense of family togetherness is *storge*, the friendship aspect is *philia*, all underpinned by *agape* altruistic attachment.

Attachment *agape* underpins love in a couple relationship. It grows in a relationship that began in an instant of *eros* attraction or over years of *philia* friendship that later became romantic. Expressions of love are culturally informed,[106] but underlying attachment is universal.[107] These distinctions help us negotiate relationship complexities and understand and celebrate diverse love expressions, including, in hyper-individualism, self-love.

Feelings of love[108] and attachment[109] are mediated in the brain by oxytocin to enhance resilience[110] and aid survival.[111] As a gross simplification, feelings of love are generated in the anterior cingulate cortex; in the insular cortex, we monitor how we interact with someone we love to regulate our behaviours to help progress to a relationship. Love's motivation and pleasure are mediated by dopamine, familiarity and comfort by serotonin, and feelings of belonging-togetherness by beta endorphin. A decision to start, maintain, or end a long-term relationship is made after orbito-frontal cortex evaluation of prefrontal values and beliefs and limbic system feelings. Less than five percent of mammals are monogamous,[112] yet long-term coupling has been the core framework for humans across most cultures across history.[113] Animals experience love, but humans experience it in "far greater complexity."[114]

Scientifically, romantic *eros* love is biological[115] and follows a lust-attraction-attachment pathway.[116] As another simplification, lust is mediated by sex hormones and pheromones, attraction by dopamine, and attachment more by oxytocin. This further differentiates attachment from sexual love.

Initial love blindness, the heady inability to think clearly as we fall in love,[117] keeps us on this pathway, even in spite of our more rational selves.

Falling in love can feel like a roller-coaster. So too can societal change feel like a hedonic treadmill[118] trying to squeeze more out of life[119] and relationships.[120] Are our desires and expectations out of control? What has changed? Biological responses change relatively slowly, but our social context can change relatively quickly. With the biological and psychological importance of surviving, thriving, altruism, attachment, and love as a background, we return to the social context.

Individualism goes hyper-

Individualism concerns people as separate units[121] rather than as a collective. It emphasizes "personal autonomy and self-fulfilment, and basing identity on one's personal accomplishments."[122] Socio-economic development, as stated, facilitates more individuals living out their individual values.[123]

Individualism is part of the top of Maslow's hierarchy. A stable, peaceful, and prosperous society is needed for the climb. Basic needs have to be in place before higher needs. Self-esteem (level 4), for example, is not a priority during war[124] and disrupted social stability (level 2). Finances will be used for food and shelter (level 1) before self-actualizing as, say, a classical musician[125] (level 5). Self-esteem (level 5) is achieved after love needs are met (level 3).[126]

In hyper-individualism, we may longingly and impatiently gaze at the summit of self-esteem and self-actualization (levels 4 and 5), but we neglect love and belonging needs (level 3) to our own demise. Attachment is biologically needed to merely survive before aiming to thrive. Someone seeking fame or riches, for example, may neglect family members, lose them, and become depressed and demoralized. I see this increasingly in my practice. Maslow's answer is to look after your relationships before pursuing your higher needs.[127]

Growing individualism adversely impacts relationships. This perception is reflected in a review article[128] concluding that increased divorce in Sri Lanka was due to industrialization, growing gender equality, relaxed divorce laws, and the influence of foreign employment. This perspective has little currency in the USA, or other nations geared towards individualism where everyone is

> a bounded, unique, more or less integrated motivational and cognitive universe of awareness, emotion, judgment, and action organized into a distinctive whole and set contrastingly against other such wholes.[129]

If individuals are "set contrastingly against" others, then couples wanting relationship longevity need to contend "against" ideals of individualism like self-achievement and self-expression. An individual ego is only for itself. It "has the task of self-preservation . . . by learning to bring about appropriate modifications in the external world to its own advantage. . . . [It] pursues pleasure and seeks to avoid unpleasure."[130]

Individualism prioritizes self above others. How much more in hyper-individualism? The growing 'me' focus is reflected in the enormously changed attitudes to sexual expression over a century, after millennia of relative stability in this area.

Changing sexual expression

Prior to the twentieth century, religions were arguably the strongest influencers to attitudes on sexual expression. Even within marriage, for example, sex was not for immediate pleasure.[131] Victorian values emphasized restraint.[132] In the early twentieth century, women were regarded as having an "anti-sexual" instinct which had to be "overcome by a process of wooing"[133] as their desire "remains latent until aroused by a lover's caresses."[134]

Into the peace, prosperity, individualism, and liberal attitudes of the roaring 1920s, flappers made their entrance. Like precocious birds wanting to fly, flappers were young females choosing to distain moral conventions, wear alluring outfits, initiate dates, enjoy alcohol and cigarettes, dance provocatively, and enjoy "petting parties."[135] They advocated for women's rights. The stock-market crash of 1929 dampened spending on glamour, smoking and drinking, and less young people could afford cars for "[sexual] rustles in the back" (Irene and Harry, 55 yrs). Liberal attitudes to sex abated, exemplifying the links among economic prosperity, individualism, and liberal attitudes.

In the 1950s, Alfred Kinsey furthered sexual liberation. Love was sexualized, and sex was eroticized.[136] At a time of rising feminism, oral contraception allowed more separation of sex and relationship. The 1962 best-seller *Sex and the Single Girl*,[137] empowering and scandalous,[138] encouraged financial and sexual independence in young females. It was, perhaps, a foreshadowing of the hook-up culture.[139]

The seventies saw more relaxed divorce laws and a continued sexual revolution. On the whole, however, people remained sexually conservative.[140] With further advances in feminism, liberation of men from stereotypes, and growing LGBTQIA+ rights, end-of-the-century first-world societies had extensively changed attitudes towards sex, gender, and relationships facilitated by growing hyper-individualism. Queer theory paved the way for acceptance of diverse sexuality,[141] and in the current zeitgeist, sex is explored within marriage and relationships, outside of these, in heterosexual, same-sex or non-binary relationships, alone, with whomever consents, or through toys, apps,[142] robots[143] and screen, techno- and cyber-sex.[144]

Sex and long-term relationships are now uncoupled. The liberal attitudes of the 1920s parallelled socio-economic development and individualism and were halted by economic depression followed by war. Hyper-individualism is now our current point-of-reference,[145] but in reality a plurality of values reigns in our developed societies.[146] Values clashes cause confusion: 'Is this a crisis of values?[147] What are the new relationship rules? Am I supposed to make someone else happy or just myself? What sort of sex is right for me? How do I put myself first while in a relationship?'

Can hyper-individualism and relationship longevity be reconciled?

Life is lived "in and through relationships."[148] According to our research, people prefer to thrive within their relationship if this is achievable. In line with hyper-individual judgement and intent to shape self-made life-stories, these can be reconciled. We argue that, for long-term self-benefit, the most self-serving thing you can do is to develop the altruism needed to nurture a secure long-term relationship.

Valuing individuals "against others" rather than in relationship "with others"[149] results in loneliness,[150] narcissism,[151] disillusionment,[152] and relationship failure.[153] This reveals a self-defeating and nihilistic side of hyper-individualism. Ideals such as judgement, autonomy, and intent[154] place extraordinary demands on individuals. Freedom requires responsible judgment and conscious choice to shape a life-story towards self-actualization rather than self-defeat. Without responsibility, however, freedom can easily lead us astray into pitfalls, binds and self-defeat. To protect against this, couples can judiciously choose to build relationship resilience and understand:

What our selfish genes are up to
How to balance selfishness and altruism
Relationship give and take
How to avoid pitfalls and binds.

A core relationship dilemma is balancing 'you' versus 'me:' couple intimacy and individual autonomy.[155] Yet exercising autonomy in a relationship for the relationship facilitates couple closeness.[156] This merits explanation. Controlling or abusive relationships self-evidently limit autonomy and deprive liberty. A free and responsible relationship, however, leads to empowerment and an increased sense of self when intimacy is freely chosen: 'when I choose you, I exercise my autonomy, so I do more of what I want to do, and am more of who I desire to be.' Achieving this takes hyper-individual judgement, choice, and intent.

Blindly seeking immediate pleasure and self-gratification above all else is perilous. It works against relationship longevity and ultimately against long-term self-benefit. A fuller awareness of the long-term self-benefits of a secure relationship is required.

Why choose relationship longevity?

A long-term relationship is a valued life-experience. Couples choosing it, however, need to know how to achieve it. A relationship is a collective identity of two: "You're 50%, the other person's 50%, but the result is the same, you become one" (Graham and Lynette, 46 years).

Relationship identity can be eroded by hyper-individual ideals[157] such as immediate self-pleasure and egocentricity, but it can be nurtured by hyper-individual judicious choice and conscious intent.

A long-term relationship protects individual physical health,[158] emotional health and wellbeing,[159] resilience,[160] and protects against unhappiness,[161] alcohol misuse,[162] anxiety, bipolar, depression,[163] and suicide.[164] It also protects against loneliness,[165] loss of identity,[166] substance addiction,[167] and decision-fatigue.[168] No medication or vitamin does all of this. From a health perspective, a relationship seems an easy decision to make, but it is not an easy choice to commit to with sustained effort.

Eating healthily and exercising regularly are also easy decisions to make from a health perspective, yet are not easy. Each takes commitment and effort: to say no to unhealthy foods and yes to nourishing foods, and no to inactivity and yes to regular exercise. A couple need to say no to relationship threats like making unconsidered unilateral decisions and being totally thoughtless and irresponsible. They need to say yes to nurturing the relationship through valuing, accepting, and understanding each other, choosing to go through adversity together, and fulfilling each other's needs.[169] Staying unfit and unhealthy affects you alone, but harming a relationship affects another human being. It takes altruism to battle placing self as the sole reference point. This clashes with hyper-individual egocentricity.

A relationship offers health and emotional benefits, mutual satisfaction, meaning-making, personal and together growth, thriving, and vitality. These are incentives to help sustain the effort needed. A healthy diet and regular exercise offer the same benefits to help sustain the constant effort needed in each.

A relationship requires balancing selfishness with altruism. This is similar to balancing screen binges with gym work-outs and balancing potato crisps and fresh vegetables. With astute choice, however, individuals can find the sweet spot in each:

> You want this to work. You want this to be a union, a couple. So then you do what makes it work. You can't be totally selfish. Everyone has to be a little selfish, but I think you can't be totally selfish when it's a partnership. (Christine and Phil, 49 yrs)

Choice is always relevant. We retain autonomy. The brain's orbito-frontal cortex makes values-based decisions to help us survive and thrive.[170] Science has shown that, in order to choose exercise, a healthy diet, or a long-term relationship over alternatives:

> Perceived or imagined rewards need to outweigh perceived or imagined costs.[171]

The rewards of a mutually supportive long-term relationship include companionship, understanding, sexual expression, dovetailing strengths, emotional security, and more. Costs include the risk of losing the relationship, risk of abuse, constricted freedom, too much effort, and the opportunity cost of exploring other life adventures. Living with another person is like living with an independent variable. They are filled with seething emotions and incongruences, 'Who knows what they'll do next?'[172] They may fill us with pleasure or wound us beyond measure.

Rewards outweigh costs for the thriving couples we interviewed and surveyed. High life expectations and the lure of myriad pleasure-filled activities may blind us to the rewards of a long-term relationship and the costs involved in pleasure. This is "error"[173] in hyper-individualism; pitfalls.

Relationship longevity involves accepting costs and rewards, give and take, pleasure and hardship, and growth and challenges. These are sprinkled with fun, arguments, pleasure, pain, comfort, and distress, all underpinned by attachment. It may be a roller-coaster or a gradual pyramid climb, but it is "not just the crossing of a field" (Alex and Alexandra, 58 yrs).

A long-term relationship is a vehicle to meet love and belonging needs (level 3) and can facilitate the climb to self-esteem (level 4) and self-actualization (level 5). Hyper-individual autonomy, conscious judgment, intent, and choice can work towards this while immediate self-pleasure-seeking and egocentricity may lead us to self-defeating pitfalls and relationship binds. These pitfalls and binds are now considered.

Pitfalls in hyper-individualism

How is it that hyper-individualism – a social ideal espousing pleasure, happiness, and self-benefit – is accompanied by so much mental illness (as seen in Chapter 2), loneliness and isolation (Chapter 3), a lack of well-being,[174] loss of identity,[175] and disillusionment?[176] These "errors"[177] or pitfalls as we call them, need to be negotiated. A pitfall is a hidden danger that one may fall into, like a covered hole in the ground to trap an unsuspecting animal. For all its promise of pleasure, hyper-individualism holds many hidden pitfalls. Other pitfalls include arrogance and egotism;[178] demoralization, paranoia, and "intoxication with power or success;"[179] manic defences such as forced happiness, busyness, and shopping therapy;[180] and decision-fatigue, denial, apathy, and impotence in the face of complex socio-economic, ecological, and ethical problems.[181]

Avoiding these pitfalls takes careful thought, considered effort, love and wisdom;[182] and knowledge, confidence, values, and skills.[183] It requires, we argue, awareness of the biological importance of attachment, love and belonging, and nurturing resilient relationships. It takes hyper-individual judgement and choice to shape a life-story that can avoid pitfalls.

Relationship binds

Hyper-individualism espouses a me-focus. Longevity in a couple relationship requires a we-focus and give-and-take compromise. Wanting a relationship in a hyper-individual age leads to binds needing to be negotiated. Eight binds are articulated here. Ways forward are explored in Chapter 6.

Bind one

Hyper-individualism, as discussed, inherently leads to values clashes which can lead to irreconcilable differences and possible separation and divorce. Irreconcilable differences can be the sole ground for divorce in Australia and Canada, but in England and Wales they must be proven through adultery, unreasonable behaviour, or desertion.[184] Here is the bind:

> Two individuals, one relationship, multiple values clashes.

In the midst of this bind, couples we interviewed and surveyed found a way to thrive (see Chapter 5).

Bind two

In hyper-individualism, resources are often channelled into self-esteem and self-actualization (Maslow's levels 4 and 5) to the detriment of belonging needs (level 3). As I have seen multiple times in clinical practice, the relationship devastation is disturbingly common:

> As an in-demand barrister, John was a wealthy high flier. Having put his career way above his partner and family, he lost them both and became depressed and suicidal.

As Maslow articulated:

> All theorists of psychopathology have stressed thwarting of the love needs as basic in the picture of maladjustment.[185]
>
> When a need has been satisfied for a long time, this need may be underevaluated.[186]

In this, Maslow states the importance of love and belonging to mental health and not taking these for granted. Can this be achieved while reaching for self-actualization? Many couples have done so:

> Christine and Ted are still together after 50 years of marriage. Each of their three daughters, however, is divorced. "Why do you still do all that for Dad?" they ask. Christine answers "Why does he do all that he does for me?"

Bind three

Hyper-individualism shames the dependency often found in strong relationships.[187] A person may, for example, freely decide to vote the way their partner does, do things they like, trust them with finances, or find their identity in their partner and the relationship. Are people 'allowed' to choose this? (A way forward is explored in Chapter 6.)

Bind four

Hyper-individualism may result from failed individuation. Parents' increased risk intolerance, individual specialness, screen technologies, and decreased socialization lead to individuation failure.[188] According to Durkheim, individuation occurs within a group.[189] Without a group, individuals may develop a fragile sense of self in a growing void rather than independence. This is exemplified in people who "lived in sin."[190] This dated term encapsulated a couple's defiance of traditional values: 'we live in sin because we're not like you.' Now that couples can be non-married without stigma, defiance does not add to their identity. Can individuation occur for couples without a group context?

Bind five

Hyper-individualism is the "psychology of affluence" in which "Instead of a concern with moral obligation to others pursued at the cost of personal desire, we have the concept of duty to self pursued at the cost of moral obligation to others."[191] In self-serving people,[192] a relationship too must serve the self.[193] The bind is that self-fulfilment becomes tyrannical and self-defeating through affluence-driven excessive choice, unrealistic expectation, and consequent anxiety and depression.[194]

Bind six

In relationship give and take, individuals enjoy shared meaning-making.[195] Altruism itself is self-satisfying,[196] but in hyper-individualism, this enjoyment is often shamed. People can often feel guilty about wanting to please their partner:

Is it okay for me to want to stop drinking because my spouse wants me to?
Is it okay for me to like looking after my spouse and family rather than having a career?
Is it okay for me to want to cook for my spouse even when I'm tired?[197]

Self-fulfilment through altruism is part of Maslow's belonging (level 3) and self-actualization (level 5); it contributes to thriving. Can one be genuinely hyper-individual and still serve others, including a partner? (This is discussed in Chapter 6.)

Bind seven

Hyper-individualism appears to complete a societal shift from 'we' to 'me' fulfilment.[198] Can a couple choose to be 'we-focussed' within the hyper-individual ideal?

Bind eight

The ultimate bind is when we pit our own wants against the relationship itself: 'why even bother trying to balance selfishness and altruism when hyper-individualism is all about me?' Solutions to these eight dilemmas are explored in Chapter 6.

Is hyper-individualism a challenge to relationship longevity?

There is no law against being in a secure, stable long-term relationship. It predicts individual happiness.[199] In this, hyper-individualism and relationship longevity are not at odds. Some hyper-individual ideals may deny couple "interconnectedness and interdependence"[200] and lead to pitfalls and binds, but others – autonomy, self-responsibility, conscious judgment, and long-term self-benefit – help individuals reach for double self-actualization in a relationship.

The real challenge, as previously stated, is for each individual needing to balance freedom and responsibility and negotiate pitfalls with little guidance. Seemingly "powerful external world influences"[201] infiltrate our private worlds to distract us from our own best interests.

Previously, marriages and long-term relationships were accepted norms, now they are a valued option. In hyper-individualism, being in a long-term relationship means confronting complex, high-stakes questions:

Should I stick with this relationship?
What if it doesn't last or something bad happens?
Can I find someone who is better in bed?
We're having problems, do I cut my losses and run?
What will I miss out on?
Can I commit to this person without narrowing down my options?[202]

These comments all pit self-benefit against committed relationship in a false dichotomy. The problem is not self versus the relationship, but instant versus delayed gratification. Self-actualization, the ultimate gratification after delay, assumes that effort has already been put into love and belonging. Through effort and delayed gratification, a couple can reach for greater fulfilment together: "There's more joy in it when you wait" (Isabella and Ben, 56 yrs). Self-actualization goes beyond self to include heightened states of love, sex, friendship, and self-transcendence.[203] In a relationship, pursuing two sets of self-actualization requires knowledge, skills, and intention. Knowledge comes from research, skills from therapists and lived experience, and intention from the couple themselves.

Couples choosing relationship longevity: the way forward

The way forward for couples choosing togetherness includes conscious intention and judicious choice to balance self-wants and relationship-needs. This shapes a life-story towards actualization, together: "Self-actualizing people are, without one single exception, involved in . . . something outside of themselves."[204] Maslow's "something outside of themselves" was present in 100% of the couples we interviewed: facing adversity, being involved in others' lives, working for a cause, caring for difficult children, caring for each other, and being committed to the relationship. This is thriving:

> Matty was a severely intellectually disabled child. We have a lot of friends with disabled children and there was only us and another couple who stayed together. The rest of them all divorced. We clung to each other. We did it out of love. (Jo and Rob, 47 yrs)

Personal and together growth comes through facing adversity together. We posit that it requires give and take to reach self-actualization together. Evidence for this is seen in Chapter 5, in thriving couple's attitudes and life journeys. "Take" helps facilitate self-actualization, and "give" altruistically facilitates a partner's actualization. "Give," however, also creates positive self-emotions[205] to an "extended sense of self."[206] Why miss out on the self-satisfaction of giving to and adding to another person? The feeling of being wanted and needed by someone is under-appreciated. This is one of the messages from interviewed couples: choosing togetherness selfishly helps yourself. The hyper-individualism – long-term relationship dichotomy disappears in what we call "together-actualization."

Together-actualization

Together-actualization is a continuous, long-term, authentic encounter in two human beings. It results in personal and relational growth, and shared meaning-making. It is greater than double self-actualization as it includes it.

Together-actualization + Self-actualization x 2 > Self-actualization x 2

This is seen in all couples we interviewed. It is a peak life experience,[207] even transcendent.[208] It is the relationship ideal of sharing, caring, and experiencing life with another person and thriving through delayed gratification for long-term self-benefits for two. These benefits are enormous and never guaranteed, but if achievable even in part, are worth the journey. Together-actualization carries burdens, past pain, and perseveres through current and on-going clashes. Overcoming or adapting to adversity adds to together-actualization. Key ingredients, to pre-empt our findings, are commitment, altruism, and sharing values to strengthen attachment:

> Sometimes you reach a point where you have to make a choice and say, "What do we want? And what do I want? And what does she want for our future?" And you have two options or three options, whatever. And you realize what is the most important to you: your relationship. (Philippe and Laure, 47 yrs)

> We always try to push one another to do better. . . . [Many] relationships degenerate to the lowest common denominator, instead of pushing up to the highest common denominator. (Peter and Rhonda, 53 yrs)

Couple relationships need not reach impossible ideals. They just need to be mutually supportive and good enough in the way that a baby's care-giver is good enough. Based on Winnicott's idea of good-enough parenting,[209] couples need only strive to be good enough. A relationship does not need to be perfect, only comfortable. Perceived rewards need to outweigh perceived costs.[210] "The relationship is not going to be Mr Perfect Mrs Perfect" (Carol and Steve, 53 yrs).

A "good enough" relationship[211] may be one that barely survives or easily thrives. It is a relationship with ongoing unresolved problems, clashes, and frustrations. Together-actualization is a good-enough relationship being "all that it can be to realize its full potential."[212] For this ideal to be realized, a relationship must have relational safety with confidence of continuing into a joint future.

Reaching for together-actualization may fly in the face of prevailing social norms, but according to hyper-individualism, any two people can selfishly choose it. Therapists, however, may need to articulate this freedom:

> If you both value each other deeply, it doesn't matter what others think.
>
> If you want to prioritize 'we' over 'me,' it's okay to ignore social media influencers.
>
> Evidence shows that sharing your lives together is a great way to go. The best.
>
> If you value together-actualization, sure, why not buck the trend?

It is, perhaps, exemplified by Olga and Raul (45 yrs):

> In that early period, we fought like cats and dogs. He was 32: a whole life of alone, doing what he wanted. And I was like a wild little pony. So we argued, we argued. We nearly separated in Rio one time, . . . but you have to get it out because then you understand each other. His family said "don't marry her." . . . Now we stand together. We never try to, for instance, be superior to the other one. We are together, same ideals. Fighting against adversity together.

Couples we interviewed each uniquely displayed together-actualization. "Great love is not the stuff of fables, but of real human experience, and therefore potentially available to anyone."[213] In twenty-first century uncertainty and competing values, this requires not only knowledge, skills, and intention, but judgment and conscious intent to continuously balance selfish genes and altruism, delay gratification, and avoid pitfalls and binds. It means seeking fulfilment through attachment and relationship resilience. This makes hyper-individualism work for you, not against you. Nurturing a strong, mutually supportive long-term relationship may just be the most self-serving thing two people could choose to do.

Part II shows that younger couples want relationship resilience, and discusses how thriving couples achieved it. Part III offers techniques to help build resilient relationships. Relationship resilience is challenged by some hyper-individual ideals but is nurtured by others. It is further challenged by mental illness and social isolation, as explored in Chapters 2 and 3.

Notes

1 See Chapter 4 and Feeney, Brooke C., and Nancy L. Collins. "A new look at social support: A theoretical perspective on thriving through relationships." *Personality and Social Psychology Review* 19, no. 2 (2015): 113–147 and Hoffnung, Michele. "Wanting it all: Career, marriage, and motherhood during college-educated women's 20s." *Sex Roles* 50, no. 9 (2004): 711–723.

2 Krug, Orah T. "James Bugental and Irvin Yalom: Two masters of existential therapy cultivate presence in the therapeutic encounter." *Journal of Humanistic Psychology* 49, no. 3 (2009): 329–354.
3 Mittelman, Willard. "Maslow's study of self-actualization: A reinterpretation." *Journal of Humanistic Psychology* 31, no. 1 (1991): 114–135.
4 See https://marriagefoundation.org.uk/half-of-todays-newlyweds-will-celebrate-their-ruby-anniversary-together/ and https://ourworldindata.org/marriages-and-divorces Retrieved 11 September 2022.
5 https://en.wiktionary.org/wiki/hyperindividualism Retrieved 7 October 2021.
6 Pakulski, Jan. "Postmodern social theory." *The New Blackwell Companion to Social Theory* (2009): 251–280.
7 Ali, Saba R., David Drustup, Yunkyoung Loh Garrison, and Duhita Mahatmya. "Economic justice and vocational psychology: Towards community change." *Journal of Career Assessment* 30, no. 3 (2022): 436–454.
8 Ogihara, Yuji, and Yukiko Uchida. "Does individualism bring happiness? Negative effects of individualism on interpersonal relationships and happiness." *Frontiers in Psychology* 5 (2014): 135.
9 Twenge, Jean M., Sara Konrath, Joshua D. Foster, W. Keith Campbell, and Brad J. Bushman. "Egos inflating over time: A cross-temporal meta-analysis of the Narcissistic Personality Inventory." *Journal of Personality* 76, no. 4 (2008): 875–902.
10 Gauchet, Marcel. "A new age of personality: An essay on the psychology of our times." *Thesis Eleven* 60, no. 1 (2000): 23–41.
11 Mărgărițoiu, Alina, and Simona Eftimie. "The lack of gratitude's practice in a hyper individualist, hyper consumer, and hyper technologized society." *Procedia-Social and Behavioral Sciences* 203 (2015): 316–321.
12 Meer, Fátima. "The global crisis – A crisis of values and the domination of the weak by the strong." *Journal of Human Values* 5, no. 1 (1999): 65–74.
13 Duffy, Bobby, Kirstie Hewlett, George Murkin, Rebecca Benson, Rachel Hesketh, Ben Page, Gideon Skinner, and Glenn Gottfried. "Culture wars in the UK: How the public understand the debate." 2021. https://www.kcl.ac.uk/policy-institute/assets/culture-wars-in-the-uk-how-the-public-understand-the-debate.pdf Retrieved 27 December 2022.
14 Baumeister, Roy F., and Michael J. MacKenzie. "The value of marriage in the era of the glorified self." *Psychological Inquiry* 25, no. 1 (2014): 53–55.
15 Gottman, John Mordechai. *The marriage clinic: A scientifically-based marital therapy*. W. W. Norton & Company, 1999, 185.
16 Maslow, Abraham H. "Personality and motivation." *Harlow, England: Longman* 1 (1954): 987.
17 Quinlan, Robert J. "Human pair-bonds: Evolutionary functions, ecological variation, and adaptive development." *Evolutionary Anthropology: Issues, News, and Reviews* 17, no. 5 (2008): 227–238.
18 Bartels, Andreas, and Semir Zeki. "The neural correlates of maternal and romantic love." *Neuroimage* 21, no. 3 (2004): 1155–1166.
19 Brown, Daniel J., Rachel Arnold, Thomas Reid, and Gareth Roberts. "A qualitative exploration of thriving in elite sport." *Journal of Applied Sport Psychology* 30, no. 2 (2018): 129–149.
20 Maslow, Abraham Harold. "A theory of human motivation." *Psychological Review* 50, no. 4 (1943): 370–396.
21 Brown, Arnold, Reid, and Roberts. "A qualitative exploration of thriving in elite sport."

22 Brown, Daniel J., Rachel Arnold, David Fletcher, and Martyn Standage. "Human thriving: A conceptual debate and literature review." *European Psychologist* 22, no. 3 (2017): 167.
23 www.bbc.com/news/world-us-canada-27610770#:~:text=%22My%20mission%20in%20life%20is,some%20humour%20and%20some%20style.%22 Retrieved 15 May 2022.
24 Shields, Brian, Ian Wacogne, and Charlotte M. Wright. "Weight faltering and failure to thrive in infancy and early childhood." *BMJ* 345 (2012).
25 Alexander, Rebecca, Oriana R. Aragón, Jamila Bookwala, Nicolas Cherbuin, Justine M. Gatt, Ian J. Kahrilas, Niklas Kästner et al. "The neuroscience of positive emotions and affect: Implications for cultivating happiness and wellbeing." *Neuroscience & Biobehavioral Reviews* 121 (2021): 220–249.
26 Ramos, Michelle C., Chia-Hsin Emily Cheng, Kathleen S.J. Preston, Allen W. Gottfried, Diana Wright Guerin, Adele Eskeles Gottfried, Ronald E. Riggio, and Pamella H. Oliver. "Positive family relationships across 30 years: Predicting adult health and happiness." *Journal of Family Psychology* 36, no. 7 (2022): 1216–1228.
27 Saphire-Bernstein, Shimon, and Shelley E. Taylor. "Close relationships and happiness." *The Oxford handbook of happiness.* Oxford University Press, 2014.
28 Fok, Hung-Kit, and Sheung-Tak Cheng. "Intimate relationships and happiness in Asia: A critical review." *Close Relationships and Happiness Across Cultures* (2018): 55–67.
29 Feeney and Collins. "A new look at social support."
30 See Luoto, Severi. "Did prosociality drive the evolution of homosexuality?" *Archives of Sexual Behavior* 49, no. 7 (2020): 2239–2244. Manzouri, Amirhossein, and Ivanka Savic. "Multimodal MRI suggests that male homosexuality may be linked to cerebral midline structures." *PLoS One* 13, no. 10 (2018): e0203189. Kanazawa, Satoshi. "Possible evolutionary origins of human female sexual fluidity." *Biological Reviews* 92, no. 3 (2017): 1251–1274.
31 Zajonc, Robert B. "Attitudinal effects of mere exposure." *Journal of Personality and Social Psychology* 9, no. 2 (1968): 1.
32 Finkel, T. and J. Eli. *The all-or-nothing marriage: How the best marriages work.* Penguin, 2019.
33 Kaur, Avneet. "Maslow's need hierarchy theory: Applications and criticisms." *Global Journal of Management and Business Studies* 3, no. 10 (2013): 1061–1064.
34 Maslow. "A theory of human motivation."
35 Comments shared in Dr Christian Heim's clinical practice.
36 Dawkins, Richard. *The selfish gene.* Oxford University Press, 1976.
37 Bargh, John A., and Julie Y. Huang. "The selfish goal." *The Psychology of Goals* (2009): 127–150.
38 Fishbane, Mona DeKoven. *Loving with the brain in mind: Neurobiology and couple therapy (Norton series on interpersonal neurobiology).* W. W. Norton & Company, 2013, xxii.
39 Dawkins, Richard. *The selfish gene.* Oxford University Press, 40th anniversary ed., 2016, 4.
40 Ibid, 8.
41 De Chadarevian, Soraya. "The selfish gene at 30: The origin and career of a book and its title." *Notes and Records of the Royal Society* 61, no. 1 (2007): 31–38.
42 Case study from Dr Christian Heim's clinical practice.
43 Sonne, James W. H., and Don M. Gash. "Psychopathy to altruism: Neurobiology of the selfish – selfless spectrum." *Frontiers in Psychology* 9 (2018): 575.

44 Decety, Jean. "The neural pathways, development and functions of empathy." *Current Opinion in Behavioral Sciences* 3 (2015): 1–6.
45 Ma-Kellams, Christine, and Jennifer Lerner. "Trust your gut or think carefully? Examining whether an intuitive, versus a systematic, mode of thought produces greater empathic accuracy." *Journal of Personality and Social Psychology* 111, no. 5 (2016): 674.
46 Weng, Helen Y., Andrew S. Fox, Alexander J. Shackman, Diane E. Stodola, Jessica Z. K. Caldwell, Matthew C. Olson, Gregory M. Rogers, and Richard J. Davidson. "Compassion training alters altruism and neural responses to suffering." *Psychological Science* 24, no. 7 (2013): 1171–1180.
47 Smith, Karen E., and Seth D. Pollak. "Early life stress and perceived social isolation influence how children use value information to guide behavior." *Child Development* 93, no. 3 (2022): 804–814.
48 Cameron, C., C. Daryl, Cendri A. Hutcherson, Amanda M. Ferguson, Julian A. Scheffer, Eliana Hadjiandreou, and Michael Inzlicht. "Empathy is hard work: People choose to avoid empathy because of its cognitive costs." *Journal of Experimental Psychology: General* 148, no. 6 (2019): 962.
49 Andreoni, James, Justin M. Rao, and Hannah Trachtman. "Avoiding the ask: A field experiment on altruism, empathy, and charitable giving." *Journal of Political Economy* 125, no. 3 (2017): 625–653.
50 Rachlin, Howard. "Altruism and selfishness." *Behavioral and Brain Sciences* 25, no. 2 (2002): 239.
51 Rand, David G., and Ziv G. Epstein. "Risking your life without a second thought: Intuitive decision-making and extreme altruism." *PLoS One* 9, no. 10 (2014): e109687.
52 Ma-Kellams, Christine, and Jennifer Lerner. "Trust your gut or think carefully? Examining whether an intuitive, versus a systematic, mode of thought produces greater empathic accuracy." *Journal of Personality and Social Psychology* 111, no. 5 (2016): 674.
53 Whiting, Beatrice B., and John W. Whiting. "Children of six cultures: A psychocultural analysis." *Contemporary Sociology* 5, no. 6 (1976): 771–772.
54 Rand, David G., et al. "Social heuristics shape intuitive cooperation." *Nature Communications* 5, no. 1 (2014): 1–12.
55 Cameron, Hutcherson, Ferguson, Scheffer, Hadjiandreou, and Inzlicht. "Empathy is hard work."
56 Marsh, Abigail A. "Neural, cognitive, and evolutionary foundations of human altruism." *Wiley Interdisciplinary Reviews: Cognitive Science* 7, no. 1 (2016): 59–71.
57 Remark by Haldane, Dugatkin, and Lee Alan. "Inclusive fitness theory from Darwin to Hamilton." *Genetics* 176, no. 3 (2007): 1375–1380.
58 Cook, Karen S., Coye Cheshire, Eric R. W. Rice, and Sandra Nakagawa. "Social exchange theory." *Handbook of social psychology*. Springer, 2013, 61–88.
59 Klimecki, Olga M., Susanne Leiberg, Matthieu Ricard, and Tania Singer. "Differential pattern of functional brain plasticity after compassion and empathy training." *Social Cognitive and Affective Neuroscience* 9, no. 6 (2014): 873–879.
60 Batson, C. Daniel, David A. Lishner, and Eric L. Stocks. "13 The empathy – altruism hypothesis." *The Oxford handbook of prosocial behavior*. Oxford University Press, 2015, 259–268.
61 Hawley, Patricia H. "Evolution, prosocial behavior, and altruism." *Prosocial Development: A Multidimensional Approach* (2014): 43.
62 Fromm, Erich. *The art of loving: The centennial edition*. A&C Black, 2000, 18–19.

63 Wolfe, Alan. "What is altruism?" *The nature of the nonprofit sector*. Routledge, 2021, 381–392.
64 Winnicott, Donald Woods. *The child, the family, and the outside world*. Harmondsworth, Penguin, 1964, 88.
65 Bowlby, John. "Forty-four juvenile thieves: their characters and home-life." *International Journal of Psychoanalysis* 25 (1944): 107–128.
66 Rowold, Katharina. "What do babies need to thrive? Changing interpretations of 'Hospitalism' in an international context, 1900–1945." *Social History of Medicine* 32, no.4 (2019): 799–818.
67 Thompson, Ross A., Jeffry A. Simpson, and Lisa J. Berlin. "Taking perspective on attachment theory and research: Nine fundamental questions." *Attachment & Human Development* (2022): 1–18.
68 Shaver, Phillip R., Cindy Hazan, and Donna Bradshaw. "The integration of three behavioral systems." *Attachment Theory and Research: A Reader* (2021): 74.
69 Oliveira, Paula, and Pasco Fearon. "The biological bases of attachment." *Adoption & Fostering* 43, no. 3 (2019): 274–293.
70 Strand, Paul S. "A comparative analysis of divergent evolutionary models of attachment and a new biobehavioral conceptualization." *The Psychological Record* (2022): 1–9.
71 Feldman, Ruth. "The neurobiology of human attachments." *Trends in Cognitive Sciences* 21, no. 2 (2017): 80–99.
72 Zayas, Vivian, and Cindy Hazan. *Bases of adult attachment*. Springer, 2014.
73 Bowlby, J. *Attachment and loss. Volume 1: Attachment*, 2nd edn. Basic Books, 1982.
74 Goldberg, Susan, Joan E. Grusec, and Jennifer M. Jenkins. "Confidence in protection: Arguments for a narrow definition of attachment." *Journal of Family Psychology* 13, no. 4 (1999): 475.
75 Dunkel, Curtis S., and Colin Harbke. "A review of measures of Erikson's stages of psychosocial development: Evidence for a general factor." *Journal of Adult Development* 24, no. 1 (2017): 58–76.
76 Gupta, Hritik, and Akriti Srivastava. "Understanding social constructivism of intimacy and isolation among heterosexuals and homosexuals." *The International Journal of Indian Psychology* 8, no. 1 (2020): 167–194.
77 Hazan, C., and D. Zeifman. "Pairbonds as attachments: Mounting evidence in support of Bowlby's hypothesis." *Handbook of Attachment: Theory, Research, and Clinical Applications* 3 (2016): 416–434.
78 Stanley, Scott M., Galena K. Rhoades, and Sarah W. Whitton. "Commitment: Functions, formation, and the securing of romantic attachment." *Journal of Family Theory & Review* 2, no. 4 (2010): 243–257.
79 Zeifman, Debra M. "Attachment theory grows up: A developmental approach to pair bonds." *Current Opinion in Psychology* 25 (2019): 139–143.
80 Kazan, Dominique, Alison L. Calear, and Philip J. Batterham. "The impact of intimate partner relationships on suicidal thoughts and behaviours: A systematic review." *Journal of Affective Disorders* 190 (2016): 585–598.
81 Wyder, Marianne, Patrick Ward, and Diego De Leo. "Separation as a suicide risk factor." *Journal of Affective Disorders* 116, no. 3 (2009): 208–213.
82 Stack, Steven, and Jonathan Scourfield. "Recency of divorce, depression, and suicide risk." *Journal of Family Issues* 36, no. 6 (2015): 695–715.
83 Liamputtong, Pranee, Zoe Sanipreeya Rice, and Dusanee Suwankhong. "Social capital and social inclusion." *Handbook of social inclusion: Research and practices in health and social sciences*. Springer International Publishing, 2021, 1–15.

84 Ward, Mary J., Shelley S. Lee, and Evelyn G. Lipper. "Failure-to-thrive is associated with disorganized infant – mother attachment and unresolved maternal attachment." *Infant Mental Health Journal* 21, no. 6 (2000): 428–442.
85 Litam, Stacey Diane Arañez, and A. Stephen Lenz. "Moderation of attachment on association between relationship status and depression." *Journal of Counseling & Development* 100, no. 2 (2022): 194–204.
86 Bowlby, John. "The making and breaking of affectional bonds: I. Aetiology and psychopathology in the light of attachment theory." *The British Journal of Psychiatry* 130, no. 3 (1977): 201–210.
87 Baumeister, Roy F., and Mark R. Leary. "The need to belong: Desire for interpersonal attachments as a fundamental human motivation." *Interpersonal Development* (2017): 57–89.
88 MacDonald, Kevin. "Warmth as a developmental construct: An evolutionary analysis." *Child Development* 63, no. 4 (1992): 753–773.
89 Long, Madison, Willem Verbeke, Tsachi Ein-Dor, and Pascal Vrtička. "A functional neuro-anatomical model of human attachment (NAMA): Insights from first-and second-person social neuroscience." *Cortex* 126 (2020): 281–321.
90 Simpson, Jeffry A., W. Steven Rholes, Jami Eller, and R. L. Paetzold. "Major principles of attachment theory." *Social Psychology: Handbook of Basic Principles* (2021): 222–239.
91 Butzer, Bethany, and Lorne Campbell. "Adult attachment, sexual satisfaction, and relationship satisfaction: A study of married couples." *Personal Relationships* 15, no. 1 (2008): 141–154.
92 Madey, Scott F., and Lindsey Rodgers. "The effect of attachment and Sternberg's triangular theory of love on relationship satisfaction." *Individual Differences Research* 7, no. 2 (2009).
93 Kachadourian, Lorig K., Frank Fincham, and Joanne Davila. "The tendency to forgive in dating and married couples: The role of attachment and relationship satisfaction." *Personal Relationships* 11, no. 3 (2004): 373–393.
94 Pistole, M. Carole. "Attachment in adult romantic relationships: Style of conflict resolution and relationship satisfaction." *Journal of Social and Personal Relationships* 6, no. 4 (1989): 505–510.
95 Quoted in Fraley, R. Chris, and Phillip R. Shaver. "Adult romantic attachment: Theoretical developments, emerging controversies, and unanswered questions." *Review of General Psychology* 4, no. 2 (2000): 132–154.
96 Crowell, Judith A., and Everett Waters. "Bowlby's theory grown up: The role of attachment in adult love relationships." *Psychological Inquiry* 5, no. 1 (1994): 31–34.
97 Imhasly-Gandhy, Rashna. "Myth, archetype and individuation." *India International Centre Quarterly* 19, no. 4 (1992): 76–87.
98 Arnett, Jeffrey Jensen. "Emerging adulthood: What is it, and what is it good for?." *Child Development Perspectives* 1, no. 2 (2007): 68–73.
99 Feeney and Collins. "A new look at social support."
100 www.pewresearch.org/social-trends/2014/11/14/chapter-2-the-demographics-of-remarriage/ Retrieved 15 May 2022.
101 Adler, Alfred. "Fundamentals of individual psychology." *Readings in the Theory of Individual Psychology*. Routledge, 2007, 37.
102 Fisher, Helen. *Why we love: The nature and chemistry of romantic love*. Macmillan, 2004, 3.
103 Heim, Christian. *The seven love-types: Navigating love in a fractured world*. Vivid Publishing, 2021.

104 Fricker, Julie, and Susan Moore. "Relationship satisfaction: The role of love styles and attachment styles." *Current Research in Social Psychology* 7, no. 11 (2002): 182–204.
105 Enright, Robert D., Jiahe Wang Xu, Hannah Rapp, Moon Evans, and Jacqueline Y. Song. "The philosophy and social science of agape love." *Journal of Theoretical and Philosophical Psychology* 42, no. 4 (2022): 220–237.
106 Razfar, Aria, and Patriann Smith. "Algorithm of love: Insights from immigrant literacies and narratives." *International Journal of Qualitative Studies in Education* (2022): 1–4.
107 Thompson, Ross A., Jeffry A. Simpson, and Lisa J. Berlin. "Taking perspective on attachment theory and research: Nine fundamental questions." *Attachment & Human Development* (2022): 1–18.
108 Neumann, Inga D. "Oxytocin: The neuropeptide of love reveals some of its secrets." *Cell Metabolism* 5, no. 4 (2007): 231–233.
109 Buchheim, Anna, et al. "Oxytocin enhances the experience of attachment security." *Psychoneuroendocrinology* 34, no. 9 (2009): 1417–1422.
110 Sharma, Samata R., Xenia Gonda, Peter Dome, and Frank I. Tarazi. "What's love got to do with it: Role of oxytocin in trauma, attachment and resilience." *Pharmacology & Therapeutics* 214 (2020): 107602.
111 Bartels and Zeki. "The neural correlates of maternal and romantic love."
112 www.livescience.com/1135-wild-sex-monogamy-rare.html Retrieved 1 March 2019.
113 Fisher, Helen. *Why we love: The nature and chemistry of romantic love*. Macmillan, 2004, 3.
114 Darwin, Charles. *The expression of the emotions in man and animals*. Appleton & Co, 1897.
115 Marazziti, Donatella, and Stefano Baroni. "Romantic love: The mistery of its biological roots." *Clinical Neuropsychiatry* 9, no. 1 (2012).
116 Fisher, Helen. *Why we love.*
117 Swami, Viren, and Adrian Furnham. "Is love really so blind?" *The Psychologist* 21, no. 2 (2008): 108–111.
118 Brickman, Philip. "Hedonic relativism and planning the good society." *Adaptation Level Theory* (1971): 287–301.
119 Diener, Ed, Richard E. Lucas, and Christie Napa Scollon. "Beyond the hedonic treadmill: Revising the adaptation theory of well-being." *The science of well-being*. Springer, 2009, 103–118.
120 Asselmann, Eva, and Jule Specht. "Changes in happiness, sadness, anxiety, and anger around romantic relationship events." *Emotion* (2022).
121 Lewis, Edwin Herbert. "Some definitions of individualism." *American Journal of Sociology* 17, no. 2 (1911): 223–253.
122 Oyserman, Daphna, and Ayse K. Uskul. "Individualism and collectivism: Societal-level processes with implications for individual-level and society-level outcomes." *Multilevel analysis of individuals and cultures*. Psychology Press, 2015, 145–173.
123 Santos, Henri C., Michael E. W. Varnum, and Igor Grossmann. "Global increases in individualism." *Psychological Science* 28, no. 9 (2017): 1228–1239.
124 Morina, Nexhmedin, and Gernot von Collani. "Impact of war-related traumatic events on self-evaluation and subjective well-being." *Traumatology* 12, no. 2 (2006): 130–138.
125 Gabor, Elena. "Turning points in the development of classical musicians." *Journal of Ethnographic and Qualitative Research* 5, no. 3 (2011): 138–156.
126 Maslow. "A theory of human motivation."
127 Ibid.

128 Ayoob, S. M. "Fundamental causes of divorce: A sociological study." Paper presented at *Promoting Multidisciplinary Academic Research and Innovation, South Eastern University*, 2019.
129 Elizabeth A. Troop. *Psychotherapy, American culture and social policy: Immoral individualism*. Palgrave Macmillan, 2009, 5.
130 Freud, Sigmund. "An outline of psycho-analysis." *International Journal of Psycho-Analysis* 21 (1940): 27–84.
131 Milhaven, John Giles. "Thomas Aquinas on sexual pleasure." *The Journal of Religious Ethics* (1977): 157–181.
132 Fee, Elizabeth. "Psychology, sexuality, and social control in Victorian England." *Social Science Quarterly* 58, no. 4 (1978): 632–646.
133 James, William. *The principles of psychology*, 1890, 438. quoted in Kelly, Gary F., ed. *Sources: Notable selections in human sexuality*. Dushkin/McGraw-Hill, 1998, 47.
134 Ellis, H. *Studies in the psychology of sex*. F. A. Davis Company, 1903, 241.
135 www.npr.org/sections/npr-history-dept/2015/05/26/409126557/when-petting-parties-scandalized-the-nation Retrieved 27 October 2021.
136 Wouters, Cas. "Balancing sex and love since the 1960s sexual revolution." *Theory, Culture & Society* 15, no. 3–4 (1998): 187–214.
137 Brown, Helen Gurley. *Sex and the single girl: The unmarried woman's guide to men*. Open Road Media, 2012. Original published 1962.
138 www.pbs.org/wgbh/americanexperience/features/pill-and-sexual-revolution/ Retrieved 27 October 2021.
139 Allison, Rachel. "Asking out and sliding in: Gendered relationship pathways in college hookup culture." *Qualitative Sociology* 42, no. 3 (2019): 361–383.
140 Laumann, Edward O., John H. Gagnon, Robert T. Michael, and Stuart Michaels. "National health and social life survey, 1992: [United States]." *Inter-university Consortium for Political and Social Research (ICPSR)[distributor]* (2008).
141 Seidman, Steven. "Queer-ing sociology, sociologizing queer theory: An introduction." *Sociological Theory* 12, no. 2 (1994): 166–177.
142 Albury, Kath. "Young people, digital media research and counterpublic sexual health." *Sexualities* 21, no. 8 (2018): 1331–1336.
143 Dubé, Simon, and Dave Anctil. "Foundations of erobotics." *International Journal of Social Robotics* 13, no. 6 (2021): 1205–1233.
144 Sundén, Jenny. "Play, secrecy and consent: Theorizing privacy breaches and sensitive data in the world of networked sex toys." *Sexualities* (2020) https://doi.org/10.1177/1363460720957
145 Quintero, Jesús Bolaño. "Post-postmodernism: Mapping out the Zeitgeist of the new millennium." *Oceánide* 15 (2022): 17–25.
146 Tsirogianni, Stavroula, and George Gaskell. "The role of plurality and context in social values." *Journal for the Theory of Social Behaviour* 41, no. 4 (2011): 441–465.
147 Meer, Fátima. "The global crisis."
148 Barrett-Lennard, Godfrey. *The relationship paradigm: Human being beyond individualism*. Macmillan International Higher Education, 2013, 19.
149 Marci, Green, and Marc Scholes. "Education for what? Attachment, culture and society." *Attachment and human survival*. Routledge, 2018, 37–51.
150 Ogihara and Uchida. "Does individualism bring happiness?"
151 Barry, Christopher T., Patricia K. Kerig, Kurt K. Stellwagen, and Tammy D. Barry, eds. *Narcissism and Machiavellianism in youth: Implications for the development of adaptive and maladaptive behavior*. American Psychological Association, 2011.
152 Mărgăriţoiu and Eftimie. "The lack of gratitude's practice."

153 Finkel, Eli J., Chin Ming Hui, Kathleen L. Carswell, and Grace M. Larson. "The suffocation of marriage: Climbing Mount Maslow without enough oxygen." *Psychological Inquiry* 25, no. 1 (2014): 1–41.
154 Pakulski. "Postmodern social theory."
155 Goodman, Catherine. "Intimacy and autonomy in long term marriage." *Journal of Gerontological Social Work* 32, no. 1 (1999): 83–97.
156 Hadden, Benjamin W., Zachary G. Baker, and C. Raymond Knee. "Let it go: Relationship autonomy predicts pro-relationship responses to partner transgressions." *Journal of Personality* 86, no. 5 (2018): 868–887.
157 Pakulski. "Postmodern social theory."
158 Wilson, Chris M., and Andrew J. Oswald. "How does marriage affect physical and psychological health? A survey of the longitudinal evidence." *IDEAS* Working Paper Series from RePEc (2005).
159 Waite, Linda J., and Evelyn L. Lehrer. "The benefits from marriage and religion in the United States: A comparative analysis." *Population and Development Review* 29, no. 2 (2003): 255–275.
160 Oswald, Ramona Faith. "Resilience within the family networks of lesbians and gay men: Intentionality and redefinition." *Journal of Marriage and Family* 64, no. 2 (2002): 374–383.
161 Easterlin, Richard A. "Explaining happiness." *Proceedings of the National Academy of Sciences* 100, no. 19 (2003): 11176–11183.
162 Leonard, Kenneth E., and Julie C. Rothbard. "Alcohol and the marriage effect." *Journal of Studies on Alcohol, Supplement* 13 (1999): 139–146.
163 Weissman, Myrna M., Roger C. Bland, Glorisa J. Canino, Carlo Faravelli, Steven Greenwald, Hai-Gwo Hwu, Peter R. Joyce et al. "Cross-national epidemiology of major depression and bipolar disorder." *JAMA* 276, no. 4 (1996): 293–299.
164 Trovato, Frank. "A longitudinal analysis of divorce and suicide in Canada." *Journal of Marriage and the Family* (1987): 193–203.
165 de Jong Gierveld, Jenny, Theo Van Tilburg, and Pearl Dykstra. "*Loneliness and social isolation.*" *The Cambridge handbook of personal relationships.* Cambridge University Press, 2006.
166 Gauchet, Marcel. "A new age of personality: An essay on the psychology of our times." *Thesis Eleven* 60, no. 1 (2000): 23–41.
167 Alexander, Bruce K. "Replacing the BDMA: A paradigm shift in the field of addiction." *Evaluating the brain disease model of addiction.* Routledge, 2022, 522–538.
168 Pignatiello, Grant A., Richard J. Martin, and Ronald L. Hickman Jr. "Decision fatigue: A conceptual analysis." *Journal of Health Psychology* 25, no. 1 (2020): 123–135.
169 Articulated as "dedication" and "restraint" in Stanley, Scott M., and Howard J. Markman. "Assessing commitment in personal relationships." *Journal of Marriage and the Family* (1992): 595–608.
170 Wallis, Jonathan D. "Orbitofrontal cortex and its contribution to decision-making." *Annual Review of Neuroscience* 30 (2007): 31–56.
171 Sellitto, Manuela, Damiano Terenzi, Francesca Starita, Giuseppe Di Pellegrino, and Simone Battaglia. "The cost of imagined actions in a reward-valuation task." *Brain Sciences* 12, no. 5 (2022): 582.
172 Multiple private clinical communications.
173 Al-Nidawi, Enas Ridha Azghar, and Shamal Abu-Baker Hussein. "Educational dilemma in a market-model global context." *International Review of Social Sciences* (2017): 9–17.
174 Ogihara and Uchida. "Does individualism bring happiness?"

175 Gauchet, Marcel. "A new age of personality: An essay on the psychology of our times." *Thesis Eleven* 60, no. 1 (2000): 23–41.
176 Mărgărițoiu and Eftimie. "The lack of gratitude's practice."
177 Al-Nidawi, and Hussein. "Educational dilemma in a market-model global context."
178 Wildman, Wesley J. "Out with the old, in with the new? From conceptual reconstruction in philosophical anthropology to a realistic theory of change." *Relational anthropology for contemporary economics*. Springer, 2022, 181–199.
179 Jakovljevic, Miro, and Zoran Tomic. "Global and public mental health promotion for empathic civilisation: The role of political psychocultures." *Psychiatria Danubina* 28, no. 4 (2016): 323–333.
180 Rudan, Dusko, Miro Jakovljevic, and Darko Marcinko. "Manic defences in contemporary society the psychocultural approach." *Psychiatria Danubina* 28, no. 4 (2016): 334–342.
181 Ibid.
182 Wildman, Wesley J. "Out with the old, in with the new?"
183 Saane, Joke van. "Personal leadership: How to change what cannot be changed: A response to Wesley Wildman's out with the old, in with the new?" *Relational anthropology for contemporary economics*. Springer, 2022, 201–208.
184 www.divorce-online.co.uk/help-and-advice/irreconcilable-differences-grounds-for-divorce-uk/ Retrieved 18 April 2022.
185 Maslow, Abraham Harold. "A theory of human motivation."
186 Ibid.
187 Feeney, Judith A. "Adult romantic attachment: Developments in the study of couple relationships." Cassidy, Jude and Phillip Shaver, eds. *Handbook of attachment: Theory, research, and clinical applications*, 2nd edn. Guilford Publications, 2008.
188 Huang, Joh-Jong, Ming-Yii Huang, and Fei-Kai Syu. "Liberated anomie in generation next: Hyperindividualism, extreme consumerism, and social isolationism." *Fooyin Journal of Health Sciences* 2, no. 2 (2010): 41–47.
189 Durkheim, Emile. *Professional ethics and civic morals*. Routledge, 2013, xiv.
190 www.collinsdictionary.com/dictionary/english/to-live-in-sin Retrieved 28 October 2021.
191 Yankelovich, Daniel. *New rules: Searching for self-fulfillment in a world turned upside down*. Random House, 1981, 189.
192 Baumeister and MacKenzie. "The value of marriage."
193 Finkel, Hui, Carswell and Larson. "The suffocation of marriage."
194 Schwartz, Barry. "Self-determination: The tyranny of freedom." *American Psychologist* 55, no. 1 (2000): 79.
195 Chang, Yen-Ping, Yi-Cheng Lin, and Lung Hung Chen. "Pay it forward: Gratitude in social networks." *Journal of Happiness Studies* 13, no. 5 (2012): 761–781.
196 Dossey, Larry. "The helper's high." *Explore* 14, no. 6 (2018): 393–399.
197 Multiple disclosures during clinical sessions.
198 Karan, Alexander, Robert Rosenthal, and Megan L. Robbins. "Meta-analytic evidence that we-talk predicts relationship and personal functioning in romantic couples." *Journal of Social and Personal Relationships* 36, no. 9 (2019): 2624–2651.
199 Diener, Ed, and Martin E. P. Seligman. "Very happy people." *Psychological Science* 13, no. 1 (2002): 81–84.
200 Harvey, Anna. "Ecology, psychoanalysis, global warming and cats: Fragmentation and interconnection." *Journal of Social Work Practice* 34, no. 4 (2020): 395–408.

201 See Introduction.
202 Comments made in Dr Christian Heim's clinical sessions.
203 Maslow, Abraham Harold. *The farther reaches of human nature*, Vol. 19711. Viking Press, 1971.
204 Maslow, Abraham. "Self-actualization and beyond." (1965)
205 Aknin, Lara B., and Ashley V. Whillans. "Helping and happiness: A review and guide for public policy." *Social Issues and Policy Review* 15, no. 1 (2021): 3–34.
206 Dossey. "The helper's high."
207 Woodward, Anne J., Bruce M. Findlay, and Susan M. Moore. "Peak and mystical experiences in intimate relationships." *Journal of Social and Personal Relationships* 26, no. 4 (2009): 429–442.
208 McLennan, Natasha Anne. *Resting in love: Intimate relationship as spiritual practice*. National Library of Canada, Bibliothèque nationale du Canada, 2003.
209 Stolzenberg, Nomi Maya. "Anti-anxiety law: Winnicott and the legal fiction of paternity." *American Imago* (2007): 339–379.
210 Ratnapalan, Savithiri, and Helen Batty. "To be good enough." *Canadian Family Physician* 55, no. 3 (2009): 239–240.
211 Rabin, Claire. *Winnicott and 'good enough' couple therapy: Reflections of a couple therapist*. Routledge, 2014.
212 Our definition in the light of Kaur. "Maslow's need hierarchy theory."
213 Sundberg, Jeffrey. "Amigeist: A new extreme love phenomenon." *International Journal of Transpersonal Studies* 31, no. 1 (2019).

Chapter 2

Resilient relationships and mental health: Attachment underlying both

In the twenty-first century, mental illness is no longer Dostoevsky's elephant in the room,[1] but Churchill's black dog[2] ruining our new sofas. Many people fear it as some random demon lurking around just waiting to rob them of personal achievement and thriving. Mental illness rates have increased over decades enough for it to be a major global concern. The facts in this chapter make for sobering reading. If the reader finds themselves reaching for comfort, and that comfort is connection to someone close, then the chapter will have served its purpose.

Public misconceptions regarding mental illnesses abound[3] and misinformation continues.[4] Scientific uncertainty regarding the cause, diagnosis, and treatment of mental illness fuels some of this. Neurologists take care of the brain, but mental illness occurs in the mind. Science has too many unanswered questions about the mind and mental illness:

How much sadness and loneliness is normal?
How does low serotonin result in feeling anxious?
How does the mind work?
How are the mind and brain connected?
How much mental illness is genetic, how much is social?
Why can't more tests be used for diagnosis?
Where is the personality?

Our knowledge-base is being updated and refined but is incomplete.[5] Psychiatry lags behind other medical specialties in understanding its illnesses.[6] This perpetuates uncertainty and leaves people questioning how much we scientifically understand mental illness. This unfortunately fuels more anxiety and distrust.

A couple dyad becomes a triad if mental illness is a strong part of their relationship. Rather than discuss mental illness in relationships, however, here we explore the scientifically-proven power of relationships to protect our mental health. Individual mental health, in turn, protects our

DOI: 10.4324/9781003263395-4

relationships. Hyper-individualism and mental illness are linked,[7] and understanding this can help couples build resilience. Nurturing a long-term relationship is self-serving, as mental health and couple relationships enhance each other.

This chapter looks at the mental health crisis and at mental illness risk and protective factors. It argues for more recognition of attachment underlying mental health to contextualize our interviewed couples' insights. That couple therapy can be used to treat individual mental illnesses points to attachment being extremely important to individual mental health. This connection seems self-evident, particularly for social creatures, but it is not emphasized in the literature. The chapter concludes by focussing on valuing relationships to value individual mental health as the two are in reciprocal relationship.

Relationships and mental health: a reciprocal relationship

Being in a reciprocal relationship means that each causes an effect in each other. Since Durkheim's insights of 1888, science has been aware of the close link between mental health and social connectivity.[8] Couple relationships are a foundational source of social connectivity, the "feelings of friendship, love, and caring that can be felt both from and toward others."[9] That supportive relationships protect mental health is a robust finding.[10] It reflects an idea central to human sciences: we are, in great part, social creatures,[11] and we are biologically dependent on each other's support[12] and adversely affected by being socially isolated.[13]

Supportive relationships[14] protect mental health at all stages of life:[15] parent-child relationships protect adolescent mental health,[16] sibling relationships promote resilience in foster care,[17] student-teacher relationships protect children in school transitions,[18] family relationships protect against youth substance use,[19] adolescent peer relationships protect against victimization[20] and mental illness,[21] and supportive families protect college students from anxiety and depression.[22] Friendship protects mental health across the lifespan[23] and into old age.[24] Like welcoming arms, human relationships protect mental health somewhere.

Last chapter we defined attachment as relational safety. It protects us from life's complexities like a harbour protects boats against rough seas. Family attachment protects children against the effects of trauma[25] and aids recovery from mental illness.[26] Psychotherapy uses professional attachment as a harbour to help someone negotiate life stress.[27] Secure attachment protects sufferers of severe mental illness,[28] severe trauma,[29] childhood psychosis,[30] and in illness recovery.[31] Relational safety is a cushion to ease the blow of the harsh "curve balls" (Rob and Jo, 47 yrs) that life often throws.

A supportive couple relationship protects against depression, bipolar disorder,[32] suicide,[33] anxiety,[34] addiction,[35] and alcohol misuse,[36] and it predicts happiness,[37] longevity,[38] and better health.[39] It protects the mental health of those who marry "too early."[40] Social isolation is a greater risk to health than either obesity or alcohol.[41] Being in a couple relationship is not a panacea,[42] but it is a major protective factor. Given the weight of these effects, it is puzzling to think that long-term coupling could ever be in decline. We would not, perhaps, shed our blankets of relational safety if we fully understood how entwined our relationships and mental health really are.

How do close relationships protect mental health?

Close relationships protect all physical and mental health through attachment and oxytocin, bringing about specific biological changes.[43] Briefly, our oxytocin level rises in response to warm interactions with someone close.[44] Oxytocin mediates our feelings of attachment and love[45] and also regulates the hypothalamic-pituitary-adrenal (HPA) axis and cortisol release. This protects against inflammation in, say, heart disease and depression.[46] Oxytocin also regulates our metabolism[47] and activates our immune system[48] to keep us mentally and physically healthy.

Attachment has beneficial effects on the brain. It decreases amygdala sensitivity and promotes prefrontal cortex function and white matter health.[49] These mechanisms begin to explain how attachment biologically protects individuals against mental and physical illness and, as discussed in Chapter 7, improves resilience.

In the real world, what a close relationship can achieve for someone's mental health is truly remarkable:

> Lachlan, in his late twenties, suffers from schizophrenia. He often required prolonged hospital admission to control psychotic symptoms and to save his life. The illness alienates him from his family. He fell in love with an old school friend and, and this led to a long, stable relationship. Lachlan's symptoms improved markedly: both medication and psycho-social strategies became more effective. He no longer needed inpatient admissions and, with Emily's encouragement, he is more engaged in fruitful outpatient management.[50]

Good relationships are biologically protective. This is not only theoretical but practical for Lachlan, our thriving couples, and for all of us. It fulfils the axiomatic idea that we are social creatures.

How does mental health protect a couple relationship?

Mental illness, the antithesis of mental health, contributes to divorce,[51] impedes finding and sustaining relationships,[52] and increases isolation and social stigma.[53] This is the reciprocal relationship between couple relationships and mental health: poor mental health leads to poor relationships, and poor relationships lead to poor mental health. Sustaining a long-term relationship takes effort and according to our findings: commitment, altruism, and shared values. A long-term relationship also involves continuous delayed gratification: great effort for great benefit. Sustaining this effort is much easier in two people enjoying mental health.

Improved relationships will improve mental health, and improved mental health will improve relationships. If the mental health of a population suffers, relationships in that population will also suffer. If relationships in a population suffer, then the mental health of that population will also suffer. This is the flow-on effect of double cause and effect. Globally, relationship longevity and mental health are both in decline. Many researchers are using the word 'crisis.'

The mental health crisis

In the past few decades, western society is said to have experienced an "age of anxiety"[54] followed by an "age of depression."[55] A mental health crisis is reported for school children,[56] tertiary students,[57] the general public,[58] adolescents,[59] and health care workers.[60] An unprecedented major global mental health crisis looms[61] with suicide rates set to rise[62] in a post-pandemic world. This section may sound particularly nihilistic. It is. There is no other way to describe it.

Increased suicide rates during the pandemic were predicted,[63] but studies showed a decrease[64] even in cities with severe lockdowns.[65] Decreases were followed by second-wave increases.[66] Anxiety and depression rates rose 25.6% and 27.6% respectively in 2020, with higher rate rises in areas hit hardest by COVID-19.[67] These fell to almost pre-pandemic levels by 2021,[68] attesting to human adaptation. Risk factors for suicide – anxiety, distress, depression, unemployment, financial loss, loneliness, and alcohol consumption – increased during the pandemic,[69] so suicide, depression and anxiety rates may yet rise tremendously. This is sobering and alarming, but it is not solely related to the pandemic. It is also related to our pre-existing mental health levels and impaired collective resilience.

Rates of mental illness have been rising for decades. During the nineties, antidepressant use in some countries tripled[70] and increased up to six-fold in others.[71] Was this increased illness, increased awareness and treatment,[72] changing definitions and attitudes,[73] or aggressive marketing?[74] Gaining a clear picture is complex. Later studies suggest, however, that rises are real: from 2013 to 2016, for example, depression in the USA rose by 63% in 12–18 year olds, 47% in 18–35 year olds, and 25% for others.[75]

In 2012, depression became the greatest contributor to global disability.[76] Why do we see such high levels of depression in a prospering world? Global anxiety rates continued to rise, more so in affluent countries.[77] In separate ten year periods, studies found that childhood anxiety rose 60%[78]

and self-harm rose 28%.[79] Why, in times of such socio-economic prosperity? Opioid deaths are at a critical all-time high,[80] anorexia nervosa is rising in children,[81] narcissism is at epidemic proportions,[82] and half of the world's population will qualify for a mental health diagnosis.[83] Why is this happening in unprecedented socio-economic progress? The UN notes that developed nations have

> . . . achieved striking economic and technological progress over the past half century without gains in self-reported happiness. . . . Instead, uncertainties and anxieties are high, social and economic inequalities have widened considerably [and] social trust is in decline.[84]

A mixed picture is seen in suicide rates. From 1990 to 2000, the UK rate declined, and has since remained steady at 10–11 per 100,000[85] with encouraging decreases for people in psychiatric care.[86] Decreases over the same period were seen in Europe and Asia with marked decreases in Eastern European, India, and China, and modest increases in South America.[87] Australia, however, saw a 30% increase from 2006 to 2017[88] and US suicide rates rose 35% from 1999 to 2019.[89] Globally, rates fell by over 30% from 1990 to 2016.[90] The global increase in female teenage suicide continues[91] and youth presentations for self-harm and suicide ideation continue to rise.[92] The exhausting topic of mental illness and suicide plagues the uncertain minds of so many young people in particular.

These statistics underscore the limits of medical science in mental illness. Astonishing advances have been made in heart disease, cancer detection, physical trauma, emergency and intensive care practices and more. Mental illness, however, is heavily impacted by all our relationships, perceived meaninglessness, social isolation, technology, and inequities. It is particularly influenced by social media, substance misuse and individual choices.[93] Doctors, psychologists and therapists have no control over these variables. I, like countless other mental health workers, have witnessed the growing suffering over 25 years: mental anguish destroying the lives of many and leaving others feeling helpless and abandoned.

But there is much hope. As a clinician in general adult psychiatry, I have seen remarkable recoveries: individuals overcoming addictions, finding meaning to come back from the brink of suicide, stabilizing major psychiatric conditions, and often, two people with mental illnesses forging a couple alliance to protect themselves. Individual solutions are easier to find and implement than large-scale societal solutions.

Like diabetes and obesity, individual mental illness and the mental health of whole countries is impacted by affluence and poor relationships.[94] Good parent-adolescent connection, measured by shared family meals, for example, protect adolescent mental health[95] and against cyber-bullying.[96] In affluence, this protection is often lost for individuals due to decreased family cohesion,[97] fast food culture, and the influence of social media.[98] These affect all of us globally. Family meal habits are also linked with obesity,[99] diabetes,[100] and metabolic syndrome[101] to further show how protective daily positive people interactions really are.

As discussed last chapter, socio-economic development, hyper-individualism and attitudes to relationships are linked. Increased divorce and decreased marriage rates run in tandem with increased rates of mental illnesses. On a societal level as on an individual level, couple relationships and mental illness are strongly connected.[102]

Before concluding that rate rises in mental illness are driven by social disconnect alone, we explore mental health risks and protective factors. This conceptual exploration highlights the growing evidence for attachment as the major protective factor[103] underlying other protective factors. Attachment conceptually connects childhood and adult relationship experiences with mental illness[104] and, it is argued, underlies the strong reciprocal link between mental illness and couple relationships.

Mental illness: a contemporary conception

The 2018 *Lancet* commission on global mental health and sustainability asserts that mental health or illness "is the unique product of social and environmental influences, in particular during the early life course, interacting with genetic, neurodevelopmental, and psychological processes and affecting biological pathways in the brain."[105] This is essentially an elaboration of the bio-psycho-social model of mental illness. Following its wording, the *Lancet* commission essentially posits that mental illness is the unique product of

1 Social and environmental factors (early life course in particular) and
2 Biological and psychological factors (and their development)

Attachment factors underlie early life course and childhood development. Allowing for safety, nutrition, and education, and conflating 'social' and 'environmental,' mental health or illness is due to

1 Social factors (plus attachment factors)
2 Biological and psychological factors (plus attachment factors)

Taking the *Lancet* commission's implied emphasis on attachment, we can further examine mental health risk and protective factors in this light.

Mental illness: risk and protective factors

Risk factors for heart and cardiovascular disease are well-known and well-defined. This is thanks to large, well-designed studies dating back to 1948.[106]

Defining risk factors for mental illness, however, is still embryonic.[107] Yet this information is sorely needed and its lack partly fuels misconceptions about mental illness. The gap is arguably filled by large think-tanks providing general information based on current best evidence.[108] This section is based on these.

The following are the commonly cited risk factors for mental illness:[109]

BIOLOGICAL: genetic predisposition, pre-birth and birth complications, chronic medical condition, alcohol and substance use, and poor nutrition

PSYCHOLOGICAL: the impact of stress and trauma, low self-esteem, poor academic achievement, meaninglessness, and perception of insignificance

SOCIAL: childhood trauma and abuse, having few friends, divorce, loneliness, personal loss, bullying, poverty and political instability, poor social skills, discrimination, lack of social supports, and lack of social engagement

Attachment *per se* is notable by its absence which is, in itself, remarkable. Its underlying importance, however, is evident. Attachment failure makes psychological stress and trauma more likely,[110] secure attachment ameliorates the psychological effects of trauma,[111] and protects against all other psychological risk factors: low self-esteem,[112] poor academic achievement,[113] and meaninglessness and perception of insignificance.[114] Attachment underpins all social factors except poverty and political instability.

Growing evidence shows that attachment underlies many biological factors. Recent mental illness rate rises are unlikely due to increased birth complications or chronic medical conditions. Poor nutrition may prove to be an important factor: poor diet and mental illness are linked[115] through the gut microbiome.[116] As previously discussed, fast food culture and socializing trends impact our daily food choices and our socializing (or not) around food.

Our genetics, the basis of biological risk, has not changed appreciably in 60,000 years. Harmful variants may have been incorporated,[117] but it is unlikely that these have suddenly expressed themselves. Decades of research have uncovered many genetic linkages for diabetes[118] and obesity[119] but very few for mental illness. Exceptions include the serotonin transporter promoter region[120] and recent markers for depression,[121] schizophrenia,[122] bipolar disorder,[123] and anorexia nervosa.[124] In this context, biological research has broadened towards epigenetics.

Epigenetics, the study of environmental factors altering gene expression, has become highly relevant to mental illness.[125] Epigenetic methylation is linked to schizophrenia and bipolar illness,[126] and childhood trauma is epigenetically linked to depression.[127] Attachment is a strong epigenetic factor[128] directly impacting methylation[129] showing attachment's strong influence on the genome.[130] Through epigenetics, and through oxytocin and the brain changes previously discussed, attachment directly influences the biology of mental health.

Evidence since Bowlby underlies attachment's biological importance in protecting all health.[131] Our attachment relationships have a large influence on the expression of other biological factors, substance misuse in particular.[132] Attachment emerges, then, as one of the most powerful biological factors to mental health.

Depression, for example, is most common in young adults experiencing a triad of parental divorce, low self-esteem, and being single.[133] These are each directly linked to attachment.[134] Many twenty-first century young adults are caught in this attachment void after emotionally leaving parents and before finding a long-term relationship. Previously, 85% of young adults went straight from one core attachment (parents) to another (marriage).[135] That an attachment void can lead to depression[136] is further evidence for attachment strongly underlying mental health.

It seems almost unacceptable for me to cite the many clinical examples that I have of young, lonely people struggling with depression, anxiety, addictions, and suicide. Hospital staff are often acutely aware of the plight of young people and their loneliness: 'Doctor, will you take them home and take care of them, or shall we?' The question always remains: who will take care of them? To whom can they attach?

In a world of increasing mobility, we make new social contacts. Increasingly we encounter people who are strangers rather than kin. In this context, social factors become more important to mental illness. That broader attachment issues impact mental health is clearly seen in the "immigrant paradox."[137]

Latino migration to the USA, for example, is paradoxically a risk and a protective factor for mental illness. Protective to the mental health of migrants is a triad of attachment factors: ethnic identity, family cohesion, and social networking.[138] Ethnic identity protects self-esteem and meaning.[139] Risk factors for mental illness in these same migrants is another attachment-related triad: discrimination, acculturative stress, and family conflict. As an oversimplification,[140] protective attachments in country of origin are disrupted by immigration.[141] Second generation migrants have higher rates of mental illness[142] to support the overwhelming importance of broader attachment in this scenario.

Attachment factors

Insecure attachment is a risk factor for depression, bipolar illness, and psychosis,[143] and for remaining single.[144] Couple relationships protect against depression,[145] PTSD,[146] and more. These further suggest that attachment underlies mental health. Genetics, epigenetics, personality, and socio-economic factors are relevant to mental health but attachment underlies even some of these.

If secure attachment underlies mental health, then treatment needs to involve not only biological and psychological approaches but also a relationship approach. This, ideally, is done for all individuals presenting to mental health services, but a societal-level approach may also be needed. Screen technology, social isolation, hyper-individualism and changing attitudes to sex and relationships impart a mental health toll. Even in mental illness, individuals can adapt[147] to make pro-relational choices. Life fortunately offered Lachlan a chance at a relationship and our treating team worked hard to support his relationship with Emily.

Due to social factors alone, the UK has stalled in improving health outcomes.[148] A couple's decision to build a resilient relationship will, in a small but significant way, improve nation-wide health outcomes. In this, couple therapy has benefits far beyond the well-being of two people. Every couple therapist aids a global preventative mental health effort[149] in a well-being model[150] of improved healthcare delivery[151] to help protect and improve global mental health. Therapists' contributions are significant.

Couple therapy treating mental illness

Couples in therapy are choosing a better relationship. Theirs is not a mental health issue, but a relationship issue, DSM Z63.0: "Relationship distress with spouse or intimate partner."[152] Because of the strong reciprocal link between mental health and relationships, couple therapy can treat individual mental illness in affected partners[153] and children.[154]

In 1990, marital therapy was shown to match individual CBT in treating clinical depression.[155] Findings were replicated[156] and couple therapy since has been shown to be effective in individual substance misuse,[157] aggression,[158] anxiety,[159] PTSD,[160] and the effects of trauma.[161] It helps partners parenting an ADHD child[162] to cope with their own illness and disability.[163] Effective modalities include cognitive-behavioural couple therapy,[164] emotion-focussed couple therapy,[165] and behavioural couple therapy.[166] Mental illness and relationship aspects are addressed synergistically. In a distressed couple, the risk of developing clinical depression rises ten-fold[167] and relational distress often triggers mental illness.[168] Couple relationships and individual mental health are inextricably connected. Fostering healthy relationships is part of the long-term solution to addressing the mental health crisis.

Couple therapy increases relationship satisfaction[169] through commitment, communication, emotional support, resolving conflict, sexual intimacy, and forgiveness to strengthen attachment.[170] A relationship becomes something of a shock-absorber as individual mental illness greatly impacts a relationship and tests relationship strength:

> When he's feeling low or depressed, if I cannot carry his intensity, well, I will just go mad. You know, I get sucked into it. So I choose. I make a

> choice. I pull away and think of other things, or I just treat the situation as "well, can't do anything about it." [I] just have to trust and pray but not get sucked into the emotional mental anguish that he goes through sometimes, because I cannot survive. (Pearl and Richard, 42 yrs)

Clinicians like myself know how protective a relationship is for someone suffering mental illness. In many cases it is life-saving. It helps beyond measure to have a partner involved to help drive management and care. Emily's support for Lachlan illustrated this. These efforts often go unappreciated: the hours of listening, the exhausting emotional toll, the perseverance. Depression, for example, imposes huge burdens on partners[171] due to symptoms such as decreased libido, lack of motivation, feelings of worthlessness, and emotional withdrawal.[172] They are hard for a partner to bear. For this reason, mental illness often triggers relationship distress.[173]

When the attachment itself is harmed, repairs need to be made. Repairs can avert mental health consequences for several people. Clinicians often see the far-reaching effects of attachment trauma and repair to individual mental health.

> Kaitlyn, married eighteen years with four children aged seven to fifteen, was diagnosed with depression. An antidepressant was commenced together with psychotherapy. Her two middle children began failing and saw school counsellors. Her eldest displayed irritability and began using THC. The family ceased attending church. Grandparents on both sides found themselves side-lined by Kaitlyn and spouse Jake. Kaitlyn stopped attending her tennis club.
>
> Jake, a company manager, had frequent interstate trips. He was having an affair. This led to arguments with Kaitlyn and threats of divorce. Antidepressants helped Kaitlyn cope, school counsellors (not knowing the issues) helped the children cope, but things moved forward when, after five months of couple therapy, Jake and Kaitlyn reconciled and included a re-commitment ceremony and large holiday. The children's grades improved, school counselling was ceased, substance use by the eldest abated and grandparents were welcomed to visit. The family attends a new church and Kaitlyn plays tennis again. Antidepressants were weaned and ceased after another year.[174]

Antidepressants and individual psychotherapy held promise for Kaitlyn only. With core attachment addressed, however, things improved for Kaitlyn, Jake, the children, and others. It took time and effort to process complex emotions. The outcome could still have been divorce or continued acrimony. This idealistic scenario is repeated surprisingly often. Repairing injured attachment in a couple can restore the mental health, function, and integration of several people.

Here, one attachment trauma adversely impacted six people. Had underlying issues not been addressed, Kaitlyn's depression would have continued, Jake's depression could have manifested later, the eldest could have become depressed and addicted, and the younger children would have grown up at higher risk of mental illness. Jake and Kaitlyn's relationship could have been another break-up: statistics gave them a fifty-fifty chance, and that is all they gave themselves. They reconciled with effort to ameliorate one incidence of clinical depression, one of substance misuse, and to potentially prevent more depression and anxiety.

Like a domino-effect, friends' and siblings' divorces and separations adversely impact a couple's relationship.[175] As a corollary, one couple working through a thorny issue and reconciling has an unknown positive impact on an unknown number of others. We are socially and emotionally connected creatures, and we are more resilient and adaptive with more people contact, if we learn information, and if we learn skills. In imparting information and developing skills, couple therapists are part of a global preventative mental health effort.

Is the mental health crisis a challenge to relationships?

The mental health crisis is a challenge to relationships, especially in the light of evidence suggesting half the world's population will qualify for a diagnosis. That means that, in the future, almost every relationship will be dealing with mental health issues. Both mental health and relationships are, however, highly desired in our society. Attachment, relational safety, underlies close relationships to protect individual mental health. Based on strong evidence, we can highlight the protective effect of attachment on mental health. The way forward for couples and individuals is to value them both.

Value mental health? Value relationships

According to the literature, for people like Kaitlyn, Jake, and the children, and couples we interviewed, valuing mental health means valuing relationships. Getting love and belonging needs met is as relevant today as it was in Maslow's 1943. Too many people, however, sacrifice love and belonging to the detriment of their own mental health and the mental health of others. As mentioned last chapter, before attachment theory was born, Maslow saw that the most important protective factor to mental health was secure attachment. This century, we may be witnessing what happens when attachment is not valued.[176]

There is a way forward for a society reeling from the mental health effects of lost attachment: to value relationships. A couple choosing relationship longevity are valuing their mental health. Couples' insights and techniques to build relationship resilience are presented in Parts II and III. To complete our contextualization, however, we turn to the effects of social isolation in Chapter 3.

Notes

1 Dostoyevsky, Fyodor. *Demons: A novel in three parts*. Trans. Pevear, Richard and Volokhonsy, Larissa. Vintage, 1994, 38.
2 https://theconversation.com/winston-churchill-and-his-black-dog-of-greatness-36570 Retrieved 28 May 2022.
3 Angermeyer, Matthias C., and Sandra Dietrich. "Public beliefs about and attitudes towards people with mental illness: A review of population studies." *Acta Psychiatrica Scandinavica* 113, no. 3 (2006): 163–179.
4 Gupta, Rohit, and Merlin Ariefdjohan. "Mental illness on Instagram: A mixed method study to characterize public content, sentiments, and trends of antidepressant use." *Journal of Mental Health* 30, no. 4 (2021): 518–525.
5 Reynolds III, Charles F., David A. Lewis, Thomas Detre, Alan F. Schatzberg, and David J. Kupfer. "The future of psychiatry as clinical neuroscience." *Academic Medicine: Journal of the Association of American Medical Colleges* 84, no. 4 (2009): 446.
6 Gurwitz, David, and Abraham Weizman. "Personalized psychiatry: A realistic goal." *Pharmacogenomics* 5, no. 2 (2004): 213–217.
7 Luthar, Suniya S. "The culture of affluence: Psychological costs of material wealth." *Child Development* 74, no. 6 (2003): 1581–1593.
8 Durkheim, Émile. "Suicide et natalité: étude de statistique morale." *Revue Philosophique de la France et de l'Étranger* 26 (1888): 446–463.
9 Hutcherson, Cendri A., Emma M. Seppala, and James J. Gross. "The neural correlates of social connection." *Cognitive, Affective, & Behavioral Neuroscience* 15, no. 1 (2015): 1–14.
10 Schwartz, Ella, and Howard Litwin. "The reciprocal relationship between social connectedness and mental health among older European adults: A SHARE-based analysis." *The Journals of Gerontology: Series B* 74, no. 4 (2019): 694–702. Ding, Ning, Helen L. Berry, and Léan V. O'Brien. "One-year reciprocal relationship between community participation and mental wellbeing in Australia: A panel analysis." *Social Science & Medicine* 128 (2015): 246–254. Won, Seojin, and Hyemee Kim. "Social participation, health-related behavior, and depression of older adults living alone in Korea." *Asian Social Work and Policy Review* 14, no. 1 (2020): 61–71.
11 Chomsky, Noam. *What kind of creatures are we?* Columbia University Press, 2016.
12 Robinson, Kelly J., Oliver J. Bosch, Gil Levkowitz, Karl Emanuel Busch, Andrew P. Jarman, and Mike Ludwig. "Social creatures: Model animal systems for studying the neuroendocrine mechanisms of social behaviour." *Journal of Neuroendocrinology* 31, no. 12 (2019): e12807.
13 Fromm, Erich. *The sane society*. Rinehart & Company, 1955.
14 Saeri, Alexander K., Tegan Cruwys, Fiona Kate Barlow, Samantha Stronge, and Chris G. Sibley. "Social connectedness improves public mental health: Investigating bidirectional relationships in the New Zealand attitudes and values survey." *Australian & New Zealand Journal of Psychiatry* 52, no. 4 (2018): 365–374.
15 Kiely, Kim M., Georgina Sutherland, Peter Butterworth, and Nicola J. Reavley. "Age and gender differences in the reciprocal relationship between social

connectedness and mental health." *Social Psychiatry and Psychiatric Epidemiology* 56, no. 6 (2021): 1069–1081.
16 Sieving, Renee E., Annie-Laurie McRee, Barbara J. McMorris, Rebecca J. Shlafer, Amy L. Gower, Hillary M. Kapa, Kara J. Beckman, Jennifer L. Doty, Shari L. Plowman, and Michael D. Resnick. "Youth – adult connectedness: A key protective factor for adolescent health." *American Journal of Preventive Medicine* 52, no. 3 (2017): S275–S278.
17 Wojciak, Armeda Stevenson, Lenore M. McWey, and Jeffery Waid. "Sibling relationships of youth in foster care: A predictor of resilience." *Children and Youth Services Review* 84 (2018): 247–254.
18 Sieving, McRee, Barbara and McMorris. "Youth – adult connectedness".
19 Trinidad, Dennis R., Chih-Ping Chou, Jennifer B. Unger, C. Anderson Johnson, and Yan Li. "Family harmony as a protective factor against adolescent tobacco and alcohol use in Wuhan, China." *Substance Use & Misuse* 38, no. 8 (2003): 1159–1171.
20 Bollmer, Julie M., Richard Milich, Monica J. Harris, and Melissa A. Maras. "A friend in need: The role of friendship quality as a protective factor in peer victimization and bullying." *Journal of Interpersonal Violence* 20, no. 6 (2005): 701–712.
21 Roach, Ashley. "Supportive peer relationships and mental health in adolescence: An integrative review." *Issues in Mental Health Nursing* 39, no. 9 (2018): 723–737.
22 Kahn, Jeffrey H., Lynda M. Kasky-Hernández, Pamm Ambrose, and Sarah French. "Stress, depression, and anxiety among transitioning college students: The family as a protective factor." *Journal of the First-Year Experience & Students in Transition* 29, no. 2 (2017): 11–25.
23 Nicolaisen, Magnhild, and Kirsten Thorsen. "What are friends for? Friendships and loneliness over the lifespan – From 18 to 79 years." *The International Journal of Aging and Human Development* 84, no. 2 (2017): 126–158.
24 Takagi, Emiko, and Yasuhiko Saito. "Older parents' loneliness and family relationships in Japan." *Ageing International* 40, no. 4 (2015): 353–375.
25 Perry, Bruce D., Maia Szalavitz, and Corey M. Snow. *Born for love: Why empathy is essential–and endangered*. HarperCollins, 2010.
26 Townley, Greg, Henry Miller, and Bret Kloos. "A little goes a long way: The impact of distal social support on community integration and recovery of individuals with psychiatric disabilities." *American Journal of Community Psychology* 52, no. 1 (2013): 84–96.
27 Slade, Arietta, and Jeremy Holmes. "Attachment and psychotherapy." *Current Opinion in Psychology* 25 (2019): 152–156.
28 Tjaden, Cathelijn D., Cornelis L. Mulder, Philippe AEG Delespaul, Arnoud R. Arntz, and Hans Kroon. "Attachment as a framework to facilitate empowerment for people with severe mental illness." *Psychology and Psychotherapy: Theory, Research and Practice* 94, no. 3 (2021): 407–425.
29 Sachs, Adah. "Through the lens of attachment relationship: Stable DID, active DID and other trauma-based mental disorders." *The abused and the abuser*. Routledge, 2019, 77–97.
30 Read, John, and Andrew Gumley. "Can attachment theory help explain the relationship between childhood adversity and psychosis?" *Telling Stories?*. Routledge, 2019, 51–94.
31 Tew, Jerry, Shula Ramon, Mike Slade, Victoria Bird, Jane Melton, and Clair Le Boutillier. "Social factors and recovery from mental health difficulties: A review of the evidence." *The British Journal of Social Work* 42, no. 3 (2012): 443–460.

32 Feder, Kenneth A., Laurie Heatherington, Ramin Mojtabai, and William W. Eaton. "Perceived marital support and incident mental illness: Evidence from the National Comorbidity Survey." *Journal of Marital and Family Therapy* 45, no. 4 (2019): 668–683.
33 Zareian, Bita, and E. David Klonsky. "Connectedness and suicide." *Alternatives to suicide*. Academic Press, 2020, 135–158.
34 Feder, Heatherington, Mojtabai, and Eaton. "Perceived marital support and incident mental illness."
35 Hoopsick, Rachel A., Katelyn R. Benson, D. Lynn Homish, and Gregory G. Homish. "Resiliency factors that protect against post-deployment drug use among male US Army Reserve and National Guard soldiers." *Drug and Alcohol Dependence* 199 (2019): 42–49.
36 Vest, Bonnie M., D. Lynn Homish, Rachel A. Hoopsick, and Gregory G. Homish. "What drives the relationship between combat and alcohol problems in soldiers? The roles of perception and marriage." *Social Psychiatry and Psychiatric Epidemiology* 53, no. 4 (2018): 413–420.
37 Lawrence, Elizabeth M., Richard G. Rogers, Anna Zajacova, and Tim Wadsworth. "Marital happiness, marital status, health, and longevity." *Journal of Happiness Studies* 20, no. 5 (2019): 1539–1561.
38 Ibid.
39 Robles, Theodore F., Richard B. Slatcher, Joseph M. Trombello, and Meghan M. McGinn. "Marital quality and health: A meta-analytic review." *Psychological Bulletin* 140, no. 1 (2014): 140.
40 Uecker, Jeremy E. "Marriage and mental health among young adults." *Journal of Health and Social Behavior* 53, no. 1 (2012): 67–83.
41 Hostinar, Camelia E. "Recent developments in the study of social relationships, stress responses, and physical health." *Current Opinion in Psychology* 5 (2015): 90–95.
42 Srivastava, Ashish. "Marriage as a perceived panacea to mental illness in India: Reality check." *Indian Journal of Psychiatry* 55, Suppl 2 (2013): S239.
43 Feder, Adriana, Sharely Fred-Torres, Steven M. Southwick, and Dennis S. Charney. "The biology of human resilience: Opportunities for enhancing resilience across the life span." *Biological Psychiatry* 86, no. 6 (2019): 443–453.
44 Nagasawa, Miho, Kazutaka Mogi, and Takefumi Kikusui. "Attachment between humans and dogs." *Japanese Psychological Research* 51, no. 3 (2009): 209–221.
45 Neumann, Inga D. "Oxytocin: The neuropeptide of love reveals some of its secrets." *Cell Metabolism* 5, no. 4 (2007): 231–233.
46 Grippo, Angela J., and Alan Kim Johnson. "Biological mechanisms in the relationship between depression and heart disease." *Neuroscience & Biobehavioral Reviews* 26, no. 8 (2002): 941–962.
47 Hostinar, Camelia E. "Recent developments in the study of social relationships."
48 Sharma, Samata R., Xenia Gonda, Peter Dome, and Frank I. Tarazi. "What's love got to do with it: Role of oxytocin in trauma, attachment and resilience." *Pharmacology & Therapeutics* 214 (2020): 107602.
49 Hostinar, Camelia E. "Recent developments in the study of social relationships."
50 Case study from Dr Christian Heim's clinical practice.
51 Butterworth, Peter, and Bryan Rodgers. "Mental health problems and marital disruption: Is it the combination of husbands and wives' mental health problems that predicts later divorce?." *Social Psychiatry and Psychiatric Epidemiology* 43, no. 9 (2008): 758–763.
52 Bartel, Ann, and Paul Taubman. "Some economic and demographic consequences of mental illness." *Journal of Labor Economics* 4, no. 2 (1986): 243–256.

53 Lauber, Christoph, Carlos Nordt, Luis Falcato, and Wulf Rössler. "Factors influencing social distance toward people with mental illness." *Community Mental Health Journal* 40, no. 3 (2004): 265–274.
54 Twenge, Jean M. "The age of anxiety? The birth cohort change in anxiety and neuroticism, 1952–1993." *Journal of Personality and Social Psychology* 79, no. 6 (2000): 1007.
55 Horwitz, Allan V. "How an age of anxiety became an age of depression." *The Milbank Quarterly* 88, no. 1 (2010): 112–138.
56 Adelman, Howard S., and Linda Taylor. "Mental health in schools and public health." *Public Health Reports* 121, no. 3 (2006): 294–298.
57 Kruisselbrink Flatt, Alicia. "A suffering generation: Six factors contributing to the mental health crisis in North American Higher Education." *College Quarterly* 16, no. 1 (2013): n1.
58 Dong, Lu, and Jennifer Bouey. "Public mental health crisis during COVID-19–19 pandemic, China." *Emerging Infectious Diseases* 26, no. 7 (2020): 1616.
59 Racine, Nicole, Jessica E. Cooke, Rachel Eirich, Daphne J. Korczak, BraeAnne McArthur, and Sheri Madigan. "Child and adolescent mental illness during COVID-19: A rapid review." *Psychiatry Research* 292 (2020): 113307.
60 Feinstein, Robert E., Sussann Kotara, Barbara Jones, Donna Shanor, and Charles B. Nemeroff. "A health care workers mental health crisis line in the age of COVID-19." *Depression and Anxiety* 37, no. 8 (2020): 822–826.
61 Ben-Zeev, Dror. "The digital mental health genie is out of the bottle." *Psychiatric Services* 71, no. 12 (2020): 1212–1213.
62 McIntyre, Roger S., and Yena Lee. "Preventing suicide in the context of the COVID-19 pandemic." *World Psychiatry* 19, no. 2 (2020): 250.
63 Reger, Mark A., Ian H. Stanley, and Thomas E. Joiner. "Suicide mortality and coronavirus disease 2019 – a perfect storm?" *JAMA Psychiatry* 77, no. 11 (2020): 1093–1094.
64 Lin, Chien-Yu, Shu-Sen Chang, and Lih-Jong Shen. "Decrease in suicide during the first year of the COVID-19 pandemic in Taiwan." *The Journal of Clinical Psychiatry* 82, no. 6 (2021): 37990. www.health.gov.au/ministers/the-hon-greg-hunt-mp/media/australian-suicide-rates-down-during-COVID-19 Retrieved 28 March 2022.
65 Radeloff, Daniel, Rainer Papsdorf, Kirsten Uhlig, Andreas Vasilache, Karen Putnam, and Kai Von Klitzing. "Trends in suicide rates during the COVID-19 pandemic restrictions in a major German city." *Epidemiology and Psychiatric Sciences* 30 (2021).
66 Tanaka, Takanao, and Shohei Okamoto. "Increase in suicide following an initial decline during the COVID-19 pandemic in Japan." *Nature Human Behaviour* 5, no. 2 (2021): 229–238.
67 www.who.int/publications/i/item/WHO-2019-nCoV-Sci_Brief-Mental_health-2022.1 Retrieved 23 March 2022.
68 Aknin, Lara B., Jan-Emmanuel De Neve, Elizabeth W. Dunn, Daisy E. Fancourt, Elkhonon Goldberg, John F. Helliwell, Sarah P. Jones et al. "Mental health during the first year of the COVID-19 pandemic: A review and recommendations for moving forward." *Perspectives on Psychological Science* 17, no. 4 (2022): 915–936.
69 Le, Hai, Burhan Ahmed Khan, Syed Murtaza, and Asim A. Shah. "The increase in suicide during the COVID-19 pandemic." *Psychiatric Annals* 50, no. 12 (2020): 526–530.
70 McManus, Peter, Andrea Mant, Philip B. Mitchell, William S. Montgomery, John Marley, and Merran E. Auland. "Recent trends in the use of antidepressant

drugs in Australia, 1990–1998." *The Medical Journal of Australia* 173, no. 9 (2000): 458–461.
71 Ihara, Hiroshi. "A cold of the soul: A Japanese case of disease mongering in psychiatry." *International Journal of Risk & Safety in Medicine* 24, no. 2 (2012): 115–120.
72 Angell, Marcia. "The epidemic of mental illness: Why." *The New York Review of Books* 58, no. 11 (2011): 20–22.
73 Moore, Thomas J., and Donald R. Mattison. "Adult utilization of psychiatric drugs and differences by sex, age, and race." *JAMA Internal Medicine* 177, no. 2 (2017): 274–275.
74 Ihara, Hiroshi. "A cold of the soul."
75 Shield, Blue Cross Blue. "Major depression: The impact on overall health." *Blue Cross Blue Shield, The Health of America Report®*. www. bcbs. com/sites/default/files/file-attachments/health-of-america-report/HoA_Major_Depression_Report. pdf (2018).
76 Murray, Christopher JL, Theo Vos, Rafael Lozano, Mohsen Naghavi, Abraham D. Flaxman, Catherine Michaud, Majid Ezzati et al. "Disability-adjusted life years (DALYs) for 291 diseases and injuries in 21 regions, 1990–2010: A systematic analysis for the Global Burden of Disease Study 2010." *The Lancet* 380, no. 9859 (2012): 2197–2223.
77 Ruscio, Ayelet Meron, Lauren S. Hallion, Carmen CW Lim, Sergio Aguilar-Gaxiola, Ali Al-Hamzawi, Jordi Alonso, Laura Helena Andrade et al. "Cross-sectional comparison of the epidemiology of DSM-5 generalized anxiety disorder across the globe." *JAMA Psychiatry* 74, no. 5 (2017): 465–475.
78 Bitsko, Rebecca H., Joseph R. Holbrook, Reem M. Ghandour, Stephen J. Blumberg, Susanna N. Visser, Ruth Perou, and John T. Walkup. "Epidemiology and impact of health care provider – diagnosed anxiety and depression among US children." *Journal of Developmental and Behavioral Pediatrics: JDBP* 39, no. 5 (2018): 395.
79 Hawton, Keith, Joan Fagg, S. U. E. Simkin, Elizabeth Bale, and Alison Bond. "Deliberate self-harm in adolescents in Oxford, 1985–1995." *Journal of Adolescence* 23, no. 1 (2000): 47–55.
80 Richards, Georgia C., Sibtain Anwar, and Jane Quinlan. "Averting a UK opioid crisis: Getting the public health messages 'right'." *Journal of the Royal Society of Medicine* 115, no. 5 (2022): 161–164. Hodder, Sally L., Judith Feinberg, Steffanie A. Strathdee, Steven Shoptaw, Frederick L. Altice, Louis Ortenzio, and Chris Beyrer. "The opioid crisis and HIV in the USA: Deadly synergies." *The Lancet* 397, no. 10279 (2021): 1139–1150.
81 van Eeden, Annelies E., Daphne van Hoeken, and Hans W. Hoek. "Incidence, prevalence and mortality of anorexia nervosa and bulimia nervosa." *Current Opinion in Psychiatry* 34, no. 6 (2021): 515.
82 www.independent.co.uk/news/science/narcissism-the-science-behind-the-rise-of-a-modern-epidemic-a6925606.html Retrieved 28 March 2022.
83 Kessler, Ronald C., Matthias Angermeyer, James C. Anthony, R. O. N. De Graaf, Koen Demyttenaere, Isabelle Gasquet, Giovanni De Girolamo et al. "Lifetime prevalence and age-of-onset distributions of mental disorders in the World Health Organization's World Mental Health Survey Initiative." *World Psychiatry* 6, no. 3 (2007): 168.
84 Helliwell, John F., Richard Layard, and Jeffrey Sachs. "World happiness report [2012]." (2012). The United Nations' Sustainable Development Solutions Network.
85 www.statista.com/statistics/282160/suicide-rate-in-the-united-kingdom-uk-since-2000/ Retrieved 28 March 2022.

86 Windfuhr, Kirsten, and Navneet Kapur. "Suicide and mental illness: A clinical review of 15 years findings from the UK National Confidential Inquiry into Suicide." *British Medical Bulletin* 100, no. 1 (2011): 101–121.
87 https://ourworldindata.org/suicide Retrieved 28 March 2022.
88 www.aihw.gov.au/suicide-self-harm-monitoring/data/deaths-by-suicide-in-australia/suicide-deaths-over-time Retrieved 28 March 2022.
89 Hedegaard, Holly, and Margaret Warner. "Suicide mortality in the United States, 1999–2019." (2021).
90 Naghavi, Mohsen. "Global, regional, and national burden of suicide mortality 1990 to 2016: Systematic analysis for the Global Burden of Disease Study 2016." *BMJ* 364 (2019).
91 McLoughlin, Aoibheann B., Madelyn S. Gould, and Kevin M. Malone. "Global trends in teenage suicide: 2003–2014." *QJM: An International Journal of Medicine* 108, no. 10 (2015): 765–780.
92 Lo, Charmaine B., Jeffrey A. Bridge, Junxin Shi, Lorah Ludwig, and Rachel M. Stanley. "Children's mental health emergency department visits: 2007–2016." *Pediatrics* 145, no. 6 (2020).
93 de Pablo, Gonzalo Salazar, Andrea De Micheli, Dorien H. Nieman, Christoph U. Correll, Lars Vedel Kessing, Andrea Pfennig, Andreas Bechdolf et al. "Universal and selective interventions to promote good mental health in young people: Systematic review and meta-analysis." *European Neuropsychopharmacology* 41 (2020): 28–39.
94 Luthar, Suniya S. "The culture of affluence: Psychological costs of material wealth." *Child Development* 74, no. 6 (2003): 1581–1593.
95 Elgar, Frank J., Wendy Craig, and Stephen J. Trites. "Family dinners, communication, and mental health in Canadian adolescents." *Journal of Adolescent Health* 52, no. 4 (2013): 433–438.
96 Goldfarb, Samantha S., Will L. Tarver, Julie L. Locher, Julie Preskitt, and Bisakha Sen. "A systematic review of the association between family meals and adolescent risk outcomes." *Journal of Adolescence* 44 (2015): 134–149.
97 Twenge. "The age of anxiety?"
98 Twenge, Jean M. "Have smartphones destroyed a generation." *The Atlantic* 9 (2017): 2017.
99 Tumin, Rachel, and Sarah E. Anderson. "Television, home-cooked meals, and family meal frequency: Associations with adult obesity." *Journal of the Academy of Nutrition and Dietetics* 117, no. 6 (2017): 937–945.
100 Mahmood, Lubna, Esther M. González-Gil, Peter Schwarz, Sandra Herrmann, Eva Karaglani, Greet Cardon, Flore De Vylder, et al. "Frequency of family meals and food consumption in families at high risk of type 2 diabetes: The Feel4Diabetes-study." *European Journal of Pediatrics* 181, no. 6 (2022): 2523–2534.
101 Park, Jung Ha, Ju Young Kim, So Hye Kim, Jung Hyun Kim, Young Mi Park, and Hye Seon Yeom. "A latent class analysis of dietary behaviours associated with metabolic syndrome: A retrospective observational cross-sectional study." *Nutrition Journal* 19, no. 1 (2020): 1–11.
102 Holt-Lunstad, Julianne, Timothy B. Smith, and J. Bradley Layton. "Social relationships and mortality risk: A meta-analytic review." *PLoS Medicine* 7, no. 7 (2010): e1000316.
103 Mortazavizadeh, Zeinab, and Simon Forstmeier. "The role of emotion regulation in the association of adult attachment and mental health: A systematic review." *Archives of Psychology* 2, no. 9 (2018).
104 Sutton, Tara E. "Review of attachment theory: Familial predictors, continuity and change, and intrapersonal and relational outcomes." *Marriage & Family Review* 55, no. 1 (2019): 1–22.

105 Patel, Vikram, Shekhar Saxena, Crick Lund, Graham Thornicroft, Florence Baingana, Paul Bolton, Dan Chisholm et al. "The Lancet Commission on global mental health and sustainable development." *The Lancet* 392, no. 10157 (2018): 1553–1598.
106 Mahmood, Syed S., Daniel Levy, Ramachandran S. Vasan, and Thomas J. Wang. "The Framingham Heart Study and the epidemiology of cardiovascular disease: A historical perspective." *The Lancet* 383, no. 9921 (2014): 999–1008.
107 Furber, Gareth, Matthew Leach, Sophie Guy, and Leonie Segal. "Developing a broad categorisation scheme to describe risk factors for mental illness, for use in prevention policy and planning." *Australian & New Zealand Journal of Psychiatry* 51, no. 3 (2017): 230–240.
108 See as examples, www.who.int/news-room/fact-sheets/detail/mental-disorders; www.un.org/development/desa/disabilities/issues/mental-health-and-development.html; www.nhs.uk/mental-health/conditions/; www.americanmentalwellness.org/prevention/risk-and-protective-factors/; www.mayoclinic.org/diseases-conditions/mental-illness/symptoms-causes/ Retrieved 7 April 2022.
109 www.americanmentalwellness.org/prevention/risk-and-protective-factors/ Retrieved 7 April 2022.
110 O'Connor, Maja, and Ask Elklit. "Attachment styles, traumatic events, and PTSD: A cross-sectional investigation of adult attachment and trauma." *Attachment & Human Development* 10, no. 1 (2008): 59–71.
111 Perry, Szalavitz, and Snow. *Born for love.*
112 Verschueren, Karine. "Attachment, self-esteem, and socio-emotional adjustment: There is more than just the mother." *Attachment & Human Development* 22, no. 1 (2020): 105–109.
113 West, Katara K., Brittany L. Mathews, and Kathryn A. Kerns. "Mother – child attachment and cognitive performance in middle childhood: An examination of mediating mechanisms." *Early Childhood Research Quarterly* 28, no. 2 (2013): 259–270.
114 Goodman, Michael L., Derrick Gibson, Thiennga T. Vo, Aaron Wang, Stanley Gitari, and Ben Raimer. "Early childhood attachment and suicidal ideation among young Kenyan men." *Advances in Life Course Research* 35 (2018): 126–134.
115 Orlando, Laura, Katarina A. Savel, Sheri Madigan, Marlena Colasanto, and Daphne J. Korczak. "Dietary patterns and internalizing symptoms in children and adolescents: A meta-analysis." *Australian & New Zealand Journal of Psychiatry* 56, no. 6 (2022): 617–641.
116 Madan, A., D. Thompson, James Chris Fowler, N. J. Ajami, R. Salas, B. C. Frueh, M. R. Bradshaw, B. L. Weinstein, J. M. Oldham, and J. F. Petrosino. "The gut microbiota is associated with psychiatric symptom severity and treatment outcome among individuals with serious mental illness." *Journal of Affective Disorders* 264 (2020): 98–106.
117 Subbaraman, Nidhi. "Past 5,000 years prolific for changes to human genome." *Nature News Nov.* (2012). https://www.nature.com/articles/nature.2012.11912 Retrieved 18 July 2022.
118 Prasad, Rashmi B., and Leif Groop. "Genetics of type 2 diabetes – pitfalls and possibilities." *Genes* 6, no. 1 (2015): 87–123.
119 Walley, Andrew J., Alexandra IF Blakemore, and Philippe Froguel. "Genetics of obesity and the prediction of risk for health." *Human Molecular Genetics* 15, no. suppl_2 (2006): R124-R130.
120 Levinson, Douglas F. "The genetics of depression: A review." *Biological Psychiatry* 60, no. 2 (2006): 84–92.
121 Mullins, Niamh, and Cathryn M. Lewis. "Genetics of depression: Progress at last." *Current Psychiatry Reports* 19, no. 8 (2017): 1–7.

122 Henriksen, Mads G., Julie Nordgaard, and Lennart B. Jansson. "Genetics of schizophrenia: Overview of methods, findings and limitations." *Frontiers in Human Neuroscience* 11 (2017): 322.
123 Gordovez, Francis James A., and Francis J. McMahon. "The genetics of bipolar disorder." *Molecular Psychiatry* 25, no. 3 (2020): 544–559.
124 Baker, Jessica H., Katherine Schaumberg, and Melissa A. Munn-Chernoff. "Genetics of anorexia nervosa." *Current Psychiatry Reports* 19, no. 11 (2017): 1–8.
125 Kular, Lara, and Sonia Kular. "Epigenetics applied to psychiatry: Clinical opportunities and future challenges." *Psychiatry and Clinical Neurosciences* 72, no. 4 (2018): 195–211.
126 Nestler, Eric J., Catherine J. Peña, Marija Kundakovic, Amanda Mitchell, and Schahram Akbarian. "Epigenetic basis of mental illness." *The Neuroscientist* 22, no. 5 (2016): 447–463.
127 Park, Caroline, Joshua D. Rosenblat, Elisa Brietzke, Zihang Pan, Yena Lee, Bing Cao, Hannah Zuckerman, Anastasia Kalantarova, and Roger S. McIntyre. "Stress, epigenetics and depression: A systematic review." *Neuroscience & Biobehavioral Reviews* 102 (2019): 139–152.
128 Darling Rasmussen, Pernille, and Ole Jakob Storebø. "Attachment and epigenetics: A scoping review of recent research and current knowledge." *Psychological Reports* 124, no. 2 (2021): 479–501.
129 Jones-Mason, Karen, Isabel Elaine Allen, Nicole Bush, and Steve Hamilton. "Epigenetic marks as the link between environment and development: Examination of the associations between attachment, socioeconomic status, and methylation of the SLC6A4 gene." *Brain and Behavior* 6, no. 7 (2016): e00480.
130 Guintivano, Jerry, and Zachary A. Kaminsky. "Role of epigenetic factors in the development of mental illness throughout life." *Neuroscience Research* 102 (2016): 56–66.
131 Stack, Steven, and Jonathan Scourfield. "Recency of divorce, depression, and suicide risk." *Journal of Family Issues* 36, no. 6 (2015): 695–715.
132 Trinidad, Chou, Unger, Johnson, and Li. "Family harmony."
133 Aro, H. "Risk and protective factors in depression: A developmental perspective." *Acta Psychiatrica Scandinavica* 89 (1994): 59–64.
134 Thomas, Marina F., Alice Binder, and Jörg Matthes. "The agony of partner choice: The effect of excessive partner availability on fear of being single, self-esteem, and partner choice overload." *Computers in Human Behavior* 126 (2022): 106977.
135 Cohn, Dvera, Jeffrey S. Passel, Wendy Wang, and Gretchen Livingston. "Barely half of US adults are married – A record low." *Pew Research Center*. www.pewsocialtrends.org/2011/12/14/barely-half-of-us-adults-are-married-a-record-low (2011)
136 Aro. "Risk and protective factors in depression."
137 Alegría, Margarita, Glorisa Canino, Patrick E. Shrout, Meghan Woo, Naihua Duan, Doryliz Vila, Maria Torres, Chih-nan Chen, and Xiao-Li Meng. "Prevalence of mental illness in immigrant and non-immigrant US Latino groups." *American Journal of Psychiatry* 165, no. 3 (2008): 359–369.
138 Leong, Frederick, Yong S. Park, and Zornitsa Kalibatseva. "Disentangling immigrant status in mental health: Psychological protective and risk factors among Latino and Asian American immigrants." *American Journal of Orthopsychiatry* 83, no. 2 pt 3 (2013): 361–371.
139 Bourguignon, David, Eleonore Seron, Vincent Yzerbyt, and Ginette Herman. "Perceived group and personal discrimination: Differential effects on personal self-esteem." *European Journal of Social Psychology* 36, no. 5 (2006): 773–789.

140 Jimenez, Daniel E., David Martinez Garza, Verónica Cárdenas, and María Marquine. "Older Latino mental health: A complicated picture." *Innovation in Aging* 4, no. 5 (2020): igaa033.
141 Alegría, Canino, and Shrout. "Prevalence of mental illness in immigrant."
142 Ibid.
143 Herstell, Simon, Linda T. Betz, Nora Penzel, Ruth Chechelnizki, Laura Filihagh, Linda Antonucci, and Joseph Kambeitz. "Insecure attachment as a transdiagnostic risk factor for major psychiatric conditions: A meta-analysis in bipolar disorder, depression and schizophrenia spectrum disorder." *Journal of Psychiatric Research* 144 (2021): 190–201.
144 Busby, Dean M., Veronica Hanna-Walker, and Jeremy B. Yorgason. "A closer look at attachment, sexuality, and couple relationships." *Journal of Social and Personal Relationships* 37, no. 4 (2020): 1362–1385.
145 Brown, George W., and Tirril Harris. *Social origins of depression: A study of psychiatric disorder in women*. Routledge, 2012. First published in 1978.
146 Britt, Thomas W., Amy B. Adler, and Jamie Fynes. "Perceived resilience and social connection as predictors of adjustment following occupational adversity." *Journal of Occupational Health Psychology* 26, no. 4 (2021): 339.
147 Arango, Celso, Covadonga M. Díaz-Caneja, Patrick D. McGorry, Judith Rapoport, Iris E. Sommer, Jacob A. Vorstman, David McDaid et al. "Preventive strategies for mental health." *The Lancet Psychiatry* 5, no. 7 (2018): 591–604.
148 Marmot, Michael. "Health equity in England: The Marmot review 10 years on." *BMJ* 368 (2020).
149 Fusar-Poli, Paolo, Christoph U. Correll, Celso Arango, Michael Berk, Vikram Patel, and John PA Ioannidis. "Preventive psychiatry: A blueprint for improving the mental health of young people." *World Psychiatry* 20, no. 2 (2021): 200–221.
150 Slade, Mike. "Mental illness and well-being: The central importance of positive psychology and recovery approaches." *BMC Health Services Research* 10, no. 1 (2010): 1–14.
151 Salmoiraghi, Alberto, and Amy Kerti. "Is attachment theory the answer to a complex healthcare system?" *BJPsych Open* 8, S1 (2022): S111–S112.
152 Foran, Heather M., Mark A. Whisman, and Steven RH Beach. "Intimate partner relationship distress in the DSM-5." *Family Process* 54, no. 1 (2015): 48–63.
153 Wittenborn, Andrea K., and Kendal Holtrop. "Introduction to the special issue on the efficacy and effectiveness of couple and family interventions: Evidence base update 2010–2019." *Journal of Marital and Family Therapy* 48, no. 1 (2022): 5–22.
154 Ibid.
155 O'Leary, K. Daniel, and Steven R. Beach. "Marital therapy: A viable treatment for depression and marital discord." *The American Journal of Psychiatry* 147, no. 2 (1990): 183–186.
156 Barbato, Angelo, and Barbara D'Avanzo. "Efficacy of couple therapy as a treatment for depression: A meta-analysis." *Psychiatric Quarterly* 79, no. 2 (2008): 121–132.
157 Hogue, Aaron, Jeremiah A. Schumm, Alexandra MacLean, and Molly Bobek. "Couple and family therapy for substance use disorders: Evidence-based update 2010–2019." *Journal of Marital and Family Therapy* 48, no. 1 (2022): 178–203.
158 Epstein, Norman B., Carol A. Werlinich, and Jaslean J. LaTaillade. "Couple therapy for partner aggression." *Clinical Handbook of Couple Therapy* (2015): 389–411.

159 Goger, Pauline, and V. Robin Weersing. "Family based treatment of anxiety disorders: A review of the literature (2010–2019)." *Journal of Marital and Family Therapy* 48, no. 1 (2022): 107–128.
160 Liebman, Rachel E., Kristen M. Whitfield, Iris Sijercic, Naomi Ennis, and Candice M. Monson. "Harnessing the healing power of relationships in trauma recovery: A systematic review of cognitive-behavioral conjoint therapy for PTSD." *Current Treatment Options in Psychiatry* 7, no. 3 (2020): 203–220.
161 Wittenborn and Holtrop. "Introduction to the special issue on the efficacy and effectiveness of couple and family interventions."
162 Lebow, Jay, and Douglas K. Snyder, eds. *Clinical handbook of couple therapy*, 6th edn. The Guilford Press, 2022, 595–614.
163 Ring, Jeffrey. "Helping couples and families navigate illness and disability: An integrated approach." *Family Medicine* 51, no. 9 (2019): 781–782.
164 Whisman, Mark A., and Steven R. H. Beach. "Couple therapy for depression." *Journal of Clinical Psychology* 68, no. 5 (2012): 526–535.
165 Dessaulles, Andre, Susan M. Johnson, and Wayne H. Denton. "Emotion-focused therapy for couples in the treatment of depression: A pilot study." *The American Journal of Family Therapy* 31, no. 5 (2003): 345–353.
166 Powers, Mark B., Ellen Vedel, and Paul MG Emmelkamp. "Behavioral couples therapy (BCT) for alcohol and drug use disorders: A meta-analysis." *Clinical Psychology Review* 28, no. 6 (2008): 952–962.
167 O'Leary, K. Daniel, Jennifer L. Christian, and Nancy R. Mendell. "A closer look at the link between marital discord and depressive symptomatology." *Journal of Social and Clinical Psychology* 13, no. 1 (1994): 33–41.
168 South, Susan C. "Pathology in relationships." *Annual Review of Clinical Psychology* 17 (2021): 577–601.
169 Ibid.
170 Diamond, Rachel M., Andrew S. Brimhall, and Michael Elliott. "Attachment and relationship satisfaction among first married, remarried, and post-divorce relationships." *Journal of Family Therapy* 40 (2018): S111–S127.
171 Benazon, Nili R., and James C. Coyne. "Living with a depressed spouse." *Journal of Family Psychology* 14, no. 1 (2000): 71.
172 Sharabi, Liesel L., Amy L. Delaney, and Leanne K. Knobloch. "In their own words: How clinical depression affects romantic relationships." *Journal of Social and Personal Relationships* 33, no. 4 (2016): 421–448.
173 Westman, Mina, and Amiram D. Vinokur. "Unraveling the relationship of distress levels within couples: Common stressors, empathic reactions, or crossover via social interaction?." *Human Relations* 51, no. 2 (1998): 137–156.
174 Case study from Dr Christian Heim's clinical practice.
175 McDermott, Rose, James H. Fowler, and Nicholas A. Christakis. "Breaking up is hard to do, unless everyone else is doing it too: Social network effects on divorce in a longitudinal sample." *Social Forces* 92, no. 2 (2013): 491–519.
176 Mikulincer, Mario, and Phillip R. Shaver. "An attachment perspective on psychopathology." *World Psychiatry* 11, no. 1 (2012): 11–15.

Chapter 3

Resilient relationships versus social isolation: effects of screen technology, atomization, and distancing

It takes a village to raise a child.[1] Individually, we were all children; collectively, we are the village. It may also take a village to help sustain long-term relationships. Maintaining a relationship is "damn hard work" (Carol and Stephen, 40 yrs) even when surrounded by supportive people.[2] Increasingly, however, we have less supportive family and friends. Can relationships grow resilient in our society's growing isolation?

In the face of interpersonal conflict, it is an enticing option to simply cut off from other people. From time to time, nations employ this policy: the "splendid isolation" of Lord Salisbury's England,[3] the US isolationism between world wars,[4] and more recently, Brexit.[5] Each was a policy solution to manage the effects of European squabbles. Historically, however, isolationism fails. The *Entente Cordiale* of 1904 ended Salisbury's isolationism and Pearl Harbour ended it for the USA. Somehow, we humans need to manage rather than avoid conflict. This is a core challenge for countries, societies, individuals and couples.

It may be difficult to remain isolated in a village, but in a city it is very easy:

> Why do people have to be this lonely? What's the point of it all? Millions of people in this world, all of them yearning, looking to others to satisfy them, yet isolating themselves. Why? Was the earth put here just to nourish human loneliness? – Haruki Marakami[6]

This chapter discusses how couple relationships are not immune to the impacts of social isolation. Atomization, social media, conflict with family and friends, and social distancing all conspire against togetherness. Being the antithesis of attachment, these adversely impact individuals and couples living in what has become a new normal: "feeling lonely and unloved is the most terrible poverty."[7] The facts again are sobering, yet hope shines in the resilience that can grow through obtaining knowledge and skills.

DOI: 10.4324/9781003263395-5

Why isolate? Hikikomori loneliness

Hikikomori is a disorder where "a person without psychosis is withdrawn into [their] home for more than six months and does not participate in society."[8] It effects over half a million people in Japan, mainly young adult males. Far from being a culture-bound syndrome, however, Hikikomori-like withdrawal is a global phenomenon; an isolation epidemic. It is the result of mental factors (social phobia, depression, and personality disorders), social factors (shame, distrust, weakened traditional values), social media and internet influence (for information and entertainment), and biological factors.[9] Sufferers disengage like isolationist countries to impede even the formation of couple relationships.

Social isolation differs from loneliness. Loneliness is "an exceedingly unpleasant and driving experience connected with inadequate discharge of the need for human intimacy."[10] It is a subjective perception directly linked to depression, alcohol misuse, and suicide.[11] Ideally, loneliness is temporary. Social isolation, however, is the "objective and quantifiable reflection of reduced social network size and paucity of social contact."[12] Loneliness can exist without social isolation, but widespread societal social isolation results in epidemic-levels of loneliness with rises in depression and suicide. Relational safety protects couples like Veronne and Wayne from social isolation and loneliness:[13]

> We could have said we didn't want to get back together. And I could have just been on an island all by myself and Veronne could have been by herself. But we're together. And that's the main thing. (Wayne and Veronne, 42 yrs)

Wayne and Veronne chose to stay together, yet why this is "the main thing" is not immediately apparent. Being in a long-term relationship is an objective, quantifiable, protective factor for health and longevity.[14] It strongly pushes against social isolation. It protects men like Wayne from suicide[15] and protects us all against loneliness, clinical anxiety and depression.[16] A couple choosing to stay together in relative peace and harmony remain individually more stable. They are attached:

You _____Me

In separation, a bond is broken, each becomes more isolated and, like separated hydrogen atoms, are subject to more volatility:

You   *Me*

Imagine this effect multiplied millions of times with each individual living more separately, more individually, and more alone. Living alone and having few contacts are markers of social isolation,[17] a major risk factor for suicide.[18] This population-level problem is entrenched in many developed societies. Mental health services treat individual loneliness and individual depression, yet it is social isolation that is more strongly associated with sickness and death.[19] Social isolation is a failure of society and social structures, not of individuals.

Social isolation has long been a problem for the elderly due to declining health and cognition, death of a spouse, losing social contacts, marginalization, income loss, and decreased social opportunity.[20] It creates a difficult twilight for people who grew up in community. Much more of a problem, however, is the recent rapid rise in social isolation and loneliness for younger people.[21] Middle-age social isolation and loneliness is now worse than old-age loneliness[22] and is directly linked with obesity,[23] alcohol misuse,[24] immune problems,[25] hypertension,[26] and early death.[27] In younger adults, it is more of a problem still: 40% of people 16–24 are lonely compared with 27% over 75.[28] This major societal concern affects relationships as social isolation is fast supplanting adult attachment.[29] This is the reality for many young adults who disclosed their plight in my office:

> I hate being alone, but so many people are so lonely, I've got to get used to it.
>
> Do you think I like being pawed by guys I don't even know? I hate it, but I hook up because I hate feeling lonely. That's what all of my friends do.
>
> I don't like casual sex. I just want to find someone who'll love me.

Due to pandemic isolation, 43% of young adults are even lonelier and 63% report being depressed or anxious.[30] In their isolation, older adults may reminisce on a youth of community as they predominantly went from family to marriage, but young adults are not even building such memories. Young adult loneliness tends to occur between core attachments: after core family time and before finding a long-term relationship. This leads, as discussed last chapter, to depression. The recent rise in middle-aged loneliness coincides with a doubling in the divorce rate in just over 20 years for those over fifty[31] and the peak age for divorce in the UK is now 45.[32]

Young adult isolation and loneliness are strongly linked with extensive screen and social media use.[33] The rise of Hikikomori in the 1990s[34] coincided with the rise of the internet; this is now being recognized.[35] This merits emphasis: a global phenomenon, the rise of the internet, coincided with another global phenomenon, heightened social isolation in young males in particular, and the emergence of a newly-described mental illness.

Other contributors to social isolation these last decades include increased mobility, marriage decline, and decreased religious affiliation.[36] A recent Harvard study recommended tackling social isolation by increasing social infrastructure in a hope to re-ignite community involvement.[37] Their findings basically suggested: 'let's rebuild our village.'

Chapter 1 articulated the links among socioeconomic development, hyper-individualism, and mental illness. Loneliness and individualism are likewise linked.[38] Socio-economic development is clearly of great benefit to humankind, but it comes with side-effects and consequences: social isolation and mental illness undermining attachment. Fewer couple relationships form, and sustaining a relationship becomes harder. When loneliness is the societal norm, separation and divorce become more accepted ways to resolve interpersonal conflict,[39] just like isolationist policies. Couples then have to justify staying together when "everyone else" divorces.[40] Separation of adults adds to growing atomization.

Living by ourselves: atomization

Atomization is the chemical process of becoming separate atoms. It also refers to individuals[41] living in smaller numbers or alone. The term infers the social alienation expounded by Emile Durkheim and Eric Fromm:[42] people lose social contact, particularly in urban rather than village environments.

Does the universe contain atoms or do atoms make up the universe? Does society contain individuals or do individuals make up society? Over half a century, our point-of-reference has shifted away from society towards the individual.[43] To many, it now sounds appallingly nationalistic and dated for a leader to suggest "ask what you can do for your country"[44] because we expect social structures to serve us as individuals.

Socioeconomic advances lead to atomized loneliness as a side-effect. In 1961, 40% of UK households contained only one or two people and by 2011 it was 65%.[45] In 1851, there were approximately five adults per English, Scottish, and Welsh household, by 2011 it was two. Similar figures are evident for the US[46] and Australia.[47] Not that everyone who lives alone is lonely, but increased prosperity and hyper-individualism has led to social isolation and atomizing *en masse*, despite increased population.

Atomization too is linked with socio-economic progress, individualism,[48] and mental illness.[49] South Korea now has over 30% single-occupied households,[50] and in large Japanese inner-cities, the figure is 50%.[51] Being single and alone becomes more usual, being in a relationship or with family becomes more unusual. Atomization increases as we climb Maslow's hierarchy: from surviving an environment (level 1), to society safety (level 2), through family and couple togetherness (level 3), to individual self-esteem and self-actualization (levels 4 and 5). The subtext becomes, 'to make it to the top, it's all about me alone.'[52] Contemplating this can be unsettling: why is this? Does success mean we have to separate as people? Are we no longer social creatures?

Social isolation decreases the opportunity for attachment, friendship, and community[53] due to increased mobility, less coupling, individualized entertainment and devalued socializing.[54] With less people interactions we socially deskill.[55] Individuals, lost among billions, then turn to their only guiding light: their (own) lonely selves. Adult children leave home later but often atomize in their bedroom. Staying securely attached, on the other hand, fosters a healthy sense of self[56] to promote resilience.[57]

We are approaching a dystopia in which "we're all islands shouting lies to each other across seas of misunderstanding"[58] and where we are "in an infinite vacuum: you can go anywhere, but there is nowhere to go."[59] Social media becomes the new meeting place as, from bedrooms around the globe, "'lonely crowds' produced by the hyper-individualism . . . coalesce"[60] to form a further "condition of atomization"[61] engendering hyper-individuality[62] to make forming and sustaining relationships even more difficult.

Social media has crept into our private lives insidiously. In the first half of the twentieth century, for example, Britons saw newsreels communally in local cinemas. British Television entered the living room, then two televisions per household and computer screens in bedrooms. Now smartphone entertainment accompanies whoever, whenever, wherever, for whatever. This facilitates atomization: less arguing about which cinema to attend or which channel to watch, but less people-interaction at all. Arguing about trivialities at least presupposes a relationship; in atomization, with whom do I argue? Benefits from internet technology hide the consequences: for many people, I, as their psychiatrist, am their only genuine person-connection.

Like the slow effects of rising water temperature on sea-life, atomization grinds away at mental health and relationships. This is not a conspiracy; it is a side-effect, an unintended consequence of economic prosperity. People innately tend to bind together, interact, and affect each other emotionally,[63] so why do we tolerate this nourishing of human loneliness? Yet there is hope. In our fast-changing social context, biological attachment drives us to psychologically adapt and strive to encounter each other in new ways.

Adapting and valuing people

For people connection, new meeting spaces emerge. In many countries, the number of cafés has exploded, more people dine out than ever before, and many more attend sporting fixtures.[64] The UK is now a "café society"[65] with almost two billion cups of coffee bought yearly[66] and, despite adverse health consequences, shisha cafés flourish thanks to the valued social interactions.[67] Going to a café is a "sensory experience . . . embodied and imaginative,"[68] a visceral encounter with fellow humans. This is adaptation, a resilient push-back from social creatures craving meaningful broader attachment.

As more evidence of how much we value relationships, we now celebrate, value and extend the right to marry. If we did not think marriage was worthwhile, why would we extend the right? If relationships were not valued, they would not form in the first place. Cafés materialize thanks to demand; marriage rights extend thanks to demand. Both are valued and the social demand is driven by our biological need for core and broader attachment. Knowing how to build resilient relationships could become a right we collectively protect, encourage, extend, and commercially promote. Like café socializing, there is an opportunity for it to replace the terrible poverty of loneliness as a valued counter to screen-centred isolation.

Internet connect, people disconnect

The amazing rise of the internet delivered more information, entertainment and new possibilities. It came, however, with side-effects, unintended consequences: social phobia,[69] extreme isolation,[70] loneliness,[71] and decreased sex and intimacy.[72] It is "hell"[73] for lonely people through insufficient likes, ostracism, and social comparison leading to depression[74] and, in cyber-bullying, suicide.[75] These are the consequences that are scientifically known, its full impact on human interactions is not.

About 87% of adults[76] and 98% of Gen Z[77] own a smart-phone. 35% of users check it more than fifty times daily[78] leading to them having less time[79] and fewer friends[80] through opportunity cost. Never in human history has the brain become so fixated on such a small device.[81] In heavy screen use, brain development is impeded[82] and IQ is lowered.[83] The WHO recommends no exposure to screens for the first year of life, then less than an hour daily for the first five years.[84]

When engaged with a screen, the brain changes:[85] being close to a screen impairs attention,[86] peripheral hearing and vision are lost as the brain's thalamus shuts out other people,[87] and dopamine reward keeps us screen-focussed[88] leading to even less people-interaction. In heavy use, the anterior cingulate cortex shrinks.[89] This is devastating: in less than two decades, social media has neurologically reduced our capacity to empathize and socialize.

People sleep with phones, find their identity in avatars, and seek out virtual realities rather than real human contact. Heavy screen use disrupts attachment brain pathways[90] and is associated with depression,[91] low self-esteem,[92] social phobia,[93] narcissism,[94] and addiction.[95] Internet[96] and social media[97] addictions[98] are mediated through dopamine.[99] Screen-induced dopamine pleasure[100] is higher than pleasure from talking with people, but it lacks people-induced oxytocin love and trust, beta-endorphin togetherness, and serotonin comfort and calm. These and other brain chemicals mediate the warm experience of socializing and connecting with people.

What does it mean to socialize? It is to participate with others through sharing ideas (talking and listening), emotions (laughing and crying together), sensations (touching and being touched), meals, drinks, experiences, and eye contact. These activate our "social brain"[101] which encompasses mind-to-mind perception, trust, and predicting others' mental states.

Socializing takes effort, but we are pleasurably rewarded by long-term serotonin, oxytocin, and beta-endorphin infusions rather than by short-term pleasure-bursts of screen-induced dopamine.

In simplified terms, we socialize with each other through our senses and generate empathy in the anterior cingulate cortex. In the amygdala, we register someone else's emotions and pain and monitor our responses in the insular cortex. In the orbitofrontal cortex we choose to hide or show our emotions and transmit these choices to the basal ganglia to subtly colour our movements and tone of voice. Through this, we show empathy or other emotions – approval, timidity, frustration or hurt – for others to read. Based on prefrontal cortex beliefs, values, judgments, and plans, other orbito-frontal cortex choices are transmitted to the motor cortex to initiate action or speech.

With a long-term love-partner, there is deeper connection still: closer mind-to-mind perception, flow[102] and "limbic resonance."[103] Intimacies – physical, emotional, and mental – involve diverse, highly-adapted brain areas and feeling states which are still poorly understood. Heightened states of flow and synchronicity occur with people who are close,[104] not with screens.

More screen use leads to less use of the social brain. People then look to screens to fulfil unmet social needs such as self-esteem,[105] acceptance,[106] and social status[107] leading to even less social engagement. The WHO's recommendation of no screens for babies encourages safe, healthy attachment in the carer-infant dyad. Who will protect the couple dyad?

> After five years together James and Lakshmi were convinced they had nothing in common and were going to break-up. To relax from busy lives, James worked out at a gym and watched world soccer and other sports. Lakshmi liked Zumba and Instagram and YouTube where her online views were growing. Emotional intimacy had waned and sex had become a battleground. I suggested their next holiday be screen-free. "At first it was painful, boring, but we started spending more time exploring the cool waterfalls and secluded beaches. We had adventures without plans, and we had to talk more. Once we lost track of time. Now, we're more into each other and we've discovered the pleasures of slow sex."[108]

Social media has brought great opportunities: people brought together, internet dating,[109] and shared entertainment. Social media, however, also influences decision-making towards divorce[110] leading to increased divorce rates:[111] "you see things on Facebook all the time about 'once a cheater, always a cheater' " (Veronne and Wayne, 42 yrs). Outside forces influence us much more than we realize[112] so awareness is needed[113] and, as stated, this places more responsibility on each individual. Individuals and couples can, however, consciously and judiciously choose to prioritize their relationship and use technology to enhance rather than detract from their intimacy. Relationships protect the brain against addictions[114] to help choose and value real-person connection even more. If, however, relationships are impeded by social media, this protection can be lost.

Social brain pathways need to be exercised, but connecting with other people often brings conflict rather than comfort. Screen technology, however, offers stimulating pleasure without any conflict. Isolating away from people towards screens is the easy option, but this too has consequences:

> We hurt people's feelings by walking away, and we often do.
> We can't hurt screens' feelings by walking away, but we often don't.

As seen next chapter, "how do you keep connected?" was a pressing question from younger people for thriving couples. One couple offered a simple answer: "Don't walk away. Hug each other every opportunity you have" (Pat and Jim, 54 yrs).

Estrangement, divorce, and separation

If people hurt us too much, we leave, divorce, separate, or become estranged. These sever attachment and increase social isolation. They can, however, be necessary steps to limit acrimony and abuse. Society has been slow to recognize and act against childhood and domestic abuses.[115] Separation is required. Abusers completing treatment programs remain at high risk of recidivism,[116] abuse crosses gender divides,[117] and abuse increased during the pandemic.[118] As seen in Chapter 5, couples will always need to reasonably tolerate each other's ranting and failings, but outright abuse is traumatizing and criminal.

Other factors, however, contribute to separation and estrangement. The internet, for example, can be misused. Social media echo chambers reinforce couple anger,[119] family discord,[120] interpersonal conflict,[121] and possibly even hate crimes.[122] Social media ideas are highly influential[123] in spurning conflict through cheap, fast broadcast of polarizing ideas,[124] even in scientific debates.[125] Through a hyper-individual focus on society's negatives,[126] social media increases isolation[127] and estrangement[128] through ideas surfacing quickly and harshly. Even in a close couple, two people may privately engage in social media ideas which slowly bring them into separate, conflicting worlds. This is a reality to be negotiated.

Estrangement is family-based separation: parent-child or sibling discord leading to loss of contact[129] driven by hyper-individualism and internet-induced[130] values clashes.[131] Maintaining a sense of family amidst discord is difficult.[132] Traditionally, a family bond was through shared biology, history, and loyalty,[133] whereas a contemporary family relies more on common values,[134] and values can often clash. Family harmony depends on choices and skills to negotiate conflict. This impacts couples: acrimony from in-laws, clashing cultural expectations, a family not accepting your spouse, values clashes, and more.

Family and friends have a powerful effect on a couple relationship for better or worse:[135] "nobody's good enough for their son or daughter" (Pat and Tony, 54 yrs). Support from others is "a significant and unique variable affecting marriage quality"[136] to undermine or help a relationship.[137] Therapists have this same influence through comments they may make.[138]

Relaxed divorce laws have positively impacted unhappy couples needing to separate. Divorce and separation can, however, become a social contagion[139] as societal values influence individual choices:[140] "if others do it, maybe we should too."[141] Knowing divorced people becomes a risk factor for divorce,[142] and knowing stable couples protects your relationship: "both our parents stayed together so we had that model and it's gone through" (Cyndy and Tony, 49 yrs). Relationship stability may be rising.[143] Marriage is no longer a social convention[144] but a valued right, and a long-term relationship is a choice towards self-actualization.[145] Staying together alleviates atomization, social isolation, loneliness, and financial disadvantage.[146] People may choose to live apart together.[147]

Inter-personal conflict has always been difficult to negotiate, and isolating is one policy choice. Realities of the human condition – separation, divorce, abuse, the strong influence of social media, friends and family, and societal trends (including atomization) – all impact decision-making for individuals and couples. Couples choosing to build resilience need to be able to embrace amazing societal influences yet be mindful of the many pitfalls.

Divorce goes viral

During COVID-19, divorce and separation rates increased internationally. Wuhan province saw a 25% increase in divorce cases with couples queueing for hours to apply for divorce.[148] A similar trend was seen in India.[149] Reasons given for divorce in Wuhan included arguing over money, screen time, chore inequity, childcare, and too much time with extended family for Chinese New Year. The government introduced a six-month cooling-off period as some couples wanted to remarry after only hours.[150] Amongst reportedly good community support,[151] 2003 post-SARS Hong Kong witnessed a 21% rise in divorces.[152] In Wuhan, however, police reported a three-fold increase in domestic violence calls during the pandemic.[153] Speculatively, arguing over domestics could have been a euphemism for abuse.

In the UK, couples' wellness apps and online relationship courses were sought at record levels.[154] To couples, lockdowns brought hardship,[155] increased connection,[156] or a mixture of both. Being in a relationship was protective to mental health.[157] Keeping distance, wearing masks, and being infection-conscious, however, combined to increase community alienation, social isolation, and loneliness[158] to undermine psychological resilience.[159] For all its deadly consequences, however, the pandemic has re-educated us on the value of people.[160] When life is at risk, we naturally re-appraise our values, priorities, and lives[161] to consider our philosophical, spiritual, and relational contentment. This was brought into sharp worldwide focus.[162]

Distancing

"Social distancing" is a term inferring "being ignored, unwelcome, left alone with one's own fears, and even excluded."[163] It has entered societal consciousness[164] when "physical distancing"[165] or "distant socializing,"[166] may have been more useful. The contra-social connotations of distancing are self-evident. Distancing, masks, gloves, and face shields changed the way we perceived each other and impacted all human interactions including couple interactions.

1.5 to 2 metres, with cultural variation, is the "public space" distance we naturally keep to strangers.[167] This distance likely evolved to minimize microbial infection[168] but also reflects the trust levels among us. We allow friends closer, and we allow our love-partner even closer, into an "intimate space."[169] Distancing and mask-wearing alienate others, impair trust, and can even trigger paranoia.[170] Less trust means less oxytocin, leading to less trust and, potentially, a downward spiral. This impacts a couple as two people perceive each other as potentially infectious rather than as intimates.

Is social isolation a challenge to relationships?

Social isolation poses a significant challenge to relationships. Isolating in bedrooms, in front of screens, separating due to conflict, physical distancing, and less socializing make forming and maintaining relationships harder. Social isolation is, unfortunately, being accepted as normal.

Social media messages inflaming values clashes, family and friends influencing us, and feelings of alienation test relationship strength. Staying together as a couple, however, is highly beneficial to individual mental health. Therapists can help couples choosing relationship longevity to build resilience and value their relationship. It is a seemingly simple solution to a complex problem. Yet realizing it will take immense effort, as seen in Chapter 5.

Valuing others to value ourselves

In a post-pandemic world, we may emerge with a renewed appreciation of relationships.[171] Self-actualization is pointless as an isolated, lonely experience; it is gratifying to celebrate it with others experiencing it too. A relationship helps weather storms but also basks in shared calm sailing. As will be

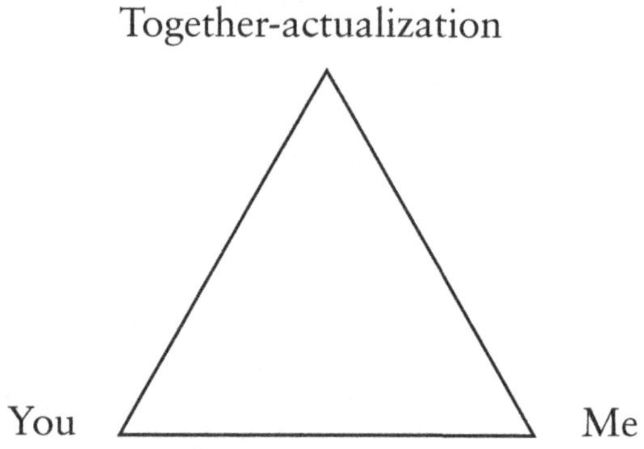

Figure 3.1

seen next chapter, for many, their relationship became a calm centre amidst the chaos of a pandemic; for others it added to the tempest. Social isolation impedes love and belonging needs, but attachment fulfils them. A couple choosing relationship resilience can reach for together-actualization even amidst increasing social isolation.

Not only did attachment connection remain for Wayne and Veronne who stayed together as "the main thing," but they can now choose to continue their climb of Maslow's pyramid together. As they ascend, they grow closer, their bond strengthens, and their relationship becomes dynamic and aspirational rather than dull and boring. Strengthened attachment and closeness can sustain and lift them to the summit ideal of together-actualization. That, perhaps, is "the main thing."

Conclusion

This chapter on contributors to social isolation and its challenges closes Part I of our book. Chapter 1 explored how certain hyper-individual ideals erode relationship longevity while others can be used help nurture it. For couples, pitfalls and binds can be avoided by shaping a together life-story and reaching for together-actualization. Chapter 2 discussed the mental health crisis. Mental health and couple relationships are underpinned by attachment, and valuing attachment helps protect individual mental health. This chapter focussed on social isolation through social media and the internet, estrangement, and social distancing. Valuing a relationship, however, becomes a much-needed push back against this unintended consequence of socio-economic development.

Having presented a context for our research, Part II presents our research findings: the Couples Surviving COVID-19 Survey in Chapter 4, and the

Couples Thriving 40+ Years Survey and Interviews in Chapter 5. Based on these, Part III presents techniques to help build relationship resilience. Consistent with the body of evidence, it will be seen that resilience is the norm, long-term relationships are valued, and the effort of maintaining a long-term relationship is often rewarded by contentment and happiness.[172] It may be "damn hard work," but the effort is beneficial and worthwhile as couples reach for resilience and together-actualization. The most self-serving thing two people can do, we argue, is to nurture their long-term relationship.

Notes

1 African wisdom, precise origin unknown.
2 Dickson-Markman, Fran, and Howard J. Markman. "The effects of others on marriage: Do they help or hurt." *Perspectives on Marital Interaction* (1988): 294–322. Rawlins, William K. *Friendship matters communication, dialectics, and the life course.* Routledge, 2017.
3 Howard, Christopher. "'Splendid isolation'." *History* 47, no. 159 (1962): 32–41.
4 Kupchan, Charles A. *Isolationism: A history of America's efforts to shield itself from the world.* Oxford University Press, 2020. Quoted in www.theatlantic.com/ideas/archive/2020/09/virtue-isolationism/616499/ Retrieved 18 August 2022.
5 Maccaferri, Marzia. "Splendid isolation again? Brexit and the role of the press and online media in re-narrating the European discourse." *Critical Discourse Studies* 16, no. 4 (2019): 389–402.
6 Cassegård, C. "7. Murakami Haruki: Loneliness and waiting." *Shock and naturalization in contemporary Japanese literature.* Brill, 2007, 162–187.
7 Attributed to Mother Teresa.
8 Kato, Takahiro A., Shigenobu Kanba, and Alan R. Teo. "Hikikomori: Experience in Japan and international relevance." *World Psychiatry* 17, no. 1 (2018): 105.
9 Kato, Takahiro A., Shigenobu Kanba, and Alan R. Teo. "Hikikomori: Multidimensional understanding, assessment, and future international perspectives." *Psychiatry and Clinical Neurosciences* 73, no. 8 (2019): 427–440.
10 Sullivan, Harry S. *The interpersonal theory of psychiatry.* W. W. Norton & Company, 1953, 260.
11 Cacioppo, John T., Mary Elizabeth Hughes, Linda J. Waite, Louise C. Hawkley, and Ronald A. Thisted. "Loneliness as a specific risk factor for depressive symptoms: Cross-sectional and longitudinal analyses." *Psychology and Aging* 21, no. 1 (2006): 140.
12 Steptoe, Andrew, Aparna Shankar, Panayotes Demakakos, and Jane Wardle. "Social isolation, loneliness, and all-cause mortality in older men and women." *Proceedings of the National Academy of Sciences* 110, no. 15 (2013): 5797–5801.
13 Lester, David. "The protective effect of marriage for suicide in men and women." *Giornale italiano di suicidologia* 4, no. 2 (1994): 84–85.
14 Rendall, Michael S., Margaret M. Weden, Melissa M. Favreault, and Hilary Waldron. "The protective effect of marriage for survival: A review and update." *Demography* 48, no. 2 (2011): 481–506.
15 Kposowa, Augustine J. "Marital status and suicide in the National Longitudinal Mortality Study." *Journal of Epidemiology & Community Health* 54, no. 4 (2000): 254–261.

16 Hald, Gert Martin, Ana Ciprić, Søren Sander, and Jenna Marie Strizzi. "Anxiety, depression and associated factors among recently divorced individuals." *Journal of Mental Health* 31, no. 4 (2022): 462–470.
17 Holt-Lunstad, Julianne, Timothy B. Smith, Mark Baker, Tyler Harris, and David Stephenson. "Loneliness and social isolation as risk factors for mortality: A meta-analytic review." *Perspectives on Psychological Science* 10, no. 2 (2015): 227–237.
18 Player, Michael J., Judy Proudfoot, Andrea Fogarty, Erin Whittle, Michael Spurrier, Fiona Shand, Helen Christensen, Dusan Hadzi-Pavlovic, and Kay Wilhelm. "What interrupts suicide attempts in men: A qualitative study." *PLoS One* 10, no. 6 (2015): e0128180.
19 Steptoe, Shankar, Demakakos, and Wardle. "Social isolation."
20 Cotterell, Natalie, Tine Buffel, and Christopher Phillipson. "Preventing social isolation in older people." *Maturitas* 113 (2018): 80–84.
21 Laursen, Brett, and Amy C. Hartl. "Understanding loneliness during adolescence: Developmental changes that increase the risk of perceived social isolation." *Journal of Adolescence* 36, no. 6 (2013): 1261–1268.
22 Penning, Margaret J., Guiping Liu, and Pak Hei Benedito Chou. "Measuring loneliness among middle-aged and older adults: The UCLA and de Jong Gierveld loneliness scales." *Social Indicators Research* 118, no. 3 (2014): 1147–1166.
23 Whisman, Mark A. "Loneliness and the metabolic syndrome in a population-based sample of middle-aged and older adults." *Health Psychology* 29, no. 5 (2010): 550.
24 Canham, Sarah L., Pia M. Mauro, Christopher N. Kaufmann, and Andrew Sixsmith. "Association of alcohol use and loneliness frequency among middle-aged and older adult drinkers." *Journal of Aging and Health* 28, no. 2 (2016): 267–284.
25 Steptoe, Andrew, Natalie Owen, Sabine R. Kunz-Ebrecht, and Lena Brydon. "Loneliness and neuroendocrine, cardiovascular, and inflammatory stress responses in middle-aged men and women." *Psychoneuroendocrinology* 29, no. 5 (2004): 593–611.
26 Hawkley, Louise C., Ronald A. Thisted, Christopher M. Masi, and John T. Cacioppo. "Loneliness predicts increased blood pressure: 5-year cross-lagged analyses in middle-aged and older adults." *Psychology and Aging* 25, no. 1 (2010): 132.
27 Lara, Elvira, Darío Moreno-Agostino, Natalia Martín-María, Marta Miret, Laura Alejandra Rico-Uribe, Beatriz Olaya, María Cabello, Josep Maria Haro, and José Luis Ayuso-Mateos. "Exploring the effect of loneliness on all-cause mortality: Are there differences between older adults and younger and middle-aged adults?" *Social Science & Medicine* 258 (2020): 113087.
28 Barreto, Manuela, Christina Victor, Claudia Hammond, Alice Eccles, Matt T. Richins, and Pamela Qualter. "Loneliness around the world: Age, gender, and cultural differences in loneliness." *Personality and Individual Differences* 169 (2021): 110066.
29 Lim, Michelle H., Robert Eres, and Claire Peck. "The young Australian loneliness survey: Understanding loneliness in adolescents and young adults." The Iverson Health Innovation Research Institute, and Centre for Mental Health, Swinburne University of Technology. 2019. https://apo.org.au/sites/default/files/resource-files/2019-10/apo-nid261896_1.pdf Retrieved 12 July 2022.
30 Weissbourd, Richard, Milena Batanova, Virginia Lovison, and Eric Torres. "Loneliness in America how the pandemic has deepened an epidemic of loneliness and what we can do about it." *Making Caring Common* (2021): 1–13.

31 Stepler, Renee. “Led by baby boomers, divorce rates climb for America’s 50+ population.” 2017. https://policycommons.net/artifacts/617987/led-by-baby-boomers-divorce-rates-climb-for-americas-50-population/1598868/ Retrieved 28 December 2022. CID: 20.500.12592/wswbh4.
32 www.nimblefins.co.uk/divorce-statistics-uk Retrieved 1 June 2022.
33 Kim, Jung-Hyun. “Getting even lonelier? Psychological well-being and problematic use of media in the over-connected society.” Coplan, Robert J. and Julie C. Bowker, eds. *The handbook of solitude: Psychological perspectives on social isolation, social withdrawal, and being alone*. Wiley-Blackwell, 2021, 240–253.
34 Kato, Kanba, and Teo. “Hikikomori: Multidimensional understanding.”
35 Tateno, Masaru, Alan R. Teo, Wataru Ukai, Junichiro Kanazawa, Ryoko Katsuki, Hiroaki Kubo, and Takahiro A. Kato. “Internet addiction, smartphone addiction, and Hikikomori trait in Japanese young adult: Social isolation and social network.” *Frontiers in Psychiatry* 10 (2019): 455.
36 Cox, Daniel A., Ryan Streeter, and David Wilde. “A loneliness epidemic? How marriage, religion, and mobility explain the generation gap in loneliness.” American Enterprise Institute. 2019. https://policycommons.net/artifacts/1295330/a-loneliness-epidemic-how-marriage-religion-and-mobility-explain-the-generation-gap-in-loneliness/1898558/ Retrieved 28 December 2022. CID: 20.500.12592/zpt025
37 Weissbourd, Batanova, Lovison, and Torres. “Loneliness in America.”
38 Barreto, Victor, Hammond, Eccles, Richins, and Qualter. “Loneliness around the world.”
39 Sieben, Inge, and Ellen Verbakel. “Permissiveness toward divorce: The influence of divorce experiences in three social contexts.” *European Sociological Review* 29, no. 6 (2013): 1175–1188.
40 McDermott, Rose, James H. Fowler, and Nicholas A. Christakis. “Breaking up is hard to do, unless everyone else is doing it too: Social network effects on divorce in a longitudinal sample.” *Social Forces* 92, no. 2 (2013): 491–519.
41 Lewis, Edwin Herbert. “Some definitions of individualism.” *American Journal of Sociology* 17, no. 2 (1911): 223–253.
42 Fromm, Erich. *The sane society*.
43 Mintz, Steven, and Susan Kellogg. *Domestic revolutions: A social history of American family life*. Simon and Schuster, 1989, 43.
44 Kennedy, John Fitzgerald. “Ask not what your country can do for you. Ask what you can do for your country.” *Inaugural Address* 20 (1961).
45 www.lse.ac.uk/social-policy/Assets/Documents/bsps/events/Explaining-changes-in-family-size.pdf Retrieved 11 April 2022.
46 www.pewresearch.org/fact-tank/2019/10/01/the-number-of-people-in-the-average-u-s-household-is-going-up-for-the-first-time-in-over-160-years/ Retrieved 11 April 2022.
47 https://aifs.gov.au/facts-and-figures/population-and-households Retrieved 11 April 2022.
48 Esteve, Albert, David S. Reher, Rocío Treviño, Pilar Zueras, and Anna Turu. “Living alone over the life course: Cross-national variations on an emerging issue.” *Population and Development Review* 46, no. 1 (2020): 169–189.
49 Smith, Kimberley J., and Christina Victor. “Typologies of loneliness, living alone and social isolation, and their associations with physical and mental health.” *Ageing & Society* 39, no. 8 (2019): 1709–1730.
50 https://koreajoongangdaily.joins.com/2021/08/03/business/economy/singleperson-household-people-living-alone-single/20210803184700342.html Retrieved 11 April 2022.

51 Ronald, Richard, Oana Druta, and Maren Godzik. "Japan's urban singles: Negotiating alternatives to family households and standard housing pathways." *Urban Geography* 39, no.7 (2018): 1018–1040.
52 Chatterjee, Arijit, and Donald C. Hambrick. "It's all about me: Narcissistic chief executive officers and their effects on company strategy and performance." *Administrative Science Quarterly* 52, no. 3 (2007): 351–386.
53 Rifkin, Susan B. "Examining the links between community participation and health outcomes: A review of the literature." *Health Policy and Planning* 29, no. suppl_2 (2014): ii98–ii106.
54 Putnam, Robert. "Bowling alone: America's declining social capital." *Journal of Democracy* 6, no. 1 (1995): 65–78.
55 Elgar, Frank J., Wendy Craig, and Stephen J. Trites. "Family dinners, communication, and mental health in Canadian adolescents." *Journal of Adolescent Health* 52, no. 4 (2013): 433–438.
56 Kawamoto, Tetsuya. "The moderating role of attachment style on the relationship between self-concept clarity and self-esteem." *Personality and Individual Differences* 152 (2020): 109604.
57 Yazdani Esfidvajani, Hamideh. "The mediating role of family functioning in the relationship between resilience and inferiority." *Journal of Psychology* 2, no. 98 (2021): 290.
58 Rudyard Kipling. *The Light That Failed*. 1891. Chapter 5. www.telelib.com/authors/K/KiplingRudyard/prose/TheLightThatFailed/chapter_5.html Retrieved 13 March 2022.
59 Schwindt, Daniel. *The case against the modern world: A crash course in traditionalist thought*. CreateSpace Independent Publishing Platform, 2016.
60 Massidda, Luca. "3. Technology is not neutral. Power dynamics and political communication in the social media era." *Changing Democracies in an Unequal World* 27, no. 3 (2020): 544–546.
61 Gerbaudo, Paolo. "Social media and populism: An elective affinity?" *Media, Culture & Society* 40, no. 5 (2018): 745–753.
62 Gold, Sharry Taylor-Efrat. "Madness and individualism: Unravelling in crazy times." *Taboo Transgression Transcendence* (2019): 135.
63 Bowlby, John. "The making and breaking of affectional bonds: I. Aetiology and psychopathology in the light of attachment theory." *The British Journal of Psychiatry* 130, no. 3 (1977): 201–210.
64 Cortright, Joe. Less in common. *City Report*. 2015. https://cityobservatory.org/wp-content/uploads/2015/06/CityObservatory_Less_In_Common.pdf Retrieved 10 June 2022.
65 Ferreira, Jennifer. "Café nation? Exploring the growth of the UK café industry." *Area* 49, no. 1 (2017): 69–76.
66 Ibid.
67 Mugyenyi, Ambrose Evarls K., Jessica E. Haberer, and Ivy O'Neil. "Pleasure and practice: A qualitative study of the individual and social underpinnings of shisha use in cafes among youth in the UK." *BMJ Open* 8, no. 4 (2018): e018989.
68 Felton, Emma. *Filtered: Coffee, the cafe and the 21st century city*. Routledge, 2019, 125.
69 Twenge, Jean M. "Have smartphones destroyed a generation." *The Atlantic* 9 (2017): 2017.
70 Teo, Alan R. "A new form of social withdrawal in Japan: A review of hikikomori." *International Journal of Social Psychiatry* 56, no. 2 (2010): 178–185.
71 Kim. "Getting even lonelier?"

72 Lei, Lei, and Scott J. South. "Explaining the decline in young adult sexual activity in the United States." *Journal of Marriage and Family* 83, no. 1 (2021): 280–295.
73 Weissbourd, Batanova, Lovison, and Torres. "Loneliness in America."
74 Nisar, Tahir M., Guru Prabhakar, P. Vigneswara Ilavarasan, and Abdullah M. Baabdullah. "Facebook usage and mental health: An empirical study of role of non-directional social comparisons in the UK." *International Journal of Information Management* 48 (2019): 53–62.
75 Vismara, Matteo, Nicolaja Girone, Dario Conti, Gregorio Nicolini, and Bernardo Dell'Osso. "The current status of cyberbullying research: A short review of the literature." *Current Opinion in Behavioral Sciences* 46 (2022): 101152.
76 https://cybercrew.uk/blog/smartphone-usage-statistics-uk/ Retrieved 29 August 2022. www.pewresearch.org/internet/fact-sheet/mobile/ Retrieved 2 November 2021.
77 https://review42.com/resources/gen-z-statistics/ Retrieved 2 November 2021.
78 https://review42.com/resources/smartphone-statistics/ Retrieved 2 November 2021.
79 Darrah, Charles. *Busier than ever!: Why American families can't slow down.* Stanford University Press, 2007.
80 Cox, D. "The state of American friendship: Change, challenges, and loss-the Survey Center on American life." *Survey Center on American Life*. 2021. https://www.americansurveycenter.org/research/the-state-of-american-friendship-change-challenges-and-loss/ Retrieved 29 August 2022.
81 Greenfield, Susan. *Mind change: How digital technologies are leaving their mark on our brains*. Random House, 2015.
82 Crone, Eveline A., and Elly A. Konijn. "Media use and brain development during adolescence." *Nature Communications* 9, no. 1 (2018): 1–10.
83 Takeuchi, Hikaru, Y. Taki, H. Hashizume, K. Asano, M. Asano, Y. Sassa, S. Yokota, Y. Kotozaki, R. Nouchi, and R. Kawashima. "Impact of videogame play on the brain's microstructural properties: Cross-sectional and longitudinal analyses." *Molecular psychiatry* 21, no. 12 (2016): 1781–1789.
84 Bull, Fiona C., Salih S. Al-Ansari, Stuart Biddle, Katja Borodulin, Matthew P. Buman, Greet Cardon, Catherine Carty et al. "World Health Organization 2020 guidelines on physical activity and sedentary behaviour." *British Journal of Sports Medicine* 54, no. 24 (2020): 1451–1462.
85 Maples, W. C., Wes DeRosier, Richard Hoenes, Rodney Bendure, and Sherl Moore. "The effects of cell phone use on peripheral vision." *Optometry-Journal of the American Optometric Association* 79, no. 1 (2008): 36–42.
86 Ward, Adrian F., Kristen Duke, Ayelet Gneezy, and Maarten W. Bos. "Brain drain: The mere presence of one's own smartphone reduces available cognitive capacity." *Journal of the Association for Consumer Research* 2, no. 2 (2017): 140–154.
87 Basso, Michele A., Daniel Uhlrich, and Martha E. Bickford. "Cortical function: A view from the thalamus." *Neuron* 45, no. 4 (2005): 485–488.
88 Cools, Roshan. "Chemistry of the adaptive mind: Lessons from dopamine." *Neuron* 104, no. 1 (2019): 113–131.
89 Montag, Christian, Zhiying Zhao, Cornelia Sindermann, Lei Xu, Meina Fu, Jialin Li, Xiaoxiao Zheng et al. "Internet communication disorder and the structure of the human brain: Initial insights on WeChat addiction." *Scientific Reports* 8, no. 1 (2018): 1–10.
90 Ibid.

91 Boers, Elroy, Mohammad H. Afzali, Nicola Newton, and Patricia Conrod. "Association of screen time and depression in adolescence." *JAMA Pediatrics* 173, no. 9 (2019): 853–859.
92 Jan, Muqaddas, Sanobia Soomro, and Nawaz Ahmad. "Impact of social media on self-esteem." *European Scientific Journal* 13, no. 23 (2017): 329–341.
93 Twenge. "Have smartphones destroyed a generation."
94 Hawk, Skyler T., Regina J. J. M. van den Eijnden, Caspar J. van Lissa, and Tom F. M. ter Bogt. "Narcissistic adolescents' attention-seeking following social rejection: Links with social media disclosure, problematic social media use, and smartphone stress." *Computers in Human Behavior* 92 (2019): 65–75.
95 Ilakkuvan, Vinu, Amanda Johnson, Andrea C. Villanti, W. Douglas Evans, and Monique Turner. "Patterns of social media use and their relationship to health risks among young adults." *Journal of Adolescent Health* 64, no. 2 (2019): 158–164.
96 Shek, Daniel T. L., Rachel C. F. Sun, and Lu Yu. *Internet addiction*. Springer, 2013.
97 Mahamid, Fayez Azez, and Denise Ziya Berte. "Social media addiction in geopolitically at-risk youth." *International Journal of Mental Health and Addiction* 17, no. 1 (2019): 102–111.
98 Weinstein, Aviv, Laura Curtiss Feder, Kenneth Paul Rosenberg, and Pinhas Dannon. "Internet addiction disorder: Overview and controversies." *Behavioral Addictions* (2014): 99–117.
99 Cools, Roshan. "Chemistry of the adaptive mind: Lessons from dopamine." *Neuron* 104, no. 1 (2019): 113–131.
100 Ikemoto, Satoshi. "Brain reward circuitry beyond the mesolimbic dopamine system: A neurobiological theory." *Neuroscience & Biobehavioral Reviews* 35, no. 2 (2010): 129–150.
101 Senju, Atsushi, and Mark H. Johnson. "The eye contact effect: Mechanisms and development." *Trends in Cognitive Sciences* 13, no. 3 (2009): 127–134. Adolphs, Ralph. "The social brain: Neural basis of social knowledge." *Annual Review of Psychology* 60 (2009): 693–716.
102 See Ramsey, Meagan A., and Amy L. Gentzler. "An upward spiral: Bidirectional associations between positive affect and positive aspects of close relationships across the life span." *Developmental Review* 36 (2015): 58–104. Graham, James M. "Self-expansion and flow in couples' momentary experiences: An experience sampling study." *Journal of Personality and Social Psychology* 95, no. 3 (2008): 679.
103 This is the premise of Lewis, Thomas, Fari Amini, and Richard Lannon. *A general theory of love*. Vintage, 2000.
104 Shehata, Mohammad, Miao Cheng, Angus Leung, Naotsugu Tsuchiya, Daw-An Wu, Chia-huei Tseng, Shigeki Nakauchi, and Shinsuke Shimojo. "Team flow is a unique brain state associated with enhanced information integration and neural synchrony." *bioRxiv* (2020).
105 Jan, Soomro, and Ahmad. "Impact of social media on self-esteem."
106 Hawk, van den Eijnden, van Lissa, and ter Bogt. "Narcissistic adolescents' attention-seeking."
107 Vogel, Erin A., Jason P. Rose, Lindsay R. Roberts, and Katheryn Eckles. "Social comparison, social media, and self-esteem." *Psychology of Popular Media Culture* 3, no. 4 (2014): 206.
108 Case study from Dr Christian Heim's clinical practice.
109 Stephure, Robert J., Susan D. Boon, Stacey L. MacKinnon, and Vicki L. Deveau. "Internet initiated relationships: Associations between age and involvement

in online dating." *Journal of Computer-Mediated Communication* 14, no. 3 (2009): 658–681.
110 Aydın, Betül, Serkan Volkan Sarı, and M. Sahin. "The effect of social networking on the divorce process." *Universal Journal of Psychology* 6, no. 1 (2018): 1–8.
111 Valenzuela, Sebastián, Daniel Halpern, and James E. Katz. "Social network sites, marriage well-being and divorce: Survey and state-level evidence from the United States." *Computers in Human Behavior* 36 (2014): 94–101.
112 Alves de Castro, Charles, Aiden Carthy, and Isobel OReilly Dr. "An ethical discussion about the responsibility for protection of minors in the digital environment: A state-of-the-art review." *Advances in Social Sciences Research* 9, no. 5 (2022): 343–370.
113 Cho, Hyunyi, Julie Cannon, Rachel Lopez, and Wenbo Li. "Social media literacy: A conceptual framework." *New Media & Society* (2022).
114 Barton, Emily A. "Understanding the brain: Grief and substance abuse." *Grief Work in Addictions Counseling*. Routledge, 2022, 49–71.
115 Jeffrey M. Masson. *The assault on truth. Freud's suppression of the seduction theory*. Farrar, Straus & Giroux; Faber, 1984.
116 Jewell, Lisa M., and J. Stephen Wormith. "Variables associated with attrition from domestic violence treatment programs targeting male batterers: A meta-analysis." *Criminal Justice and Behavior* 37, no. 10 (2010): 1086–1113.
117 Warburton, Emma, and Georgia Raniolo. "Domestic abuse during COVID-19: What about the boys?" *Psychiatry Research* 291 (2020): 113155.
118 Rengasamy, Emma R., Sarah A. Long, Sophie C. Rees, Sioned Davies, Torsten Hildebrandt, and Emily Payne. "Impact of COVID-19 lockdown: Domestic and child abuse in Bridgend." *Child Abuse & Neglect* 130 (2022): 105386.
119 Wollebæk, Dag, Rune Karlsen, Kari Steen-Johnsen, and Bernard Enjolras. "Anger, fear, and echo chambers: The emotional basis for online behavior." *Social Media+ Society* 5, no. 2 (2019).
120 Powers, Elia, Michael Koliska, and Pallavi Guha. "Shouting matches and echo chambers": Perceived identity threats and political self-censorship on social media." *International Journal of Communication* 13 (2019): 20.
121 Baughan, Amanda, Justin Petelka, Catherine Jaekyung Yoo, Jack Lo, Shiyue Wang, Amulya Paramasivam, Ashley Zhou, and Alexis Hiniker. "Someone is wrong on the internet: Having hard conversations in online spaces." *Proceedings of the ACM on Human-Computer Interaction* 5, no. CSCW1 (2021): 1–22.
122 Salojärvi, Eero, Matti Rantanen, Emilia Nieminen, Alina Juote, and Heidi Hanhela. "The 'incel' phenomenon in the digital era–How echo chambers have fueled the incel movement." Amadae, S. M., ed. *Computational transformation of the public sphere*. University of Helsinki, 2020, 195–210.
123 Bastick, Zach. "Would you notice if fake news changed your behavior? An experiment on the unconscious effects of disinformation." *Computers in Human Behavior* 116 (2021): 106633.
124 Zeitzoff, Thomas. "How social media is changing conflict." *Journal of Conflict Resolution* 61, no. 9 (2017): 1970–1991.
125 Arnold-Forster, Agnes. "Polarisation, incivility, and scientific debate during COVID-19 – an essay by Agnes Arnold-Forster." *BMJ* 374 (2021).
126 Mărgăriţoiu, Alina, and Simona Eftimie. "The lack of gratitude's practice in a hyper individualist, hyper consumer, and hyper technologized society." *Procedia-Social and Behavioral Sciences* 203 (2015): 316–321.

127 Gauchet, Marcel. "A new age of personality: An essay on the psychology of our times." *Thesis Eleven* 60, no. 1 (2000): 23–41.
128 Ogihara, Yuji, and Yukiko Uchida. "Does individualism bring happiness? Negative effects of individualism on interpersonal relationships and happiness." *Frontiers in Psychology* 5 (2014): 135.
129 Scharp, Kristina M., and Elizabeth Dorrance Hall. "Family marginalization, alienation, and estrangement: Questioning the nonvoluntary status of family relationships." *Annals of the International Communication Association* 41, no. 1 (2017): 28–45.
130 Ibid.
131 Gilligan, Megan, J. Jill Suitor, and Karl Pillemer. "Estrangement between mothers and adult children: The role of norms and values." *Journal of Marriage and Family* 77, no. 4 (2015): 908–920.
132 Baxter, Leslie A., and Kristina M. Scharp. "Dialectical tensions in relationships." *The International Encyclopedia of Interpersonal Communication* (2015): 1–6.
133 Scharp, Kristina M., and Lindsey J. Thomas. "Family "bonds": Making meaning of parent – child relationships in estrangement narratives." *Journal of Family Communication* 16, no. 1 (2016): 32–50.
134 Ibid.
135 Dickson-Markman, and Markman. "The effects of others on marriage."
136 Dehle, Crystal, Debra Larsen, and John E. Landers. "Social support in marriage." *American Journal of Family Therapy* 29, no. 4 (2001): 307–324.
137 Abbas, Jaffar, M. Aqeel, Jaffar Abbas, B. Shaher, A. Jaffar, J. Sundas, and W. Zhang. "The moderating role of social support for marital adjustment, depression, anxiety, and stress: Evidence from Pakistani working and nonworking women." *Journal of Affective Disorders* 244 (2019): 231–238.
138 Doherty, William J., and Steven M. Harris. "Relationship-undermining statements by psychotherapists with clients who present with marital or couple problems." *Family Process* 61, no. 3 (2022): 1195–1207.
139 Duato, Rubén, and Lucas Jódar. "Mathematical modeling of the spread of divorce in Spain." *Mathematical and Computer Modelling* 57, no. 7–8 (2013): 1732–1737.
140 Schwartz, Shalom H. "Values: Individual and cultural." van de Vijver, F. J. R., Chasiotis, A., and Breugelmans, S. M., eds. *Fundamental questions in cross-cultural psychology*. Cambridge University Press, 2011, 463–493.
141 McDermott, Fowler, and Christakis. "Breaking up."
142 Ibid.
143 https://ifstudies.org/blog/why-is-divorce-declining-in-the-uk Retrieved 17 March 2022.
144 Ibid.
145 Finkel, Eli J. *The all-or-nothing marriage: How the best marriages work*. Penguin, 2019.
146 Smyth, Bruce, and Ruth Weston. "Financial living standards after divorce." *Family Matters* 55 (2000): 10–15.
147 De Jong Gierveld, Jenny. "Remarriage, unmarried cohabitation, living apart together: Partner relationships following bereavement or divorce." *Journal of Marriage and Family* 66, no. 1 (2004): 236–243.
148 Prasso, Sreridan. China's divorce spike is a warning to the rest of lock-down world. *Bloomberg*. 31/03/2020. www.bloomberg.com/news/articles/2020-03-31/divorces-spike-in-china-after-coronavirus-quarantines Retrieved 5 May 2020.

149 Shehadi, Sebastian and Partington, Miriam. Why lockdown's toll on relationships could be a public health issue. *Newstateman*. 11/6/2020. www.newstatesman.com/science-tech/coronavirus/2020/06/why-lockdown-s-toll-relationships-could-be-public-health-issue Retrieved 10 July 2020.
150 Wray, Meaghan. China's divorce rates rise as couples emerge from coronavirus quarantine. *Global News*. 2/4/2020. https://globalnews.ca/news/6767589/china-divorce-rates-coronavirus/ Retrieved 10 July 2020.
151 Lau, Joseph T. F., Xilin Yang, H. Y. Tsui, Ellie Pang, and Yun Kwok Wing. "Positive mental health-related impacts of the SARS epidemic on the general public in Hong Kong and their associations with other negative impacts." *Journal of Infection* 53, no. 2 (2006): 114–124.
152 Prasso, *China's divorce spike.*
153 Ibid.
154 Shehadi and Partington. *Lockdown's toll on relationships.*
155 Ahuja, Kanika K., and Dhairya Khurana. "Locked-down love: A study of intimate relationships before and after the COVID lockdown." *Family Relations* 70, no. 5 (2021): 1343–1357.
156 Kallová, Nikola, Denisa Hnatkovičová, and Ivan Lukšík. "A misfortune or a benefit? Young people's quality of life and romantic relationships during the COVID-19 pandemic." *Human Affairs* 32, no. 2 (2022): 241–266.
157 Till, Benedikt, and Thomas Niederkrotenthaler. "Romantic relationships and mental health during the COVID-19 pandemic in Austria: A population-based cross-sectional survey." *Frontiers in Psychology* (2022): 2094.
158 Williams, Simon N., Christopher J. Armitage, Tova Tampe, and Kimberly Dienes. "Public perceptions and experiences of social distancing and social isolation during the COVID-19 pandemic: A UK-based focus group study." *BMJ Open* 10, no. 7 (2020): e039334.
159 Gundogan, Selim. "The mediator role of the fear of COVID-19 in the relationship between psychological resilience and life satisfaction." *Current Psychology* (2021): 1–9.
160 Sadani, Aachal. "A Different Point of View about Corona Pandemic." *Psychology and Education Journal* 58, no. 2 (2021): 423–429.
161 van Gurp, Jelle L. P., Liza G. G. van Lent, Nicole Stoel, Carin C. D. van der Rijt, Maja J. A. de Jonge, Saskia M. Pulleman, Julia van Weert, and Jeroen Hasselaar. "Core values of patients with advanced cancer considering participation in an early-phase clinical trial: A qualitative study." *Supportive Care in Cancer* (2022): 1–9.
162 Diener, Ed, and Martin E. P. Seligman. "Very happy people." *Psychological Science* 13, no. 1 (2002): 81–84.
163 Wasserman, Danuta, Rutger van der Gaag, and Jan Wise. "The term 'physical distancing' is recommended rather than 'social distancing' during the COVID-19 pandemic for reducing feelings of rejection among people with mental health problems." *European Psychiatry* 63, no. 1 (2020).
164 Aminnejad, Reza, and Rosa Alikhani. "Physical distancing or social distancing: That is the question." *Canadian Journal of Anesthesia/Journal canadien d'anesthésie* 67, no. 10 (2020): 1457–1458.
165 Kumar, Satyendra. "Corona virus outbreak: Keep physical distancing, not social distancing." *Not Social Distancing* (2020).
166 Pandi-Perumal, Seithikurippu R., Sophie R. Vaccarino, Vijay Kumar Chattu, Nevin F. W. Zaki, Ahmed S. BaHammam, Dilshad Manzar, G. J. M. Maestroni et al. " 'Distant socializing,' not 'social distancing' as a public health strategy for COVID-19." *Pathogens and Global Health* 115, no. 6 (2021): 357–364.

167 Brown, Nina. "Edward T. Hall: Proxemic theory, 1966." *Center for Spatially Integrated Social Science. University of California, Santa Barbara*. www.csiss.org/classics/content/13
168 Farboodi, Maryam, Gregor Jarosch, and Robert Shimer. "Internal and external effects of social distancing in a pandemic." *Journal of Economic Theory* 196 (2021): 105293.
169 Layden, Elliot A., John T. Cacioppo, and Stephanie Cacioppo. "Loneliness predicts a preference for larger interpersonal distance within intimate space." *PLoS One* 13, no. 9 (2018): e0203491.
170 Wasserman, van der Gaag, and Wise. "The term 'physical distancing'."
171 Golightley, Malcolm, and Margaret Holloway. "Unprecedented times? Social work and society post-COVID-19." *The British Journal of Social Work* 50, no. 5 (2020): 1297–1303.
172 Diener and Seligman. "Very happy people."

Part II

Our study

Chapter 4

Survey findings: couples surviving COVID-19

As argued in Part I, hyper-individualism, social isolation, and the mental health crisis are major twenty-first century socio-cultural conditions affecting relationships. It is in the context of these that building resilient relationships can be considered. Couples married 40+ years interviewed for this book were cognisant of this: "The way you think about [relationships] now seems to be a bit different . . . the world has changed so much" (Inno and Tiiu, Estonia, 66 yrs). It is vital that ideas passed on from these couples are contextualized for twenty-first century couples. To keep findings applicable, we surveyed couples that had been in a relationship for 3+ years. The survey included this question:

> If you could ask someone married for 40+ years a relationship question, what would it be?

Answers to this and other questions informed both the 40+ Years Married Survey and the Thriving Couples Interviews to be discussed next chapter.

This chapter begins Part II of this book, in which we present our findings. It gives a brief overview of relationship studies during COVID-19 and outlines our Surviving COVID-19 Survey, before detailing the findings of the survey. The chapter concludes with a discussion of the findings in the context of issues surfacing in Part I. It starts, however, with an overview of the three arms of our study.

Three arms to our study

To our knowledge, this is the largest multi-national, cross-sectional study of long-term relationships ever undertaken. Over 1400 people across 52 countries were surveyed or interviewed. As detailed in the methodology section of the Introduction, results presented in Part II of this book were drawn from three study arms:

1 The Thriving Couple Interviews
2 The Surviving COVID-19 Survey
3 The Married 40+ Years Survey

DOI: 10.4324/9781003263395-7

This chapter focusses on study arm 2: The Surviving COVID-19 Survey. This survey of individuals in a committed relationship for 3+ years was undertaken in 2020 when surveyed couples were either in lockdown or had experienced some form of lockdown. The 290 respondents were from 21 countries representing 37 ethnicities and included married and non-married couples in a relationship for at least three years. Questions from couples in The Surviving COVID-19 Survey informed the other two arms of the study.

The Surviving COVID-19 Survey aimed to capture a glimpse into the relationship landscape during the pandemic. Individuals were isolating, many were experiencing mental health issues, and hyper-individual aspirations were being challenged. Relationship issues were brought into sharp focus. We were able to sample couples and glean from their concerns and what they learnt about their relationship: their learnings.

We had not originally planned to include this study arm. The pandemic, a worldwide disaster, however, presented us with the opportunity to survey aspects of couple adaptability and resilience. Many of those surveyed had experienced job insecurity and loss, mental illness, health anxiety, fear of death, and the actual death of loved ones. These acute stressors tested relationship resilience.

The health consequences of the pandemic are multifarious. Its ramifications on divorce and general effects were considered last chapter. Here we focus on specific relationship issues experienced by couples at that time and their impacts on relationship resilience.

Studies on relationships during COVID-19

Global epidemics, war, and weather-related and technological disasters create additional challenges for individuals and relationships.[1] During the pandemic, many isolating couples experienced increased conflict[2] and decreased relationship satisfaction,[3] while others experienced increased relationship satisfaction or no change.[4] Variation can be explained by differences in relationships' pre-existing conditions and underlying attachment.[5]

Based on our Surviving COVID-19 Survey, we posit that one of the "pre-existing contextual vulnerabilities"[6] exacerbated by lockdown or isolation was pressures brought on by hyper-individual values. Autonomy, for example, is considered a "significant negative predictor of marital problems"[7] and our research broadly supports this. During lockdown, individual autonomy was constricted. Other stress-inducing factors included having children at home,[8] conflict over division of labour,[9] lowered optimism,[10] constricted social networks, and mental health issues. Values clashes led to couples arguing more[11] and existential fear of being single[12] also contributed to conflict.

Underlying the studies cited earlier are some significant assumptions: that being in a supportive relationship is preferable to being single, that holding certain values can undermine relationship health, and that relationship health is worth protecting. We too hold these assumptions. They are based on the axiomatic idea that we are social creatures who need close attachment and have a strong desire for broader relationship. Assumptions such as these, however, are being eroded in the current zeitgeist to increase complexity and confusion for individuals wanting to know how to secure relational safety. Individuals we surveyed had to negotiate these complexities.

The Surviving COVID-19 Survey

Our Surviving COVID-19 Survey amassed information regarding relationship satisfaction and dissatisfaction: problems, benefits and learnings. It collected questions from respondents for us to then ask couples thriving 40+ years. An outline of the survey's methodology is found in the Introduction and the survey questions can be found in Appendix 2.

Respondents were dealing not only with the pandemic but with the sociocultural context of hyper-individualism, the mental health crisis, and social isolation brought to an intense peak. The questions respondents wished to ask couples together 40+ years emerged as the most efficacious aspect of this survey. These revealing questions, informed by the pressures they were experiencing and the hopes they retained, provided pertinent material for the other two study arms. What follows is an overview of our findings finishing with a discussion of these questions.

Relationship happiness

Our survey asked about happiness rather than satisfaction. "Satisfaction" has a specific meaning in couple research,[13] but to couples, the term may often connote fulfilment with a functional, consumerist, or sexual focus. Our couple interviews, for example, revealed more passion and enthusiasm than the word "satisfied" captures and the word was used by only one of 180 interviewees; that person happened to be an academic. "Happiness" or "happy," in contrast, were terms used by 142 interviewees and became more apposite descriptors for our research.

Happiness can be Hedonic pleasure seeking,[14] but respondents' use of the term was Eudaimonic as their fulfilment described was gained from activities harmonizing with their values[15] rather than from appetitive pleasures. Happiness in couples is predominantly measured in terms of personal happiness,[16] but to gain more of a relationship focus, we asked respondents to rate their perception of their partner's *relationship* happiness levels as well as their own *relationship* rather than personal happiness.

69% of respondents rated their relationship happiness levels as high or very high during lockdown, and 66% rated their pre-COVID-19 happiness levels as high or very high. 68% ranked their partner's happiness levels during lockdown as high or very high, and 68% rated their partner's pre-COVID-19 happiness levels as high or very high. Consistent with other research[17] responses to open-ended questions revealed that some couples grew closer while others drifted apart. Partner and children proximity during lockdown also adversely impacted relationship happiness levels.

Respondent relationship happiness

	Very low	*Low*	*Average*	*High*	*Very High*
Pre-COVID-19	1%	7%	27%	37%	29%
In COVID-19	2%	10%	21%	39%	30%

Partner relationship happiness

	Very low	*Low*	*Average*	*High*	*Very High*
Pre-COVID-19	2%	5%	25%	38%	30%
In COVID-19	2%	7%	23%	39%	29%

Relationship problems during COVID-19 and what helped

While relationship problems were not the focus of our research, we needed to enquire about these to contextualize couple's resilience and adaptability. These relationship problems, like the pandemic itself, were adversities which needed to be overcome during "these unprecedented times" (50–59 yrs). The survey revealed marked differences in coping and adapting to adversity for couples across age brackets.[18] 74% of respondents articulated relationship problems. Significantly, the largest reported problem was mental health issues. The major five issues were, in order:

Mental health issues
Finances
Arguing with partner
Parenting issues
Constricted space

Mental health issues

As seen in Chapter 2, mental health issues escalated during COVID-19:

> Persistently high levels of stress and anxiety regarding external factors seeped into our internal relationship dynamic. COVID-19 prompted

> deep existential reflection leading to re-evaluation of the relationship. (3–5 yrs)
>
> Covid has been a trying time and has affected our mental health a lot. I've had two breakdowns during COVID-19. . . . The depression was awful and lucky there were caring, understanding doctors who told me I was not alone. (31–40 yrs)

We also asked, "If you had relationship problems, what helped?" The majority of the couples dealing with mental health issues replied "nothing." Others noted: "Getting a counsellor that we both liked and trusted" (6–10 yrs), "doing a ton of chores to keep the house clean and relaxing for her" (16–20 yrs), and "have conversations around mitigation strategies" (16–20 yrs).[19] Some responses were detailed:

> Initially, at the very start of lockdown, having more time together allowed for an increase in meaningful communication and a renewed sense of bondedness: experiencing the crisis together, supporting each other. However, as time progressed and the realities of the situation set in, intense work load/work environments, mental health issues within family and communities, anxiety about the future . . . became overwhelming and destabilizing. (3–5 yrs)

Our findings highlight that the pandemic exacerbated the already high levels of mental health issues impacting relationships. As articulated previously, initial mutual support could revitalize a relationship. As the crisis continued, however, limits to this couple's coping mechanisms became apparent.

Did mental health issues contribute to relationship unhappiness?

	Not at all	*A little*	*Average*	*More than average*	*A lot*
Pre-COVID-19	53.88%	24.14%	12.93%	5.6%	3.45%
In COVID-19	21.93%	8.33%	52.19%	12.28%	5.26%

Finances

Finances were the second largest problem reported by couples in the Surviving COVID-19 Survey.[20] Couples had "financial issues due to hours being cut at respective jobs" (11–15 yrs), many couples "fought about finances" (6–10 yrs), some "never did get past the financial problems" (6–10 yrs) which "became worse" (21–30 yrs). Others worked to find solutions deciding to "budget more closely and make some sacrifices" (11–15 yrs). One couple sought a counsellor to discuss financial conflicts.

Did financial stress contribute to relationship unhappiness?

	Not at all	*A little*	*Average*	*More than average*	*A lot*
Pre-COVID-19	20.69%	30.6%	29.31%	12.93%	6.47%
In COVID-19	13.79%	13.79%	40.95%	24.14%	7.33%

Arguing

During this time of heightened tension, our survey showed that arguing became more of a problem for couples during COVID-19. Couples, particularly those married for 3–5 or 6–10 yrs, commented on "lots of arguing" and "constant arguing." Some were cognisant of the source of their arguments: "Fear of bad things happening, leading to stress, leading to arguing" (6–10 yrs) or "I can be aggressive when I argue and understandably my wife doesn't like that" (6–10 yrs). This respondent saw a therapist and was helped greatly.

For one respondent, "constant arguing" was the problem and "constant communication" was the solution. Many couples "talked things out" to "see things from the other person's perspective" (11–15 yrs) and understand "the issue [they] were facing" (3–5 yrs). Some couples distanced themselves from each other. One couple in the early stages of their relationship played video games together to help dissipate tensions and help build bridges.

Did arguing contribute to relationship unhappiness?

	Not at all	*A little*	*Average*	*More than average*	*A lot*
Pre-COVID-19	33.91%	37.39%	19.57%	6.52%	2.61%
In COVID-19	16.52%	18.26%	50%	13.48%	1.74%

Parenting issues

The stress of having children at home and learning remotely was, for some, the "Biggest stressor" (21–30 yrs) causing arguments. In isolation, children at home "Intensified family responsibilities of doing work, caring for children, being like business partners and not being able to find the time and space for connection and intimacy as a couple" (11–15 yrs). Disagreements over "boundaries for our kids" (16–20 yrs) created high tensions for some. To cope, the majority of couples were "Taking long walks and talking" (21–30 yrs) and "Being open minded, listening, working together" (21–30 yrs), spending time away from children or "both respectively connected with new interests, hobbies, exercised more, and started volunteering. By finding a sense of purpose as individuals, [they] had more capacity to give to each other" (11–15 yrs). This balancing of self-wants and altruism resulted in more togetherness. Other couples coped with humour[21] or by dividing chores more equitably. For couples dealing with the needs of children during COVID-19, communication and pursuing individual and/or together aspirations were prominent coping mechanisms.

Did children's needs contribute to relationship unhappiness?

	Not at all	*A little*	*Average*	*More than average*	*A lot*
Pre-COVID-19	53.68%	16.02%	16.88%	9.96%	3.46%
In-COVID-19	20.44%	6.09%	51.3%	16.52%	5.65%

Constricted space

To suddenly live in close proximity 24 hours a day after much separation became a challenge. In this, lockdowns mirrored the adjustments retiring couples need to make but with added stress and without years of considered planning. "Not getting self-time" (20–29 yrs) or "Too much time together . . . realizing I don't like certain things about [them]" (16–20 yrs) led to arguing.

The primary coping mechanism was to have planned separate time or for some younger couples, "Going back to the office" (3–5 yrs). Increased humour and communication were other common strategies:

> Being able to laugh and try to understand each other helped get through problems. (16–20 yrs)
>
> It helped to communicate our feelings more freely, with an open air of understanding that we were working together during this unprecedented time. (11–15 yrs)

Did constricted space contribute to relationship unhappiness?

	Not at all	*A little*	*Average*	*More than average*	*A lot*
Pre-COVID-19	53.25%	21.21%	18.62%	4.33%	2.6%
In COVID-19	16.38%	5.17%	50.86%	20.69%	6.9%

Other problems articulated by respondents included, in order, division of chores, lack of sexual expression, restricted freedom, value clashes, wanting to separate, distrust and infidelity:

> We would argue about the division of chores. (11–15 yrs)
>
> Could never have sex. The house was always occupied and we could not go away. (21–30 yrs)
>
> Less sex with kids home all the time. (31–40 yrs)
>
> The lack of space (having [had] the house to myself) was difficult for me, and my partner's anxiety heightened things. (16–20 yrs)
>
> Can't share the household work. Can't go out. Can't get self time. (3–5 yrs)
>
> More time together so . . . some values caused more clashes. (31–40 yrs)
>
> I need a break from him. There is no escape. (21–30 yrs)
>
> Lack of trust and communication. (16–20 yrs)
>
> We had infidelity on both ends; trying to work to stay together. (21–30 yrs)

These responses reflect not only the stress of constricted space, but the importance of sex, trust, and open communication in a relationship. Societal pressures, present long before the pandemic, significantly contributed to relationship problems as articulated in these five major issues. The problems which led to arguing in our respondents may have led to divorce in Wuhan.

Breaking up

In our survey, 9% of the respondents were considering breaking up. Most of these had been together for 11–15 years and were 30–39 years of age. This group experienced the most problems overall. Factors contributing to this were, in order: financial issues, personality clashes, mental health issues, arguing, too much time together, and in-law interference. Parenting issues were only cited by two respondents as a reason to contemplate breaking up. Half of the 24 respondents considering break-up were working on staying together through talking, counsellors, taking time apart, and through forgiveness.[22] This reflects their valuing of their relationship. Almost a third did not move forward in resolving the issues, and two respondents wrote that they had decided to break up. As we were surveying individuals, we do not know if this represented one couple or two.

COVID-19 actually saved at least one relationship:

> Prior to Covid, [breaking up] was a consideration, but during, after Covid, it no longer became the solution to anything. Being able to spend more time together allowed us to have many deeper, longer discussions. (6–10 yrs)

Gaining an overview of respondents' relationship problems during COVID-19 helped understand the adversity they needed to overcome. Learnings are adaptations. In considering benefits and learnings, we see how many couples adapted to and maintained relationship well-being in adversity to not only build resilience but discover something new and surprising in their relationships.

Relationship benefits from COVID-19

In keeping with a salutogenic approach, the Surviving COVID-19 Survey asked: Were there benefits for your relationship during isolation? 64% of the respondents reported benefits. The following, in order, were the major benefits reported:

More time together
Being closer and valuing each other more
Forced us to work on our problems and values
More emotional support
More time with children and family

All of these benefits more or less resulted from having more time together. By considering these separately, however, we can glean some of the meaning from the respondents of the time spent together: relational, problem solving, emotional, or basking in being a family unit. Each benefit reported highlighted one of these.

More time together

By far, the most widely reported benefit was time spent together. This led to the other benefits: being closer, forcing couples to work on their problems, more emotional support, and time spent as a family unit. Our findings in this are consistent with those in other studies.[23] Interestingly, constricted space, a major problem for some couples (23%), emerged as the primary benefit for others (54%). Isolating together was an opportunity for these couples to grow closer.

Younger couples appear to have benefitted the most from the time together:

> We got a lot closer and were able to help each other with mental health struggles. (3–5 yrs)
>
> More time together with our son. (3–5 yrs)
>
> Much more time spent together which has been lovely. (3–5 yrs)

Couples together 21 years plus also benefitted:

> Time to discuss us and who we are. (21–30 yrs)
>
> Time to learn about each other and [our]selves. (31–40 yrs)

More time together with less distractions was experienced as a benefit by more than half of the respondents. In the fury and hurry of twenty-first century life, with its consumer and achievement focus, a couple often becomes time poor and robbed of the time needed for strengthening their attachment bond. Time away from the relationship became known as "distractions:" work, busyness, coping with the logistics, socializing, working away from each other, and even "stupid things." Having had time to reflect, some couples described these distractions as a negative force "interrupting" and "stealing focus from each other" (16–20 yrs). This "forced" time together "helped [many couples'] overall relationship improve" (11–15 yrs) and for people to "be there more fully" (11–15 yrs) for each other and "Get to know each other again" (6–10 yrs). These couples valued their relationship.

Some respondents said that time together became "relationship-focussed bonding" (16–20 yrs) and "more bonding" (11–15 yrs). This is the language of attachment. Time and proximity, as Bowlby explained, naturally strengthens the attachment bond. This is particularly the case when proximity is untainted by mental illness or distractions. Proximity to another human being is the antithesis of loneliness. These couples were isolating, but they were not lonely; they were together.

Being closer and valuing each other more

30% of the respondents reporting benefits stated that time together drew them closer leading to valuing each other more. COVID-19 gave couples time for "us to focus on us" and to be "who we are" to "learn about ourselves" and "time to discuss us." It drew people "closer as a couple:" "we are more in love now than we were before" (3–5 yrs) with "deeper understanding of each other's needs, wants, goals, ambitions" (11–15 yrs) and "time to reconsider values" (6–10 yrs). Some learnt "new things about one another" (6–10 yrs) and "solidified [their] relationship" (21–30 yrs), while others had "more meaningful conversations" (11–15 yrs). In close proximity, social beings naturally bond together and grow close to rediscover and value each other more.

Forced us to work on our problems and values

In lockdown, 16% of the respondents "worked through problems" (11–15 yrs), "helped each other with mental health struggles" (3–5 yrs), "talk[ed] about issues more" (16–20 yrs), or just "talked a lot of stuff out" (11–15 yrs) to "work out our differences" (11–15 yrs). Couples did "become closer as a result" (11–15 yrs) of "enforced time together to work through problems" (11–15 yrs):

> Sharing a negative experience that was clearly outside of our relationship brought us together. Too often we can make problems about the relationship rather than using the relationship to address problems. Covid was so clearly not about us that we could work side by side more easily. (16–20 yrs)

This was a time of hardship for some couples, but many couples thrived: "More time together facing a difficult situation made us closer" (16–20 yrs) and learning to "lean on each other to cope with all the bullshit" (3–5 yrs). This "us-against-the-world" attitude is consistent with "blame the pandemic" studies showing that some people became "more forgiving and less blaming of their partner's negative behaviours"[24] during isolation. For these couples, time together meant being able to rekindle teamwork and using each other as cognitive resources.

More emotional support

During these stressful times, many couples found more emotional support in each other: "We are a team and we worked together to get through the financial stress of my husband being out of work" (3–5 yrs). The benefit was "[my] partner being present physically to support [me] emotionally (11–15 yrs)," "More time together, less stress [in] conflicting work schedules" (11–15 yrs), and "being together and not being stressed" (3–5 yrs). 10% of respondents reported benefits mentioning emotional support.

More time with children and family

More time with children and family was a problem for some, but a benefit for others (5%). Reported benefits included "more time with our kids and together. . . . Not running around . . . left more time to actually all spend together" (11–15 yrs). "Much needed time" (11–15 yrs) created more "family togetherness" (21–30 yrs). "Valu[ing] each other more" (6–10 yrs) and not "taking things for granted anymore" (11–15 yrs) also emerged as benefits. This too was consistent with other studies.[25] The benefits were both in the logistical running of a household and in that feeling of belonging-togetherness as a family, which is an expression of *storge* love.

It is noteworthy to find how many couples benefited from time together. This is consistent with the idea that couples essentially wanted their relationship to succeed and were happier when it did. The busyness of twenty-first century life gets in the way of couples being close, appreciating and valuing each other, emotionally supporting each other, and remembering what they first saw in each other. Busyness in work and individual pursuits versus time together reflects balancing selfishness and altruism. Life's current complexity may hinder us from finding this balance.

Positive relationship learnings

The brain is wired to learn through adversity, so in our survey we asked, "What did you learn about your relationship during COVID-19?" 90% of respondents answered the question. Of these, 87% reported a positive learning predilection, 13% reported negative. Almost seven times as many couples had positive as opposed to negative learnings. A positive bias is expected but such a strong positive result is noteworthy. Closeness to a partner as a primary attachment figure likely led to increased quality of life, increased sense of self, and increased trust, leading to optimism.

Numerous, diverse positive learnings were reported. The following were the top five:

> Together we are stronger than we thought
> I now know more about my partner's strengths and weaknesses
> Communication is important
> Enjoying time together is important
> Enjoying time apart is important

Together we are stronger than we thought

This was the overwhelmingly largest positive learning, cited by 42% of respondents reporting positive learnings:

> We survived COVID-19, we can survive anything. (3–5 yrs)
>
> Together we can get through anything as long as we pool our resources and work together as partners on a team. (3–5 yrs)
>
> When the going gets tough, we stick together. (11–15 yrs)

Couples could "handle any problem [they] face, even financial difficulties" by "work[ing] together through it" (16–20 yrs). Some noted they could now "work through anything" (6–10 yrs) and can "conquer a lot if we stick together" (11–15 yrs). Teamwork was emphasized:

> We are together. We are a team. We've got each other's back. (16–20 yrs)
>
> Although sometimes we might hit some rough spots we can overcome them if we work together. (3–5 yrs)
>
> We are strong, committed, a team and true best friends. We make great partners. (16–20 yrs)

These comments encouragingly reflect relationship resilience as these couples faced adversity together and came out stronger. "Strong" was cited 20 times, other terms included "solid as a rock," "tough," "adapt," "determined," "overcome," "survive," and "flexibility." Relatedly, couples said they learnt about relationship survival, longevity, relational security and relationship priority.

One couple together 3–5 years said of their relationship: "it's going to last." Another assured:

> we will stand the test of time because we actually like each other and, thanks to work stresses and rat race kind of life subsid[ing], we are

> more relaxed and understanding of each other. We give each other time and lots of love. (3–5 yrs)

Couples such as this stepped off the twenty-first century "rat race" treadmill, to discover not only that they "actually like each other" but that the closeness and togetherness helped them grow in love. Sometimes it takes a pandemic to recognize the gold we have right in front of us.

Others stated that "This is a long haul deal" (31–40 yrs). These and similar comments confirmed to us that people want relationship longevity and actively worked towards it. Many couples were surprised to find that that they actually liked each other, and this assuaged previous relationship insecurities. Many couples emerged more secure in their relationship, being "better off than we thought," "stronger than we realized," "closer than we gave ourselves credit for being," and "love each other more than we thought." COVID-19 gave some previously insecure individuals a much-needed opportunity to cement and appreciate their relationship.

Prioritizing a relationship was part of being "stronger together." One couple consciously prioritized their relationship:

> As two registered nurses going to work through a pandemic, the stress and anxiety we both felt could have easily worn away at our new marriage. . . . We learned that the foundation of our relationship is, indeed, as strong as we thought. We prioritized our marriage and sat down to talk through our feelings before/after work. We wanted to make sure we did not project our stress/anxiety/frustration on our partner but acknowledge each other's feelings. It allowed us to be understanding of each other when one of us might be short-worded, "moody," or withdrawn for a short period of time. COVID-19 has been a real test of our relationship foundation, but with our active effort to preserve our relationship at its pretty-COVID status, no cracks suspected! (6–10 yrs)

And further from other respondents:

> You have to find ways to make your relationship stronger no matter what is happening outside of your relationship. You have to make your relationship a top priority. (11–15 yrs)

> The relationship has had many downs, but I have seen that we are both determined to make it work. (6–10 yrs)

> We love each other and we need to make more time for just us and not always be so focused on working and making money. (11–15 yrs)

> You don't really know someone until you see how they cope with adversity. (3–5 yrs)

That COVID-19 was expected to produce cracks in relationships was a reasonable supposition. Some couples broke up. These comments, however, displayed resilience through valuing and prioritizing their relationship, being in it for the "long haul," and working together to overcome adversity. These helpful attitudes find their way into the techniques to build resilience presented in Part III of this book.

I now know more about my partner's strengths and weaknesses

Testing times reveal strengths and weaknesses: "Because we spent more time together than usual, there were some positive aspects of my partner that I'd overlooked, i.e.: his accommodation of things and humour. But there were also negative characteristics that I noticed more" (31–40 yrs). Others discovered "very similar values and world views, which really became apparent during isolation" (11–15 yrs) and "deep layers of motivations, desires and priorities that we kind of knew about but didn't really understand how deeply they play out in day to day life" (16–20 yrs). People evaluated their strengths and weaknesses:

> During the beginning of the pandemic [our] relationship started getting really rocky. . . . We have started focusing more on what each of our strengths and weaknesses are and we have tried to let that round us out. We will do things that help us to help fill out deficits that the other person might have. (11–15 yrs)

It is tempting to jump to thinking 'strengths are helpful, weaknesses are not.' The real relationship benefit is, however, that couples actually came to know each other more. Getting to know someone more deeply strengthens the attachment bond for the long-term.

The importance of communication

Some couples struggled while others came up with a communication style that worked:

> We learnt that when we are unsure within the relationship we become brittle and cautious. We are happier when we are a little rougher with each other – making fun, being demanding, saying no etc. . . . Trying to 'be polite' because we have friction only drains the play from our relationship and makes everything more strained. (16–20 yrs)

Some couples "learned how to communicate better. . . . It is definitely better to talk about things" (16–20 yrs). Others reached an impasse: "We both hate conflict and don't know how to express ourselves well verbally" (31–40 yrs). Couples learning the benefits of communication still bemoaned the "emotional labour" (3–5 yrs) amidst "talking about your feelings" (6–10 yrs).

It is interesting that a couple together almost twenty years now learn that it is "better to talk" whereas a young couple bemoan the "emotional labour" of communicating. Good communication in a relationship is a lifetime ideal. It emerges as a goal that both younger and more established relationships strive for to preserve relationship longevity.

Enjoying time together and time apart

The last two major relationship learnings were enjoying time together, without distractions, and enjoying time apart:

> We are really happy just being us for a while. (3–5 yrs)
>
> Isolation does not bother us at all, we prefer our own company. (16–20 yrs)
>
> We are all we need. (11–15 yrs)
>
> We learned that we like spending more time together, . . . we actually do LIKE each other's company more than we thought. (16–20 yrs)
>
> We like spending more time alone and just with each other, not with friends. (3–5 yrs)

Liking each other's company again emerges as a surprise as couples discover "we are all we need." This underlines the idea that, given the chance away from distractions, relationships likely flourish.

Conversely, many respondents discovered that "time together is great, but there is such a thing as too much time together. We need more space" (11–15 yrs) and "We do need space apart sometimes" (6–10 yrs) as "We have to be a team completely while allowing each other to have space and their own identity as well" (16–20 yrs).

The balance of time together and apart is reflected in being "apart-together." Informed by personality and cultural backgrounds, each couple will find their own balance in time together and time apart. This too reflects the selfishness-altruism balance in relationship give and take: both time together and time apart are needed to balance individuality and relationship identity. Finding the balance requires negotiation. One couple united the two seeming opposites: "We . . . give each other space even when being around each other more" (6–10 yrs).

Negative relationship learnings

Just as many couples were surprised by their relationship strengths, some were confronted by their relationship vulnerabilities. These appeared through close proximity and increased time together. The following were the top five negative learnings:

> Our relationship is not as stable as we thought
> We shouldn't be together

Working together is tough
We have nothing in common
We have trust issues

These five learning can be seen to stem from the first, which is represented by the following:

> [Our relationship] is not as stable as we thought. (11–15 yrs)
>
> [It] is even more fragile and weak than we had feared. (16–20 yrs)
>
> My wife goes to pieces quite easily during a crisis and . . . my mental health is too weak to deal with it. (6–10 yrs)

Some of these respondents considered breaking up: "I'm better off alone" (3–5 yrs), "we shouldn't be together" (11–15yrs), "he married the wrong person and I did too" (11–15 yrs).

For some respondents "it was tough to work in home" (3–5 yrs), "we don't work well together" (3–5 yrs) or "my husband drives me crazy" (31–40 yrs). Division of labour also "caused some resentment" (21–30 yrs). Other respondents found that they "really have too many different interests and ideas" (16–20 yrs) or their partner "doesn't trust" them (16–20 yrs).

Negative learnings in adversity are expected. At least one couple's negative experience was directly impacted by mental illness. Questions then arise:

How will a couple respond to what has been learnt?
Will they work on this or walk away?
What resources could they mobilize to help them?

Information, skills, therapy, and more may be needed. Much depends on the choices two individuals make together and separately for themselves. Negative learnings become growth opportunities for some, but other couples remain stuck. The valued responses in this survey help inform our present study so that this book may join the many others as a resource for couples choosing to move forward together. Others may choose to move apart. Encountering each other in the confines of close proximity leads people to realizations: positive and negative.

Couples encountering each other

After decades of growing hyper-individualism, growing prosperity, and pervasive social isolation, COVID-19 tested the resilience of relationships. It threw many couples into close and intense proximity to encounter each other and the reality of their relationship in a new way: away from distraction and many twenty-first century life logistics. This strengthened many relationships and left others more vulnerable. It made couples pause to think about and appraise themselves through each other.

In this, couples were given the prized opportunity to encounter each other more fully. The encounter, in which we see ourselves more fully by being known more fully by another, has been discussed by philosophers,[26] artists,[27] and psychiatrists[28] alike. These couples we surveyed here encountered more than each other as people, they encountered themselves, their relationship, what the relationship was, and what it meant. This led to surprise for some, and disappointment or exaltation for others. If, as McGilchrist argues, "both parties evolve and are changed through the encounter [to] become more fully what [they] are,"[29] me-ness can evolve into we-ness, opening a pathway to individual- *and* together-actualization. It is positive relationship adaptation through overcoming adversity together.

Together-actualization, we posit, is authentic, genuine, long-term encounter in the couple dyad to encompass individual and relational growth and shared meaning-making. If the growth and shared meaning-making is not enough, and if the perceived cost of togetherness outweighs perceived benefits, a couple may choose to break up. If the relationship is perceived to include at least the potential of personal and together growth and worthwhile life experience, couples in their surprise will embrace the gift of each other more deeply. They will deepen their encounter.

According to our survey, less than 1% of couples had major issues that led to breaking-up with 9% overall considering a break-up. Another 6–15% were feeling "stuck." About 16% recognized they had strengths and weaknesses that needed work, and it appears that somewhere between 60% and 70% felt that they were strong as a couple. Without the encounter of lockdown closeness, couples may not have been confronted with the reality of their relationships, be it positive, negative, or a mixture of both.

Surveyed couples encountered each other to expose problems, surprises, and strengths. Depending on how the encounter is handled, the positive and negative learnings can help reach for together-actualization rather than meandering through the day-to-day with hope but without understanding. Building relationship resilience needs conscious effort and time and resource investment. The COVID-19 pause offered time and the gift of encounter.

In lockdown, resilience is tested, but overcoming adversity increases resilience. Couples married 40+ years have, as presented next chapter, overcome much adversity. They possess insights from which younger couples can benefit. Before discussing these we consider the questions younger couples wanted to ask couples married 40+ years.

Questions asked by young couples

After reflecting on relationship happiness, problems and benefits experienced, and positive and negative learnings, respondents were invited to formulate questions to ask couples married 40+ years. Of the 290 respondents, 266 articulated 283 questions. To capture the concerns of couples most affected by the hyper-individual zeitgeist, we were particularly interested in questions from younger couples, those in relationship 3–15 years. Unsurprisingly, the majority of questions came from this group. Their top five questions were:

> What is your secret to staying together?
> Is the spark still there?
> How do you stop arguing and get through hard times?
> How do you keep your marriage fun and not boring?
> How do you keep connected and communicate well?

What is your secret to staying together?

That this question was asked by 70% of younger respondents who formulated a question for couples thriving 40+ years merits emphasis. It is evidence that these couples want to stay together, they want relationship longevity, and they want to resolve the me versus we dilemma posed in today's societal context if they possibly can. Their actual questions included "How did you last so long?", "How is it even possible?", "What made you stick around for so long?", and "How did you make it work so long?" Myriad questions were asked regarding a "special secret," "key tip," "Secret to long marriage," "Key to staying together," and "secret for being happy."

The question encapsulates the core aim of this book. It was the first question asked of the couples married 40+ years in the in-depth interviews. It took the following form:

> What is your secret to staying married for such a long time; what is the glue that has kept your relationship together?

Is the spark still there?

The second-most asked question exemplified how keenly interested younger respondents were in lasting sexual intimacy: "How do you keep the fire going when you are old and grey?" (3–5 yrs). The term 'spark' or some iteration alluding to the combustible nature of sex was used frequently. How to "maintain the spark," "Keep the spark going," and "keep the fire burning" alluded to passion and sex. "Do you still have sex?" and "Is the sex still good?" were other articulations of the question. Some younger respondents appeared convinced that "the spark goes" after "60." Others wanted "Tips for keeping the romance alive" (3–5 yrs) or how to keep "affection alive and thriving" (3–5 yrs), or "do you still get the same butterflies when they smile or walk in a room or when they kiss you or when you both say that you love each other?" (3–5 yrs).

This reveals how important sex is in relationships. Based on these, interviewed couples thriving 40+ years were asked "is the spark still there?" This question was often answered with much passion and pride as discussed next chapter.

How do you stop arguing and get through hard times?

Respondents sought advice on how to manage conflict:

> How do you keep from fighting all the time? (3–5 yrs)
>
> How many times did you almost divorce and how did you come back together stronger? (3–5 yrs)
>
> Do the arguments over small petty issues ever really go away? (11–15 yrs)

Others asked for specific techniques on how to "handle the extreme differences," "resolve arguments," "let go of hurt," "come back together faster after a fight," "keep your temper," or "how do you deal with financial issues without accusations and yelling?" (11–15 yrs).

These questions revealed how arguing is very much part of relationships and that it is a concern to couples. It also reveals the resilience of these younger relationships as they evidently bounce back from conflict. Finally, it reveals how much relationship peace is valued as couples seek to find it. Handling conflict so that two people in a relationship can live together peacefully is a major concern. How thriving couples argue and handle conflict is discussed in the in-depth interview analysis next chapter. Arguing techniques and techniques to help handle conflict are presented in Part III.

How do you keep your marriage fun and not boring?

"How did you keep the fun alive?" (11–15yrs) and "How do you not get bored" (3–5 yrs) were frequently asked questions by younger couples. Some respondents could not understand how couples "keep it interesting after being with someone that long, and that person basically knowing everything about you" (11–15 yrs). Respondents wanted to know if people together 40+ years were "a little bored with [their] relationship" (6–10 yrs), "How do you keep from getting bored in, like, year 30?" (6–10 yrs) or "get tired of being with the same person day in and day out for that long" (11–15 yrs). Maintaining "freshness" and "keeping it interesting" and "alive" were also enquired after. A question on what couples 40+ did for fun was asked in the Thriving Couples Interviews.

How do you keep connected and communicate well?

Couples asked questions about what thriving couples did to "keep" or "stay" connected. Staying connected was a particular concern for those in relationships 11–15 years; some respondents in this bracket were considering breaking up. Others wanted to "learn how best to communicate" (6–10 yrs) or "how the hell do you learn to communicate inadequacies about your partner to them without offending them?" (6–10 yrs). This rather desperate comment reflects the delicate balance needed in expressing self-needs and considering partner-needs. It requires a degree of altruism. We present interviewed couples' ideas on connection and communication next chapter.

Me-focus or we-focus?

Each of these questions aim at ensuring a good quality long-term relationship. They encapsulate, in some way, the dilemma between self-wants versus partner-needs in a relationship; selfishness versus altruism, and a me- versus a we- focus. We infer from the questions that some hyper-individual ideals – autonomy, immediate self-gratification, and reaching for self-achievement over togetherness – may have contributed to a relationship's pre-existing vulnerability in the COVID-19 crisis.[30]

Respondents asked, "how do you make sure to not lose yourself?" (3–5 yrs) or "How do you maintain time for yourself?" (11–15 yrs). These questions likewise seek to balance me-ness and we-ness. The same can be said of the following:

> How can you possibly love the same person for that long of a period of time when you change and grow as a person over the years? (11–15 yrs)
> How do you stay committed to your spouse as you, yourself grow and change? (11–15 yrs)
> How do you make sure to grow together as a couple instead of individually? (6–10 yrs)

As contributors to this field of couple therapy, we declare our bias towards wanting to enhance we-ness connection in couple relationships. Each individual, however, is a free, autonomous agent. Some respondents, for example, had already made the decision to prioritize their me-ness to preserve their individual needs: "I'm doing better financially than my partner and it's better that I'm alone cos I'll have myself to look after rather than the both of us on one income" (3–5 yrs). This female made a conscious decision for herself.

Others were grappling with the dilemma:

> With the definition of a relationship changing so much and now being so amorphous how do you manage your own understanding of what

> your relationship is? I.e. if you started your relationship under one set of assumptions but now see different ways your relationship could function how do you discuss and/or explore those new formations without damaging the foundations of what you have? (16–20 yrs)

This insightful question hits at the heart of one hyper-individual dilemma: that each individual becomes their own guiding light. From where does our understanding of what a relationship is come? In hyper-individualism, each individual must answer this for themselves or at least choose their guiding lights. This will naturally lead to the question of values which, as couples tell us next chapter, is so important, and therefore, becomes the subject of Chapter 6.

Using scientific understanding of the biological role of relationships and the importance of attachment to surviving and thriving as our guiding lights here, pitting self against a coupled relationship invokes a false dichotomy. As discussed in Chapter 1, hyper-individualism and relationship longevity can be reconciled. Although in long-term self-interest, on a practical, day-to-day basis, this involves much altruism and compromise. It also includes much frustrating, worthwhile effort as well as contented comfort and pleasure as explored next chapter.

Conclusion

COVID-19 increased adversity for some individuals in relationship: mental health concerns, financial pressures, and partner and children proximity in particular. The majority of respondents, however, reported benefits, particularly in more time spent together, discovering strengths, and being more resilient. Most learnt they were "in a surprisingly good place" and "stronger together than ever!!" as lockdown became "a positive shift" which "helped [their] relationship" as they "really bonded" and discovered things such as: "I love my wife, a wicked lot!" Still, even contented couples wanted to know more: how to ensure relationship quality and longevity in particular.

Our survey findings indicate that, during COVID-19 isolation, many couples learnt the need for time together, communication, time apart, teamwork, emotional support, and they learnt about each other. Many reflected on their relationship and set new goals. Teamwork, we-ness, and togetherness emerged as the backbone for many couples:

> I fell apart due to work. My husband picked me up and nursed me back to health. After 21 years of marriage I think he finally felt needed, as I am very independent. (21–30 yrs)

Questions for thriving couples revealed the basic assumption that a supportive long-term relationship is desired and that couples are happier when their relationship flourishes. This is consistent with theoretical considerations discussed in Part I. We also infer the following:

Most couples want relationship longevity and want to know how to achieve it
Couples encountered each other intensely during isolation
Surprisingly few people are dissatisfied in their relationship
Constricted space can increase togetherness and teamwork or increase tension
Having a supportive relationship is an asset

Most specifically, the five questions from younger couples revealed that couples

Keenly want relationship longevity
Find sex very important and want it to last
Want to know how to minimize arguing and conflict
Want fun in their relationship
Want to stay emotionally connected

These affirm the science of attachment: that we crave close proximity and togetherness to help us survive and thrive. Relationships, however, are difficult. Next chapter we discover the answers given by couples thriving 40+ years to the questions posed by younger couples previously. Many of these thriving couples have survived great personal adversity. Their insights were used to help shape the techniques of Part III, all of which are aimed at building resilient relationships.

Notes

1 Lowe, Sarah R., Jean E. Rhodes, and Arielle AJ Scoglio. "Changes in marital and partner relationships in the aftermath of Hurricane Katrina: An analysis with low-income women." *Psychology of Women Quarterly* 36, no. 3 (2012): 286–300.
2 Alexopoulos, Cassandra, Elisabeth Timmermans, Liesel L. Sharabi, David J. Roaché, Alyssa Croft, Elizabeth Dorrance Hall, Laurie James-Hawkins, Veronica Lamarche, and Maximiliane Uhlich. "Settling down without settling: Perceived changes in partner preferences in response to COVID-19." *Journal of Social and Personal Relationships* 38, no. 6 (2021): 1901–1919.
3 Pollard, Agnieszka E., and Ronald D. Rogge. "Love in the time of COVID-19: A multi-wave study examining the salience of sexual and relationship health during the COVID-19 pandemic." *Archives of Sexual Behavior* 51, no. 1 (2022): 247–271.
4 Leonard, Michelle T., Charles Giraud, and Christen Abraham. "Coupling with COVID: The role of dyadic coping in relationship satisfaction and psychological distress during the COVID-19 pandemic." *Journal of Family Issues* 43, no. 8 (2022): 2234–2252; Walsh, Alison R., and Rob Stephenson. "Positive and negative impacts of the COVID-19 pandemic on relationship satisfaction in male couples." *American Journal of Men's Health* 15, no. 3 (2021).

5 Pietromonaco, Paula R., and Nickola C. Overall. "Implications of social isolation, separation, and loss during the COVID-19 pandemic for couples' relationships." *Current Opinion in Psychology* 43 (2022): 189–194.
6 Ibid.
7 Goodman, Catherine. "Intimacy and autonomy in long term marriage." *Journal of Gerontological Social Work* 32, no. 1 (1999): 83–97.
8 Twenge, Jean M., and Thomas E. Joiner. "Mental distress among US adults during the COVID-19 pandemic." *Journal of Clinical Psychology* 76, no. 12 (2020): 2170–2182.
9 Waddell, Nina, Nickola C. Overall, Valerie T. Chang, and Matthew D. Hammond. "Gendered division of labor during a nationwide COVID-19 lockdown: Implications for relationship problems and satisfaction." *Journal of Social and Personal Relationships* 38, no. 6 (2021): 1759–1781.
10 Merolla, Andy J., Christopher Otmar, and Carlos Ruvalcaba Hernandez. "Day-to-day relational life during the COVID-19 pandemic: Linking mental health, daily relational experiences, and end-of-day outlook." *Journal of Social and Personal Relationships* 38, no. 8 (2021): 2350–2375.
11 Feeney, Judith A., and Jennifer Fitzgerald. "Autonomy – connection tensions, stress, and attachment: The case of COVID-19." *Current Opinion in Psychology* 43 (2022): 18–23.
12 Alexopoulos, Cassandra, Elisabeth Timmermans, Liesel L. Sharabi, David J. Roaché, Alyssa Croft, Elizabeth Dorrance Hall, Laurie James-Hawkins, Veronica Lamarche, and Maximiliane Uhlich. "Settling down without settling: Perceived changes in partner preferences in response to COVID-19." *Journal of Social and Personal Relationships* 38, no. 6 (2021): 1901–1919.
13 Javadivala, Zeinab, Hamid Allahverdipour, Mohammad Asghari Jafarabadi, Somaye Azimi, Neda Gilani, and Vijay Kumar Chattu. "Improved couple satisfaction and communication with marriage and relationship programs: Are there gender differences? – a systematic review and meta-analysis." *Systematic Reviews* 10, no. 1 (2021): 1–14. Sternberg, Robert J., and Mahzad Hojjat, eds. *Satisfaction in close relationships*. Guilford Press, 1997.
14 Seligman applies these Greek forms of pleasure to studies of happiness. Seligman, Martin EP. *Authentic happiness: Using the new positive psychology to realize your potential for lasting fulfillment*. Simon and Schuster. 2002. www.aithentichappiness.sas.upenn.edu/de/content/pleasure-meaning-eudaimonia-0 Retrieved 1 June 2018.
15 Wirth, Werner, Matthias Hofer, and Holger Schramm. "Beyond pleasure: Exploring the eudaimonic entertainment experience." *Human Communication Research* 38, no. 4 (2012): 406–428.
16 Hilpert, Peter, Guy Bodenmann, Fridtjof W. Nussbeck, and Thomas N. Bradbury. "Improving personal happiness through couple intervention: A randomized controlled trial of a self-directed couple enhancement program." *Journal of Happiness Studies* 17, no. 1 (2016): 213–237.
17 Vowels, Laura M., Rachel R. R. Francois-Walcott, Rhia E. Perks, and Katherine B. Carnelley. " 'Be free together rather than confined together': A qualitative exploration of how relationships changed in the early COVID-19 pandemic." *Journal of Social and Personal Relationships* 38, no. 10 (2021): 2921–2943.
18 Years together in relationship are noted after each response.
19 This is consistent with Donato, Silvia, Miriam Parise, Ariela Francesca Pagani, Margherita Lanz, Camillo Regalia, Rosa Rosnati, and Raffaella Iafrate. "Together against COVID-19 concerns: The role of the dyadic coping process for partners' psychological well-being during the pandemic." *Frontiers in Psychology* 11 (2021): 578395.
20 Stevenson, Clifford, Juliet R. H. Wakefield, Mhairi Bowe, Blerina Kellezi, Beth Jones, and Niamh McNamara. "Weathering the economic storm together:

Family identification predicts future well-being during COVID-19 via enhanced financial resilience." *Journal of Family Psychology* 36, no. 3 (2022): 337–345.

21 Lillie, Helen M., Skye Chernichky-Karcher, and Maria K. Venetis. "Dyadic coping and discrete emotions during COVID-19: Connecting the communication theory of resilience with relational uncertainty." *Journal of Social and Personal Relationships* 38, no. 6 (2021): 1844–1868.

22 Fitzgerald, Jennifer, ed. *Foundations for couples' therapy: Research for the real world*. Routledge, 2017, 155.

23 Hamermesh, Daniel S. "Life satisfaction, loneliness and togetherness, with an application to Covid-19 lock-downs." *Review of Economics of the Household* 18, no. 4 (2020): 983–1000.

24 Williamson, Hannah C. "Early effects of the COVID-19 pandemic on relationship satisfaction and attributions." *Psychological Science* 31, no. 12 (2020): 1479–1487.

25 Jiang, Da, Ming Chiu, and Shuang Liu. "Daily positive support and perceived stress during COVID-19 outbreak: The role of daily gratitude within couples." *Journal of Happiness Studies* 23, no. 1 (2022): 65–79.

26 Sartre, Jean-Paul. *Being and Nothingness: An Essay on Phenomenological Ontology*. Trans. Hazel E. Barnes. Routledge, 2003, 260.

27 Jerzy Grotowski and Eugenio Barba, *Towards a Poor Theatre*. ed. Eugenio Barba. Routledge, 2002, 57–58.

28 See McGilchrist, Iain. *The matter with things: Our brains, our delusions, and the unmaking of the world*. Perspectiva Press, 2021.

29 Ibid.

30 Pietromonaco and Overall, "Implications of social isolation, separation, and loss during the COVID-19 pandemic for couples' relationships," 189–194.

Chapter 5

Interview and survey findings: couples thriving 40+ years

Away from the screaming screens and the treadmill of twenty-first century aspirations, in the quiet of homes, some filled with the timelessness of dark wood furniture and vintage ceramic tea sets, or in a cosy local coffee shop or other quiet space, 90 couples married 40 to 73 years shared with me their relationship stories. The questions asked in the 45 to 120 minute interviews[1] evoked memories and feelings that caused some to weep uncontrollably, laugh with abandon, or argue. Laughter and crying are contagious[2] so it is unsurprising that we shared these emotions as professional trust was built. Couples contributed what they were comfortable sharing, and were often surprised by their own candour, or their partner's responses. Many encountered new aspects of their relationship even though married for decades. These encounters became an opportunity to grow and affirm love.

The Thriving Couples Interviews, 90 in-depth interviews of couples married 40+ years, is the core study arm. It is supported in this chapter by the largest study arm: the Married 40+ Survey of 932 respondents. Other couple insights not included here can be found in Appendix 1. The aim of the survey was to get a larger sample size to confirm, refute, or put into a broader perspective ideas covered in-depth and responses given in the interviews.

Interview questions were proffered to both spouses; responses mostly aligned, but sometimes conflict was stimulated. The interviews aimed to capture something of the essence of each unique thriving relationship. Couples' rich, diverse responses form the argument of this chapter: that relationship resilience is built over many years of living out shared values together. This, we found, was present in all interviewed couples.

A long-term relationship is "not a walk down a primrose path. It's very dynamic and ever-changing, and it's like a dance more than a walk" (Barbara and Lance, Aus. 52yrs).[3] Interviewed couples danced along a path with many turns, rough patches, victories, disappointments, and triumphs. They thrived despite affairs, the deaths of children, severe mental illness, and more. Some couples never argued, others argued almost every day. All built a relationship resilient enough to survive the heartaches, trials, and contentment of 40+ years. Boris (100 yrs old) and Veselina (96 yrs old) from Bulgaria are still together

DOI: 10.4324/9781003263395-8

after 73 years. Couples "not only coped, but [trials] made us stronger" (Beti and Clive, Wales 60 yrs). We are honoured to provide a glimpse into these couples' time-tested relationships supported by the 932 survey respondents. For couples in our Surviving COVID-19 Survey who asked, this chapter aims to show how relationship longevity may still be possible in a world of hyper-individual ideals, mental illness, and increasing social isolation.

This chapter firstly gives a brief overview of extant studies on long-term relationships. It then describes the interview process before presenting the findings. Findings are presented as

'Glue-secrets' couples told us helped keep them together
Aspects of their relationship we asked about
Threats: things that threatened to tear them apart
Answers to questions of younger couples
Relationship happiness: what couples told us about this.

Previous long-term relationship studies

Compared to the literature on young couples and relationship problems, far fewer studies consider the positive aspects of long-term relationships. One of the first, however, was by Terman et al.[4] assessing Marital Happiness. Its lengthy findings were presented in a hefty tome amidst the relationship stability of the 1930s. Surveys of 1133 individuals in relationships of an average of 11.5 years revealed the primary factors of marital happiness to be, in order:

Affection
Philosophy of life
Friendship

Stinnett et al., 1972[5] measured marital satisfaction in a time of shifting attitudes to sex and coupling. It surveyed 408 couples married 40+ years and found the key determinants of long-term relationship success to be:

Love
Determination
Common interests

A proliferation of small studies on long-term relationships followed in the 1980s, a time of increasing divorce rates. The largest of these is the often quoted study by Lauer and Lauer, 1986.[6] It included surveys and interviews of 351 couples married for 15+ years and found that marriages endure due to

Being best friends
Commitment
Valuing marriage as sacred

Three smaller studies from the 1980s found the following key ingredients to relationship longevity:

Commitment[7]	Love[8]	Flexibility[9]
Companionship	Family	Acceptance
Caring	Commitment	Commitment

Alford-Cooper's oft-cited "Long Island Study" of 1994[10] surveyed and interviewed 1152 married people to ask "what makes marriages last." Findings during this time of peaked divorce rates were:

Trust
Love
Compromise

Four smaller studies from the 1990s found the following to be key ingredients for lasting relationships:

Commitment[11]	Commitment[12]	Feel respect[13]	Conflict contained[14]
Liking partner	Loyalty	Feel cherished	Sharing decisions
Best-friends	Shared values		Communication

Before our present study, the largest study of long-term relationships was by Sharlin, Kaslow and Hammerschmidt, 1998.[15] Their rigorous study across eight countries surveyed 1220 individuals in long-term relationships of 20–46 years. The main ingredients to relationship success were found to be:

Mutual trust
Mutual respect
Mutual give and take
Mutual support

In the twenty-first century, Pillemer, 2015[16] surveyed and interviewed 700 people married 30+ years to find the hallmarks of successful marriage to be:

Communication
Knowing your partner
Commitment

Table 5.1 outlines large cross-sectional studies on long-term relationships since Terman, 1938. Studies including under 100 participants or without adequate or described methodology are not included.

Table 5.1 Studies Assessing Relationship (Marital) Longevity

Year	*Sample size*	*Researchers*	*Type*	*Years together*	*Countries represented*
1938	1133	Terman et al.	Surveys	1–27+ 11.5 av.	USA
1972	408	Stinnett et al	Surveys	40+	USA
1980	100	Roberts	Interviews and surveys	50–65 55.5 av.	USA
1982	200	Rowe and Meredith	Surveys	25–62	USA
1985	200+	Klagsbrun	Interviews	15+	USA
1986	702	Lauer and Lauer	Interviews and surveys	15+	USA
1990	200	Lauer, Lauer and Kerr	Surveys	45–64 54.5 av.	USA
1992	294	Fennel	Surveys	20+	USA
1994	1152	Alford-Cooper	Interviews and surveys	50+ 52 av.	USA
1994	100	Wallerstein and Blakeslee	Interviews	10–40	USA
1995	120	Mackey and O'Brien	Interviews	20+	USA
1992–98	1220	Sharlin, Kaslow, Hammerschmidt	Surveys	20–46	USA, Canada, Israel, Germany, Chile, Netherlands, Sweden, South Africa
2015	700	Pillemer	Interviews and surveys	30 + 44 av.	USA
2021	331	Abreu-Afonso et al	Surveys	Unspecified	Portugal
2023	1402	Heim and Heim	Interviews and surveys	40+ 50 av. (interviews)	52 countries

Most studies, as can be seen, were conducted in the United States and represented a middle-high socio-economic demographic. Few used mixed methodology and sample sizes were relatively small. We aimed to ameliorate these limitations in our study.

From the 1980s onwards, the prominent finding was "commitment" as a key to long-term relationship success. This is consistent with findings in longitudinal studies on relationship quality.[17] Commitment may have been taken for granted in studies prior to the relaxing of divorce laws. "Communication" and "containing conflict" may have entered as key ingredients in the 1990s as couples began to reflect ideas learnt from relationship researchers, but this is speculation.

Our present study, combining interviews, surveys, and participant observation, was undertaken between 2017 and 2022 to include 1402 individuals across 52 countries. We primarily sampled couples married 40+ years. Many of these couples, as they told us, witnessed the relationship struggles of their children and grandchildren: "in the technology generation, parents are pushed further away from the coalface and so, you know, these kids are struggling" (Peter and Rhonda, Aus. 53 yrs).

The interviews

Our aim in the in-depth interviews was to allow couples to lead us to their ideas of what helped their relationship longevity. In a small sense, we were asking this on behalf of younger couples from our Surviving COVID-19 Survey who posed questions. Details of this quasi-inter-generational dialogue and methodology are found in the Introduction.

The first question was an open-ended invitation: "So what is *your* secret to staying together . . . years? Could you describe the glue? It may be one thing, it may be many . . ." After an often lengthy discussion of the glue-secrets, the interview became more directed. Informed by young couples' questions from the Surviving COVID-19 Survey, and Dr Christian Heim's clinical experience, couples were asked about specified relationship 'aspects': arguing, friendship, romance and physical intimacy, time spent together and separately, division of labour, and finances; "So how does [this aspect] work in your marriage? It would be great if you could think back to early in your relationship . . . and also describe how that has changed over time." Discussing these aspects allowed couples to impart relationship stories for warmer and friendlier engagement and to disclose more of their personal journeys.

Sometimes significant couple issues arose to direct the course of the interview. Later, after building more trust and understanding, couples were invited to talk about things that threatened their relationship: "Was there anything that threatened to tear your relationship apart but didn't?" This often heralded a time of poignant and affect-laden disclosure. As the interview progressed, we touched on the happiness of each relationship several times. Towards the end, couples were asked to proffer specific insights to pass on to couples starting out or struggling in their relationships, and a relationship affirming-question finished the interview.

Findings: couple's glue-secrets

The first and most critical question was:

What is your glue-secret to staying together so long?

Answers to this question informed our main findings. The couples did not choose from a list nor were suggestions proffered. The five most important glue-secrets we found were, in order:

Commitment
Altruism
Shared values
Communication
Compromise: give and take

Commitment as a key ingredient has been the prominent finding in studies since 1980. Altruism was found to be a key ingredient in only one longitudinal study of 100 couples by Mudd and Taubin, 1957–79.[18] Shared values as a key ingredient reflects earlier studies if "seeing marriage as sacred" and "moral values" (Fennel 1992) and "philosophy of life" (Terman et al., 1938) are seen as quasi-synonymous to shared values. Communication and compromise as major ingredients to longevity are consistent with studies dating back to 1994.

The top 17 glue-secrets of our Thriving Couple Interviews were:

1 Commitment
2 Altruism
3 Shared values
4 Communication
5 Compromise: give and take
6 Love
7 Never give up
8 Patience/forgiveness/tolerance
9 Teamwork
10 Respect
11 Family focus
12 Common interests and backgrounds
13 Separate time
14 Friendship

15 Opposite personalities
16 Modelling (replicated or rebelled against)
17 Humour

Some expected glue-secrets are notable by their absence: compatibility, similar personalities, conflict resolution, no arguing. Some are surprises: opposite personalities when having similar personalities predicts relationship longevity.[19] Others are absent to the chagrin of younger couples: sex, novelty, fun, financial independence. These may still be important to couples but, for relationship longevity, may need to be underpinned by other key ingredients.

These couples' glue-secrets have been forged in trials and pleasurable experiences, and through individual and together-growth in long-term relationships. We discuss details of the top five glue-secrets: commitment, altruism, shared values, communication, and compromise. Couples' own words help capture some of their journeys and ideas.

Glue-secret one: commitment

Commitment is

> to each other, . . . it's a process, it's when you know that you're committed to each other: it's a love relationship and it's a depth of relationship that is unconditional. We make that commitment . . . based on our capacity to love one another. (Monte and Jeneen, USA 45 yrs)

This embeds the idea of "process" into commitment: initial commitment, then unconditionally committing to the relationship itself. The majority of interviewed couples said that commitment was "essential," "150% important," or "the number one thing." Commitment was frequently spoken about in relation to marriage vows and working at it:

> A promise to commit made when we got married. (Linden and Hermann, Aus./Germany 54 yrs)
>
> A promise – you can't break it. (Bruce and Jan, New Zealand 57 yrs)
>
> I promised in front of a big congregation. Come what may I have to stay. (Margaret and Ian, Aus. 57 yrs)

I made a marriage vow, I made a commitment publicly . . . I firmly believe in that, and that's what I've lived by for all these years. (Malcolm and Jeanette, UK 64 yrs)Carol and Stephen both experienced childhood sexual abuse, and worked through infertility issues and workplace trauma. They have "been through hell and back again. . . . Many times I had to go back to our vows and through thick and thin you keep them. . . . It would have been easy to walk away" (Aus. 40 yrs). Culture is relevant: "We came from our country where marriage should last forever. Till death do us part. So it's something that we embrace, that it's not going to be easy" (Nicia and Juanito, Philippines 48 yrs).

"Working through it" and "sticking at it" express ongoing commitment as "adversity strengthens commitment" (Graeme and Anjelika, Aus./Germany 46 yrs). Commitment is to the relationship for the long-term. "Never give up" (glue-secret 7), also articulated as "sticking at it," is more related to the immediate expression of underlying commitment when needed to get through tough times. Lucy had cancer three times, but "[we] got even more committed [each time] . . . no matter how angry you are at that person, you take care of each other through thick or thin. That's commitment" (Lucy and Frank, USA 55 yrs). Ultimately "you commit for better or for worse. We've seen the best and the worst" (George and Franky, Aus./UK 44 yrs).

Though currently counter-cultural, including marriage vows as "intention to be together, to have a future"[20] helps endure tough times.[21] Commitment and attachment walk hand in hand[22] to help build resilience.[23] As such, they underlie love, relationship satisfaction, and resilient togetherness to celebrate victories over adversity as well as anniversary milestones. Commitment is foundational for relationship identity[24] and longevity.

Glue-secret two: altruism

The Estonian word for marriage is *abielu*: "a compound word of two words, 'help' and 'life'. What it means is that we have to live and help each other" (Inno and Tiiu, Estonia 66 yrs). Altruism is helping each other. The thriving couples described altruism as:

> Putting yourself on the backburner. (Anjelika and Graeme, 46 yrs)
>
> Putting yourself in the other person's shoes. (Marilyn and Gerry, Aus. 49 yrs)
>
> Getting your ego out the equation. (Steven and Chuck, USA 30 yrs)
>
> Promoting your partner. (Gary and Ruth, USA/Aus. 54yrs)

"It's really hard, you have to work at it" (Sharon and Bob, Aus. 46 yrs) as there are "so many common pitfalls" (Gary and Ruth, 54yrs). "It's not easy these days. There are too many distractions" (Dorothy and Gaetano, Italy 49 yrs) and "most people tend to be more selfish than altruistic" (Yin-Leng and Mike, China/Canada 48 yrs).

Wayne coped with Frances's severe depression for over 42 years, Wendy forgave Andy's affair (UK 43 yrs), Shirley stuck with Patrick in spite of his interfering family (Hong Kong 48 yrs), and Lunesa nursed Romeo through thyroid cancer and a heart attack (Philippines 48 yrs). Altruism is also expressed, as couples shared, through day-to-day thoughtfulness: protecting a spouse's sleep, having meals prepared in advance, notes of how to handle finances, and much more.

Early in their marriage, Gary and Ruth were keen to "turn the normal selfishness that we know we have, upside down" by outdoing each other in chores: "taking out the garbage, . . . but sometimes she still beats me in making the bed. I say, 'Okay, you beat me to it, I lost' " (54 yrs). Their competitive altruism is fun. Altruism boosts wellbeing[25] and strengthens attachment.[26]

Altruism includes sacrifice:

> When our first son was born, she stayed home for 17 years sacrificing her career. (Romeo and Lunesa, 48 yrs)
>
> Annette who has a tremendous brain wanted to study. . . . When we had kids I took two years off all my music activities. It made me look at her side of the fence. (Annette and Bernie, Netherlands/Aus. 60 yrs).

Bill was a Freemason but he "just simply left" as "it didn't mean as much to me as my relationship" (Bill and Fay, Netherlands/Aus. 57 yrs). Sacrifice increases trust[27] and relationship longevity.[28] It is a core part of commitment[29] but is unhealthy if motivated by guilt.[30]

'Sacrifice' as a word may have little currency in hyper-individualism, but in the survey it was mentioned 18 times. The survey included numerous comments about altruism including: "Always put her first no matter what pain it causes you" and "Rather than look at the other person for what they can offer you, look at yourself and ask what you can offer [them]" or "selfishness breaks up marriages." Altruism upsets our selfish genes for relationship longevity.

Glue-secret three: shared values

Shared values, as couples told us, are vital to relationship longevity:

> Values are important. If you don't have the right value system you're . . . not going to value the intimacy, companionship, friendship, communication. [That] somebody will commit themselves to you is absolutely incredible. What a value! (Monte and Jeneen, 45 yrs)

"Shared values are what drew us together in the first place" (Steven and Carol, 53 yrs) and are "part of what causes us to be able to continue our relationship" (Frank and Lucy, 55 yrs). "Without shared values you wouldn't be together" (Bruce and Jan, 57 yrs) as "values are the basis of any good relationship" (Tiiu and Inno, 66 yrs) but "it's no good having shared values if you can't enact them" (Allan and Carol, Aus. 55 yrs).

Shared values, we were told, abrogate apparent risk factors for divorce such as having opposite personalities:

> Whilst we're different in personalities, our values are the same. (Christine and Ted, Aus. 50 yrs)
>
> Even though we seem very opposite, our values have been almost the same. (Pat and Jim, USA 54 yrs)
>
> We have more shared values than . . . common interests. (Stella and Fred, Aus. 42 yrs)

Chuck and Steven (30 yrs) share religious values, having met through their church. Shared religious values emerged strongly for some couples:

> Our religious beliefs are the bedrock of our foundation. Everything else is peripheral to that. (Michael and Jennifer, Canada 43 yrs)
>
> Religion has been something that I questioned. But the older I got, religion became much more important to me. So Anjelika and I are in a much tighter togetherness on that value now. (Graeme and Anjelika, 46 yrs)

Keith and Stephen attend a "predominantly gay and lesbian church" because they needed a "safe haven" (30 yrs). Spirituality is an "equally important" value for them. For one couple, "spiritual connection is evidenced in the fact that we love going into the bush walking" (Christine and Phil, Aus. 49 yrs). Some had different beliefs but still valued their togetherness: "I'm very religious. George believes, but he's not religious. Because we've been together forever, he's still his own person and I'm my own person. It works" (Lana and George, 50 yrs).

Differing political values can cause much rancour. Some couples choose to "Not talk politics. Otherwise it's a lot of arguments" (Mary and Brian, USA 50 yrs) especially when "one is a Republican and one a Democrat. It creates a tremendous amount of difficulty" (Steve and Avima, USA/Israel 41 yrs). Political values can change over time:

> We have changed our values, dramatically. When we got married, we were extremely conservative, politically, religiously, and socially. We . . . are now both very much left wing. (Peggy and Howard, USA 48 yrs)

Heather and Lyle shared parenting values. They have eight children: "we didn't bring them up, we told them to get up or else" (Aus. 69 yrs). Jennifer has a Masters in Early Childhood Education, so Michael "often deferred to her" (43 yrs). William and Mildred "didn't always have the same values as far as discipline and order" for their boys (USA 40 yrs). Several men regretted not playing more of a role in bringing up their children.

Altruism, for many couples, was itself a shared value: "our shared value is empathy. Both of us have . . . empathy for people less fortunate. . . . We stand up for the underdog" (Rob and Jo, Scotland/Aus. 47 yrs). Be "kind to your neighbours. Do things for people" (Christine and Phil, 49 yrs) and "do unto others how you wish others would do unto you" (Veronne and Wayne, Aus. 42 yrs) was a shared value that featured highly. Some couples feed the homeless, help people from low-income families, volunteer at a domestic violence refuge, take in homeless international students, help the house-bound and seriously ill, help tourists, volunteer at their local hospital, feed street kids, or visit the lonely. Cyndy and Tony (49 yrs) drive from the south of England to London and back to deliver kosher food for incapacitated people, and Judy and Gordon (Aus. 66 yrs) "do concerts in nursing homes" because they "like to give pleasure to others." Maslow noted that self-actualized people are invariably altruistic:

> Our shared value is helping someone in need. If one of us sees somebody in need we discuss it. I don't mean just financially but it can be socially: we need to spend time helping someone. (Yin-Leng and Mike, 48 yrs)

Integrity-related values were also important:

> Moral values, loyalty, effort, hard work, do the best you can all the time and things will turn out in a positive manner. (Steve and Carol, USA 53 yrs)
>
> I wouldn't have married Ted unless he had certain values of integrity, honesty, commitment and truth. (Marge and Ted, Aus. 56 yrs)
>
> Those basic values: truth, sincerity, honesty are the values that I respect the most in Ergun . . . if you don't have the trust you don't have anything. (Anne and Ergun, France/Turkey, 41 yrs)

Commitment, faithfulness, hard work, family, friends, art, culture, and saving the planet were valued by interviewed couples. Boris and Veselina, married 73 years, valued their marriage itself. In the online survey, shared values almost equalled the number one glue-secret, commitment. Recent studies attest to the importance of shared values to relationship longevity;[31] our study adds to this evidence.

Glue-secret four: communication

Some couples, such as Barbara and Lance (52 yrs), do actually finish each other's sentences. For others, frustratingly, "communication is still a work in progress" (Sharon and Bob, 46 yrs). Interviewed couples reported that

> Communication improves with the decades
>
> Non-verbal communication becomes more important
>
> Cultural and personality clashes are ameliorated by communicating

"[Avima] used to be a lot more upfront and sometimes confronting . . . [and has] mellowed out over the years" (Steve and Avima, 41 yrs). Clive would "just have a gut feeling and then verbalize it . . . [but is now] more inclined to give it a lot more quiet thought" (Clive and Beti, 60 yrs).

Some couples became "quicker to say what [they] need and quicker to listen" (Peggy and Howard, 48 yrs). They reminisced that "When we were young, you think it in your head, but you don't say it. You've got to learn along the way to talk it out" (Debby and David, Aus. 48 yrs). Yet "sometimes it takes some degree of courage to say what I think" (Stella and Fred, 42 yrs). Articulating needs is particularly important, as no-one can mind-read:

> I was always assuming that I knew either what [Paula] was thinking, wanted or cared about. I have learned that my assumptions are usually wrong, and then to talk about it. (Don and Paula, USA 57 yrs)

> Early on, I didn't talk to Peter at all when there was an issue. I'd just shut my head and not talk. I was terrified. I grew up afraid. I got over that, because it's now safe. (Elizabeth and Peter, Aus. 60 yrs)

Communication is "not just talking, it's listening" (George and Franky, 44 yrs):

> Understanding the meaning behind the words and the emotion behind the words is very important. (Keith and Stephen, 30 yrs)

> I've grown better over time at actually listening to whether he is upset . . . I've learned to listen. (Christine and Phil, 49 yrs)

Other communication improvements over time included giving more time and space, being more honest, trying not to be overbearing or reactive, and being more patient and tolerant.

Communication is more than verbal:

> [We] felt each other's presence. (Patrick and Shirley, 48 yrs)

> We communicate by certain looks and certain gestures. If I get her mad, I can see the hairs on the back of her neck stand up. (Tony and Pat, USA 54 yrs)

> Body language always kind of tells the story with my wife and me. I can tell when things are irritating her a lot and she can tell when things are irritating me a lot. So that way we've improved on our communication over the years. (William and Mildred, USA 40 yrs)

Communication between spouses can reach beyond words and reading body language and tone of voice to border on flow states,[32] which, like love and attachment, are mediated by oxytocin.[33] After spending 30 years in

Japan working together, for example, Ruth and Gary became much quieter in their interactions to "feel as a group what everyone is thinking" (40 yrs). Judy "still feels the tingle when [she] sees him" (Judy and Gordon, 66 yrs). In long-term couples, heart rates can begin to synchronize.[34]

Through social-brain interactions, flow may be the "electric air"[35] between spouses:

> [It's] unconscious telepathy. (Bruce and Susan, Rhodesia 49 yrs)
>
> We just know what needs to be done. And it gets done. (Ben and Isabella, Germany 56 yrs)
>
> We can almost hear [each other's] answers and know what each other is going to say. (Eve and Graham, Aus. 65 yrs)
>
> I know what he's thinking before he does and vice versa. (Cyndy and Tony, 49 yrs)

At first, Ruth and Ken, from different countries, could not speak each other's language: "we took the exceptional step of getting married after only nine months of seeing each other only on weekends. [We] both knew we had deep feelings for each other and communication was often by looks" (Switzerland/UK 54 yrs). Chinese Yin-Leng is a visual thinker and Canadian Mike is a more abstract thinker. This causes much tension between them. Previously frustrated, Yin-Leng will now "sit patiently and wait" (48 yrs). Conversely, Pearl "came from a shame-based culture" and could never correct her husband in public. She has now learnt to "become more free in correcting" him (Pearl and Richard, Philippines/UK 42 yrs).

In the literature, good communication has been considered a primary indicator of relationship satisfaction,[36] but this is being challenged.[37] Communication, number four glue-secret for thriving couples interviewed, was also number four in answer to the survey question "what makes a good relationship?" It was always proffered as advice in the interviews and surveys for younger relationships.

Glue-secret five: compromise

Compromise is mutual give and take:

> Compromise is a very good tool to use in a relationship because you never, ever agree on every single thing. (Margaret and Ian, 57 yrs)
>
> We've learnt over the years to compromise, that's probably the most important thing. A marriage is a joint thing, you've got to work together and you may have to give some things up here and there. (Gregory and Merilyn, 50 yrs)

In relationship give and take, couples balance selfishness and altruism:

> It's give and take. Being prepared to put some work into a marriage and to listen to each other and support each other. Always checking "can I feel, well, on an equal level here?" (Pauline and Denis, 44 yrs)
>
> It's give and take, it's compromise. And if one's feeling down well the other one's got to get the other one up. Through the hard times you support each other. (Samantha and Timothy, Aus. 51 yrs)
>
> There was a lot of give and take at different times: Allan did one degree after another for a very, very long time, and then it changed. (Carol and Allan, 55 yrs)

The survey included numerous comments on compromise including: "compromise meets in the middle, no one is always right," "try to understand the other person's point of view, and move on from there to reach a compromise" and, "be willing to compromise if the issue isn't worth the grief."

Findings: relationship 'aspects' we specifically asked about

Building on issues of interest arising from the Couples Surviving COVID-19 Survey and from clinical practice, we asked couples thriving 40+ years specifically about the following relationship aspects:

Commitment
Friendship
Separate time
Communication
Arguing
Romance and physical intimacy
Shared values
Division of labour
Finances

As we later found that commitment, communication, and shared values were identified by couples as prominent glue-secrets, these have been discussed and will not be revisited here. The interviews were more than just a dialogue; they were an encounter, so much information was conveyed through body language, eye contact, or felt tensions and comfort levels. Observations and impressions of these are noted hereafter to convey a fuller understanding of the couples and discourses.

Aspect: friendship

Couples are happier and healthier than singles, and this benefit is multiplied if they consider themselves best friends.[38] 68% of the interviewed couples said that friendship was very important, and 46% said they were best friends. 50% said that their friendship had "deepened," "grown stronger" or "matured" over time.

Friendship is confiding, accepting and sharing some fun:

> We can be silly and have fun and enjoy silly things that other people say. (Carol and Brien, Aus. 50 yrs)
>
> It is just lovely to have someone accept me as I am, as a friend. (Laura and Russell, 50 yrs)
>
> I know Hermann's secrets and he knows all my secrets, and we share them. (Linden and Hermann, 54 yrs)

Friendship is also "someone who's going to be there" (Stephen and Keith, 30 yrs). Some couples were so close to each other that the word friendship had negative connotations. For them it implied "a more apart relationship" (Lance and Barbara, 52 yrs). They preferred terms such as "lifetime companion," "intimate other half," "working partner," "team," or "part of me."

There were many varied perceptions of 'best' friendship in a couple relationship:

> He's my closest and best friend and the only person who understands me and still loves me as I am. (Marge and Ted, 56 yrs)
>
> I classify him as my best friend. Not necessarily my most exciting friend or my most compatible friend. (Chuck and Steven, 30 yrs)
>
> It's more gratifying to be able to stand back and say we've become better friends because we've become better people. (Steve and Carol, 53 yrs)
>
> That's what brought us together, friendship. Friendship was really important. You can love a lot of people, you can love everybody and everything but only if you're a friend can you live with them as far as I'm concerned. (Jim and Pat, 54 yrs)

For many couples, friendship meant deep disclosure and trust: "what creates friendship is really the trust that you can talk about anything and everything" (Anne and Ergun, 41 yrs). In a relationship, you can "trust and rely on and discuss things and reveal your feelings" (Bruce and Susan, 49 yrs). "If my friends are telling me something, but I cannot tell other people, the first thing that I say is, 'Can I tell Patrick? If not, don't tell me'" (Shirley and Patrick, 48 yrs). Friendship is for "binding the relationship together" (Ruth and Gary, 40 yrs). Several couples saw it as disloyal to their relationship-friendship to withhold information from each other.

Observations: Friendship was also reflected in couple's comfort with each other, their banter, and their laughter during these disclosures. Many angled towards each other, used touch often, and gently spoke to each other to reflect the years of built-up understanding. They often graciously left space for the other and much was communicated through comfortable silences. Familiarity with each other's personality was a mark of timeless friendship: Gerry and Marilyn's effortless ease in each other's presence, Barbara and Lance's sensitivity and respect for each other's displays of emotion, and Wendy and Harry's talking over the top of each other while making gentle jokes at each other's expense. Friendship ran deep and started in some of these relationships, as I found out, in couple's teen years.

Aspect: separate time

Separate time and interests were very important to 32% of the interviewed couples and to 28% of the surveyed respondents:

> We don't have to always do the exact same thing. We each can be our own person and do the things that we each like to do. We do things together but we also are individuals and have different likes. (Kathy and Jim, USA 43 yrs)
>
> Coming back from Vietnam, I didn't go near an RSL [Returned and Services League] for 20 years, but I was very into sport. And that helped me emotionally get through. And so I get the space for that. (Gerry and Marilyn, 49 yrs)
>
> We're so different, so we've just allowed the other space to pursue what they enjoy. That's who I am, and that's who he is. It's really just accepting that. (Pearl and Richard, 42 yrs)
>
> We share our time together and then give ourselves space to have our "me" time. (Online survey)

Three couples said they "don't have or want separate time" (Keith and Kay, Aus. 52 yrs). Most struck a balance between together and separate time:

JENEEN We respect each other's time. Monte is a backpacker, there's no way I could do what he does. But because I love him I let him do whatever he would like and he lets me do what I'd like to do. So we have freedom in that.

MONTE We do, we respect it. Because we have freedom and that comes from the commitment. . . . She's secure that I love her no matter what I'm doing, and vice versa. (45 yrs)

Just as secure attachment in the carer-infant dyad facilitates freedom for a child to explore, commitment facilitates security and freedom in the couple dyad: "Respecting each other's separate time and interests is one factor that contributes to longevity" (Romeo and Lunesa, 48 yrs).

The currently highly-valued girls' or guys' night's out[39] is something that many interviewed couples "would never have thought of" (Elizabeth and Peter, 60 yrs): "We almost thought it would have been disloyal to prefer the company of your friends for a holiday or a weekend" (David and Trish, Aus. 48 yrs). Others "can't think of anybody I would rather spend time with . . . it's just more fun to be with her" (Michael and Jennifer, 43 yrs). Whether celebrating time together or "giving each other space to do our own things" (Trevor and Sandra, 43 yrs), couples enjoyed each other: "If you asked 30, 40 years ago, I probably would not have predicted that this time spent always together would have given me so much insight, so much enjoyment" (Steve and Avima, 41 yrs). Doing things together increases relationship satisfaction.[40]

Observations: Separate/together time appeared to be a superficial thing for interviewed couples to discuss. Some couples were, however, very quick to confirm that they needed their own space. As I entered into their homes the couples often pointed out their separate time sanctuaries: Christine's orchid garden, Ted's bees, Timothy's shed, Irene's porcelain doll collection. What was most notable, however, was the warmth and contentment that spread across the faces of partners as their spouses described their interests. They celebrated the accomplishments together. Couples' answers appeared to be grounded in deeper security allowing them to be "separate but together" (Jennifer and Michael, 43 yrs).

Aspect: arguing

The vast majority of interviewed couples argued, some even daily. When asked about communication, a quarter immediately brought up arguing. Consistent with previous research,[41] 70% of the couples said that arguing had changed over time. In the surveyed couples, 37% said arguing had not brought any discontentment at all and 3% said it had brought much discontentment.

Interviewed couples said they argued over (in order): little things, the children, money, in-laws, and division of labour. They argued more when they were tired or stressed, when one was travelling away, because of childhood abuse, or when personality or values clashed. In arguing, couples generally aimed to express, understand, and reconnect rather than 'win.'

Responses to conflict

Arguing is a response to conflict. Other responses to conflict in the couples included: talking, the silent treatment, slamming doors, and avoiding:

> Because of my anxiety, I am a runner. I just want to run somewhere. But I'm also a silencer. I just shut down, I don't want to talk about it. (Jo and Rob, 47 yrs)

> The longest we would have the silent treatment will be two days. It hurts me when we don't talk. After that, we come back to normal. (Romeo and Lunesa, 48 yrs)
>
> A cold war can last a few days. (Clare and Albert, Hong Kong 40 yrs)

Jim is a Vietnam veteran with PTSD. His spouse Pat said, "I just internalize everything and we still fight that. I go out and slam a cupboard door and I feel much better when I do that" (Pat and Jim, 54 yrs). Alexandra used to throw "always the worst cup and always into the kitchen sink . . . I knew what I was doing. It was an emphasis I had to make" (Alexandra and Alex, Russia 58 yrs). For Carol, it was a visceral response: "my body says, 'oh God, how can I put up with this? I don't like this. I don't like this feeling that it's giving me.' So I will do anything to avoid it" (Carol and Steve, 53 yrs). Sometimes one partner "just won't argue" (Margaret and Merv, Aus. 59 yrs), and it's "like speaking to a brick wall" (Trish and David, 48 yrs): "how can you have an argument with somebody who just wanders off?" (Merilyn and Gregory, 50 yrs).

Responses may reflect childhood modelling:

> In our family everybody was interrupting and shouting all the time. In his family I don't think they interrupted. So that's the big problem. I'm aware of it, but I'm not really able to change it. (Ruth and Russell, USA 40 yrs)

Stella, a litigation lawyer, said, "[In conflict,] I'm paralysed, I can't think or do another thing until its finished. Sometimes that sort of paralysis goes on for days . . . Fred has the ability to leave it alone and go and do a Sudoku or something" (42 yrs). Personalities play a part: "[We] bring both strong personalities into an argument and both dig heels in" (Stephen and Keith, 30 yrs). One couple were humoured by the "opposites don't attract" myth: "A lot of people didn't think that we'd last two years let alone fifty" (Christine and Ted, 50 yrs).

Olga and Raul (Paraguay) "fought like cats and dogs [for the first five years] . . . arguing was pure hell . . . [we] would sometimes have lively arguments until two or three o'clock in the morning." Theirs has been turbulent life with two sets of in-laws working to sabotage their marriage. Against an initial back drop of extreme poverty, family rejection, and later, a fire that destroyed their furniture business, they have persevered "as a team" for over 45 years.

The importance of arguing

For ten interviewed couples: "Arguing is important in our marriage, . . . It would be really horrible if one or the other would never argue. If you don't argue there's something wrong. It is just a necessary part. It's a closer relationship" (Steve and Avima, 41 yrs). Others concurred:

> You have to be able to express it. If you hold it in a while, a little tiny thing become a big deal . . . then, it's going to be just a big burst. Then trust leaves. We respect each other enough that we can get mad. (Chuck and Marion, USA 44 yrs)

> If you don't argue the worst situation is that you don't have a relationship. . . . Sometimes I'll say 'shout, okay?' because you need to get that gas out of you. And sometimes releasing it helps to get the other person to realize how sincere you are with your point of view. (Arnie and Liz, UK 51 yrs)

Several couples told us they would raise voices, yell or shout, even to "very high decibels":

> I get very angry, very angry. We haven't ever hit one another. But with words I have hit him. (Tiiu and Inno, 66 yrs)

> When we argue I don't worry that it's going to harm our relationship. (Marion and Chuck, 44 yrs)

> If you don't argue, there's something wrong. (Jack and Judy, USA 60 yrs)

Eleven couples stated that they never argued, but had "disagreements," "differences of opinion," "bickering," "reasoning," "debates," "strong discussions," or "disputes." Those that did not argue "saw it as a sign of weakness" (David and Trish, 48 yrs), or were "allergic to raised voices" (Gaetano and Dorothy, 49 yrs). "Avoidance was a cultural thing" (Juanito and Nicia, Philippines 48 yrs), and because of "Chilean loudness, [Patty and Jorge] go for it." They are confused by the "Australian and British tendency to keep cool" (47 yrs). Modelling contributed to approaches to conflict:

> I have so many memories of my mum and dad just standing there shouting at each other that I just decided it wasn't going to be part of my marriage. (Fay and Bill, 57 yrs)

> Mum and dad argue all the time . . . so painful to watch . . . occasionally, I've worried – shouldn't we be having some kind of disagreement? (Candy and Gregg, USA 49 yrs)

The question "Do you argue in front of the children?" was met with strong and often conflicting opinions: "You don't argue in front of children because they don't need to know those sorts of things that you are arguing about, it sets a standard" (Kay and Keith, 52 yrs). Yet "I don't think my kids ever saw us really having arguments or disagreements. And so they sometimes feel like it's been difficult in their marriages, because they haven't seen us struggling with that" (Paula and Don, 57 yrs). Marge and Ted (56 yrs) talked to a young couple who had never heard their parents argue. "[When they] had their first argument, [one] came in tears saying 'our marriage is over.' "

Arguing changes over time

Time mellows and matures us:

> When we were younger, we wanted to get our own way. Whereas as you mature, that's just not that important. (Christine and Ted, 50 yrs)
>
> When we were just married we did a lot of arguing, but mostly because of my insecurities and trust issues. (Jeneen and Monte, 45 yrs)
>
> The rough spot we went through made me more insecure and think, 'I don't know if this is gonna work.' I don't have any of those feelings any more, we worked through all that. (Peggy and Howard, 48 yrs)

Interviewed couples shared their changed approaches to arguing over time:

> I can be incredibly offensive without knowing it. I used to go down that road. And I realized you don't talk to your wife that way. So I now understand and remember that. (George and Helen, Canada 48 yrs)
>
> You mellow and you're more compromising. (Franky and George, 44 yrs)
>
> If we have any sort of argument, we can laugh about it. (Wendy and Harry, UK 50 yrs)
>
> We resolve it quick. And I think we're a little more mature about it: not wanting to get our own way. (Christine and Ted, 50 yrs)
>
> I think I'm more accepting of the arguing. I've learned that I'm not going to change my wife and maybe I'm not going to change either. So I just let it go, let it pass. (Russell and Ruth, 40 yrs)
>
> I've learned to be forceful. I don't think I started out like that. Yeah, but now I feel that it's made me more assertive. (Liz and Arnie, 51 yrs)

As seen in the previous comments, through compromise, listening, relaxing, tolerating, letting go quicker, being more assertive, using humour, and through hindsight and insight, couples became more accepting and more valuing of what was important to them.

Observations: Three couples argued during the interview but they were comfortable with this. There were no apologies and there was no embarrassment. Although the air was thick with tension, it often dissipated quickly. There appeared to be no need for repairs to the relationships, although Mike and Ying-Len said they would "talk about it later" so as not to interrupt the flow of the interview. Contrastingly, the 11 couples that "never argue" (Gunter and Lee, 52 yrs) were all proud to never have argued.

Aspect: laughter and humour

The vast majority of interviewed couples laughed together more over time, 19% laughed less. 73% of surveyed respondents said laughter improved relationship contentment a great deal, for 11% it did not matter. In response to the survey question "What little things do you do, even daily, that help keep your relationship together?" laughing and joking together was number three behind affectionate touch and acts of service. Laughter is an indicator of relationship well-being.[42]

Approaches to humour changed over time: "We've learnt to laugh because it wasn't part of our modelling," "we've learnt to relax with each other more," "we value [humour] more," and "we've become more bold [in humour]." Laughter was absent from five couples' lives due to learnt behaviour, cultural issues, communist censoring, or when surviving a war left little place for laughter.

Scottish humour helped ease the pressure of raising a severely intellectually disabled child who had up to 1800 seizures a day: "If I get in a cranky mood Rob always makes me laugh" (Jo and Rob, 47 yrs). Laughter helped alleviate suffering:

> Laughter is a huge part of our marriage. Absolutely. We laugh a lot. Even though we've had severe tragedy in our home. We lost our middle boy to melanoma cancer a few years ago and it was hard, but the laughter has come back. (Monte and Jeneen, 45 yrs)

> Laughter is just a great way of overcoming. If you're laughing 95% of the time, and you have 5% of an argument, then, the reality is, it's not going to be a big problem. (Graeme and Anjelika, 46 yrs)

Humour re-enforces shared values:[43] years of running jokes or making fun of each other "in a playful way. Not in a mean, or a put down way" (Howard and Peggy, 48 yrs), or

> we can be in a room full of people and somebody might be talking . . . nonsense and we'll give each other a look. I'll try desperately to avoid looking at him because it'll set us off. (Carol and Brien, 50 yrs)

Jennifer and Michael have "a lot of laughs" by blaming everything on their little Maltese Terrier that "had to be put down about a year ago, and it was hard. Winston still gets blamed for everything" (43 yrs). Laura works tenaciously on scientific papers, so Russell says: "I try to get her to laugh as many times a day as I can" (50 yrs). They were up to 15 times the day of the interview. Interestingly, the word 'joy' surfaced only rarely: "We learnt a certain joyfulness and capacity to make painful things humorous" (Richard and Pearl, 42 yrs). After horrific trials, many couples attested to laughter's healing properties.

Observations: In the interviews I contagiously laughed along with couples who laughed at the questions, humorous memories, at each other's emotions, or to nervously cover up insecurities. Laughter at the beginning of the interviews often relaxed some of the couples who were a little apprehensive regarding personal questions. Couples would sometimes use well-worn adages to answer questions: "You know, happy wife, happy life." This may have reflected this couple's reality or it may have covered deeper truths. In half of the couples, each spouse had about the same level of humour and only one couple had vastly differing levels. Each couple's humour language was unique and when it emerged, they would often share a quick glance with me to ensure I was on side. A jokester's partner would laugh along or apologize for them: "He's the funny one, . . . we all have our strengths" (Marion and Chuck, 44 yrs). Liz and Kevin laughed together throughout the interview in loud belly laughs (New Zealand 40 yrs). A few couples did not smile at all.

Aspect: romance and physical intimacy

In response to the question "is the spark still there?" 84% of the interviewed couples indicated they were still sexually active, with 25% volunteering that they were still very active, including one couple in their eighties. The majority, however, said that their frequency and drive had decreased over time. 55% of the survey respondents noted that satisfying sexual intimacy improved their relationship contentment a lot or a great deal, and 9% said that dissatisfying sexual intimacy affected their relationship a lot or a great deal. In response to the online survey question "Looking back, what made this person a good love-partner for you?" physical attraction/great sex/romance was the number five response. In survey questions regarding sexual activity, 25 respondents left comments such as "my own business," "not telling nosy surveys about it," "that's private," and "no comment."

Younger couples feel a need to succeed in sex,[44] but "Sex is not the full story of what a marriage is all about" (Margaret and Merv, 59 yrs). Time leads to "deeper and better sex . . . that is built on deep love" (Isabella and Ben, 56 yrs). A few couples revealed that they had a "wonderful" and "passionate" sex life.

Sexual problems

Just under a quarter of interviewed couples reported sexual problems, including infertility and pain during intercourse. Three couples disclosed that mental health and childhood abuse adversely affected sexual function. Due to medical issues, several couples had to adapt. Pearl and Richard, had to redefine "normal sexual activity. . . . Being caring" became very important (42 yrs). Couples worked together in this:

> We grow stronger as a couple, more understanding. (Pauline and Denis, UK 44 yrs)
>
> [We found a] different form of intimacy . . . with more love and more affection. (Phil and Christine, 49 yrs)
>
> Romance was a big issue. But I'm always there for her. Whatever she needs, I try and do. (Stephen and Carol, 40 yrs).

The love is in the trying. Even for couples facing sexual difficulties, a healthy sex life was reported to be important.

Romance

"Romance conjures up a lot of different things: saying nice things, being loving, being lustful, a whole range of adjectives come to mind" (David and Trish, 48 yrs). For all couples, there were "different ways of showing your love" (Jack and Judy, 60 yrs):

> Lots of hugs and kisses during the day. (Wayne and Veronne, Aus. 42 yrs)
>
> When we go shopping or when we are doing nothing, we hold hands. That, to me is sort of a sexual relationship . . . always a kiss in the morning and a kiss at night. (Wendy and David, Aus. 41 yrs)
>
> A "very loving" [relationship is] . . . eight hugs a day. (Annette and Bernie, 60 yrs)
>
> Many times when I travelled, . . . I stretched out my arm to touch her and she was not there, I started to panic. I feel much stronger and more secure when she's next to me. (Gaetano and Dorothy, 49 yrs)
>
> Romance is having that security there, still sleeping in the same bed, cuddling up. (Kay and Keith, 52 yrs)
>
> Romance to me means love, feeling safe, feeling secure. (Lana and George, 50 yrs)

Some couples still enjoyed date nights, flowers, and Valentine's cards, but these were not important to the majority of interviewed couples, even early in their relationship: "I don't like receiving flowers because I have to watch them die. . . . So I do not want flowers. I'm not into jewellery. I'm not into gifts. Just be there [for me]" (Beverly and Allen, 46 yrs). Laure "didn't want flowers dying in the house" (Laure and Philippe, France 47 yrs). Eight other women disdained flowers and some couples felt that the expectations of "trying to find a particular day to celebrate" was "contrived" (Patrick and Shirley, 48 yrs). Many chose to express their togetherness every day: "Valentine's Day means nothing . . . that's once a year. That's not enough. It's got to be something that's 365 days a year" (Ben and Isabella, 56 yrs).

Ten men said that they were not "good on the romance side of things" (Gary and Ruth, 54 yrs). Yet this was always countered: "But I think you are romantic. There's a gentle, consistent, really important thing with you that's precious" (Elizabeth and Peter, 60 yrs). The timelessness of generational courtesies as expressions of love were discussed:

> He opens the door, pulls out the chair and walks on the outside of the sidewalk . . . that's very important, that shows respect. (Kay and Keith, 52 yrs)
>
> [I've kept] every single [letter from Jack's army days] and want to be buried with them. (Jack and Judy, 60 yrs)

Many couples wrote and saved letters. The tactile, memorial experience[45] of reading and re-reading a timeless expression of romance, signifies commitment security. Young adults are now beginning to appreciate this.[46]

"Her poetry" attracted Inno to Tiiu (66 yrs), or for others it is the "beautiful things he writes in cards" (Elizabeth and Peter, 60 yrs). "Pleasing each other not only sexually but visually" (Peter and Sharon, Aus. 57 yrs) was also important as was appreciating: "there's never a day goes by that I don't tell her how much I love her and how important she is to me and how much I adore her" (Brien and Carol, 50 yrs).[47] Other modes of romantic expression included spending time, doing favours, walks, respect, compliments, travelling, sharing things spiritually, talking intensely, watching stars and sunsets together, renewing vows, massages, dancing, and going to concerts together.

Lawyers Ruth and Russell find working together romantic:

RUTH When we're working on a serious trial, we have fun doing it, seeing the clients together and even at the settlement conferences.

RUSSELL Fellow lawyers, always wonder "why are you always with your wife"?

RUTH I think we're a romantic couple but not in a soupy kind of way. (40 yrs)

Many couples were not openly "soupy," they had their own private romance.

Observations: Some couples were comfortable expressing their love by holding hands, patting laps, or stroking arms. I noted how Gaetano and Dorothy, and Veselina and Boris were immaculately dressed for the occasion of the interview and how important visual pleasing each other was for them. Peter, who had been relatively reflective and considered throughout the interview at one point spontaneously exuded: "I've always been madly in love with her and I still am!" (Peter and Elizabeth, 60 yrs). For some, however, embarrassment levels were understandably high during this question. This was the aspect where couples checked with each other the most to preserve, presumably, trust and loyalty. Having grown up in an age of relative modesty most couples did not touch at all during the interviews, yet an occasional knowing look reflected something of their private intimacy.

Aspect: division of labour

Household and gendered roles have changed significantly.[48] Of the interviewed couples, 72% of females took care of the inside of the house, and men the outside. 21% practiced equality in division of tasks from the beginning of their relationship. Couples discussed breadwinning, homemaking, providing, and the liberating and oppressive aspects of these roles. 11% of surveyed respondents' relationship discontentment was affected a lot or a great deal by division of labour and 75% none at all or a little.

The concept of the 'provider' attenuated in the late 1970s[49] when females took on more of the provider role:[50]

> He's always been a wonderful provider. (Barbara and Lance, 52 yrs)
>
> Peter was always very conscious of being able to provide for the family. (Peter and Rhonda, 53 yrs)

In the twenty-first century, gendered roles are being dramatically rearticulated and disarticulated.[51] Interviewed couples witnessed these struggles: "you're quite sorry for the young people. They seem to be really tense over roles" (Keith and Lana, New Zealand 49 yrs).

Studies show that couple contentment is highest "in male-breadwinner, female-homemaker households,"[52] but many exceptions exist. Division into "inside work and outside work" (Timothy and Samantha, 51 yrs) was "traditional" but "We have different strengths. Steve is a great cook, I'm very good mechanically. So I fix whatever" (Avima and Steve, 41yrs). Three other couples inverted the traditional roles. Judy, for example, was "the handyman, a Miss fix-it" (Judy and Gordon, 66 yrs).

The division of household chores had evolved greatly during the time of the thriving couples' marriages, reflecting the move towards gender equality.[53] Many couples valued equality. In response to "what is the glue in your relationship?" Veselina and Boris both said "equality" (73 yrs). Although

Veselina did most of the cooking, Boris would stand beside her when he came home from work always eager to help. Others re-defined the division of labour construct:

> Sharing labour and division of labour has been vital to our survival. We don't divide, we share. (Laura and Russell, 50 yrs)
>
> I still believe in [gender] equality, . . . but essentially we've got our gifts. We just divided things by the role we thought we did best. (Jeanette and Malcolm, 64 yrs)
>
> There were chores we naturally gravitated to. (Beverly and Allen, 46 yrs)
>
> It just sort of evolved that we each have strengths or just a task that has to be done and it gets done. (Paula and Don, 57 yrs)

Some females described their homemaker role with enthusiasm:

> I love doing house chores, taking care of my family, being there for my husband. That gives me the greatest joy. (Lynette and Graham, Aus. 46 yrs)
>
> I just love doing it. I love keeping home and cooking. (Samantha and Timothy, 51 yrs)
>
> It fulfils me. (Lucy and Frank, 55 yrs)
>
> I find housework very relaxing. (Pat and Tony, 54 yrs)

Culture plays a part: "I just followed what my mother did. The woman, especially from an Italian family, cooks and does everything for the husband" (Dorothy and Gaetano, 49 yrs). Maria from Italy still cooks a lunch every fortnight for the children, grandchildren, and great-grandchildren; (42 relatives in all) "and sometimes their friends" (Maria and Gennaro, 65 yrs).

Some females, however, felt trapped in the homemaker role:

> Sometimes I'd get jealous of Ted being out all the time. (Marge and Ted, 56 yrs)
>
> I have a college degree and here I am sitting in a one-bedroom apartment bored out of my skull. I wasn't very good at housecleaning. Yeah. And finally, I just said to him, "I'm wasting my education." So, I wrote a newspaper column and finally eased myself into a full time job. (Mary and Brian, 50 yrs)

While Bruce from New Zealand travelled a lot selling packaging and cosmetics, Jan "felt lonely. It was a wee bit tough" (57 yrs). Some men felt "regret . . . I should have done more . . . to my shame, I was pretty selfish" (Bill and Fay, 57 yrs). While there was often regret for "not being there enough" or "not helping enough" that was well-founded, some females retorted, "I didn't really want him to cook. I liked my kitchen" (Anjelika and Graeme, 46 yrs). Beyond the resentment and regret, nearly all couples made light of division of labour and had a good-humoured chuckle about it. No interviewed couple argued about division of chores.

Aspect: attitude to finances

There was not as much joviality shared when discussing finances: 16% of the interviewed couples were poor at one stage or for most of their relationship, 6% experienced extreme poverty. 90% had joint accounts and 55% of the females managed the finances, but only 10% of couples regularly argued over finances. In 13% of the surveyed couples, financial stress contributed to relationship discontentment a lot or a great deal. Finance-driven discontent is known to be higher in younger couples.[54]

Inno and Tiiu arrived in Australia from Estonia "with nothing, totally penniless" (66 yrs). Olga "saved for [her] wedding dress by not eating." She became anaemic and had a breakdown on her wedding day. While explaining, Olga wept: "We bury painful stuff. It's painful just to remember" (Olga and Raul, Paraguay to USA 45 yrs). Steve and Carol "had to start all over [after losing their business] . . . and did nothing for about four years: didn't go to dinner, didn't buy anything, no clothing . . . it brought us much, much closer together" (53 yrs).

Joint bank accounts were discussed:

> It wasn't my money, and it wasn't her money, it was our money. (Malcolm and Jeanette, 64 yrs)
>
> My bank account belongs to her. (Albert) And mine belongs to him (Clare). We see it as a whole. (Albert and Clare, 40 yrs)

This meant "trusting each other implicitly" (Anjelika and Graeme, 46 yrs) and "trust[ing] the other person would never go do anything rash with money" (Lance and Barbara, 52 yrs). Trust, couples told us, was an integral part of commitment and the foundation for attitudes towards finances.

Aspects summary

These questions stirred memories, often pleasant and often painful. Couples telling stories frequently wept or laughed at their mistakes. Questions regarding arguing, physical intimacy, and friendship were confronting. Couples enjoyed discussing domestics: "it's the little things that are important. Not big things. They're all part of the picture. The important things are all the little details that make the mosaic" (Ben and Isabella, 56 yrs).

Much of this may sound strange to many younger couples: joint accounts, poverty bringing couples closer together, indifference to gender roles and chores, not wanting much separate time, vastly different attitudes to sex and romance, or the acceptance of arguing. It is, perhaps, in these relationship aspects that the cohort effect of our research is most clearly seen. Yet these are the couples who 'made it,' the ones who stayed together. Their comments represent evidence and documentation of some ideas which may keep a relationship together.

These couples also encountered obstacles that threatened to tear them apart. During these discussions of the relatively light relationship aspects, much trust and rapport was built. The interviews then took an uncomfortable turn.

Findings: things that threatened to tear couples apart

Many interviewed couples experienced significant hardship, yet remained together. We are very grateful to these couples for their courage in sharing some of the pain in their journeys as well as their elation and insights. In the interviews, the penultimate question was "Was there anything that threatened to tear your relationship apart but didn't?" Asking this question leant on the trust built up earlier to create enough safety for honest and safe disclosure. Couples often checked with each other as if to ask 'should we tell her?'

One third of the couples did not identify a threat, two thirds did: "I don't think anything could tear us apart, I honestly don't, but they've come close" (Carol and Brien, 50 yrs). The issues that came close are, in order:

1. Death or severe illness of a child
2. An affair
3. Major physical issues
4. In-law issues
5. Living away from home
6. Major mental health issues
7. Financial issues
8. Employment-related issues
9. Someone else in love with a spouse

We discuss the first six before turning to the question of divorce in interviewed couples' lives.

Threat 1: death or severe illness of a child

> Our son was 18. He was an apprentice, still living at home. One Wednesday night he came home, showered, changed clothes, went to his mate's place which he did quite often because he had an Xbox or Gameboy. Four men broke into the house and shot him

through the head. And it was absolutely terrible, terrible. Home invasion. . . . David was the rock and I was the mess. Then after 12 years, [David] collapsed. He was on the brink of suicide, and that's when he started on anti-depressants. . . . You battle through it. . . . Lots of support from friends. The homicide victim support group was wonderful. (Debby and David, 48 yrs)

Our daughter went to Adelaide with this guy she met in rehab and was in a domestic violence situation. He bashed her. He almost killed her. We sent her an airfare from Adelaide to come straight back home. . . . We got a call on the 25th of May two years ago at midnight. *Crying*. The doctor rang me from Emerald hospital to say she had a fall horse-riding, she's not going to survive the night, the bleeding on the brain was so bad. She died from the fall. . . . We needed each other. We sat down and hugged each other saying, "look, come on. We're going to get through this together." (Samantha and Timothy, 51 yrs)

We lost our middle boy to melanoma cancer a few years ago and it was hard. You're never going to be okay with it. If you don't have a close relationship these things can hit you without you even preparing for it. And if you don't have a good relationship a lot of couples can split because of this. I don't like it. I don't have to like it, nobody said you have to like what you go through in life. But it's happened. So now, how do we deal with it, how do we go on? Let's talk through this, let's work through this. Because of our faith we also respected each other to grieve in our own personal way. . . . That was the hardest thing in our marriage and we're stronger together because we're the only two people that went through that tragedy with our son. . . . Yeah. That was a big one. (Monte and Jeneen, 45 yrs)

We started off with three children but one was killed in a shooting accident. He was 18. . . . It was quite amazing because we've always had a very strong relationship but I felt that during that time, we just felt so much closer together and so much more love flowing around. I was given a verse just before Peter was killed from my sister-in-law "when you walk through the fire, you won't be burned. When you walk through the water, you won't be drowned." That was a really fiery and deep-water experience. (Margaret and Ian, 57 yrs)

Our oldest son passed away and that was a very difficult time for us, it was so painful. I would usually wake up in the middle

> of the night to go to the bathroom and then I would think about our son being gone and I would just be filled with so much grief and despair. How am I going to make it? It was really a hard time. But I think it kind of helped us to grow closer together because we had to experience that, and to go through the most difficult thing either one of us have ever had to experience. (Mildred and William, 40 yrs)

These deaths of children are shocking. How do parents cope? Couples told us that they coped together. In severe illness of a child, coping is likewise needed; day in, day out, often from infancy:

> Matty was about seven months old when we realized something was very wrong. He had caught a germ at the hospital. He's severely intellectually brain damaged. So that was a real hard knock for me at 24 and by the time I reached 30 I had a breakdown. . . . I grieved and blamed myself for what happened to Matt, that I didn't do enough to save him. For seven years I didn't go out of the house. . . . It's a lot of pressure on the marriage having a disabled child. If Rob hadn't been the husband that he was we would have been a split family. . . . We committed to doing this together. And we're going to do it to the last breath together no matter what. (Jo and Rob, 47 yrs)

> Our only son was a very bright young fella. . . . Unfortunately, in schools in our area, when you stand out for any reason you tend to become a target, and this is what happened to him. When he got to be about 13 or 14 kids started to pick on him and make his life miserable. . . . He started dodging school and taking drugs. He was becoming violent. He'd be gone for nights. I'd go out and look for him. Sometimes I'd find him and sometimes I wouldn't, and I'd beg him to come home. And it got to a stage where it was starting to impact our relationship. I had no doubt that this had the capacity to tear our relationship apart. It reached a point where rather than put our son first, as we had since he was born, we had to put ourselves first and just hope that he could find his own way out of this. It was the hardest decision that we've ever made. (Brien and Carol, 50 yrs)

> When our son was twelve weeks old the doctor took the baby off me and said "go and get your husband. You need to go to the Mater hospital now, they need to do a lumbar puncture." At the hospital they said "He's got meningitis, and he's going to die." He didn't die, but he was intellectually handicapped. He would scream for eight hours non-stop. He used to just break everything. He used to pull [our other son's] hair out. We had to teach him to sleep by holding him down. It was survival

for the whole family. . . . If anything, it has probably brought us more closer together, because we had to look out for it together. . . . Our intellectually handicapped son was the best thing that could have happened to us. (Kay and Keith, 52 yrs)

We have a son that's diagnosed bipolar and schizophrenic. He probably weighs close to 300 pounds. He's very, very, very unhappy and that makes us unhappy. . . . I know, it's mental and he can't help it. But I hate the problem. . . . We deal with it by talking it through with each other, open communication, not swallowing our emotions. And through our situation we have empathy for what other people are going through. (Marion and Chuck, 44 yrs)

Observations: I felt like holding my breath as I heard these stories. The deep pain of loss and years of exhausting struggle was etched on faces re-living these journeys, often crying and shaking. During these, I witnessed gentle rescuing: a soft pat on the leg, a warm hand massaging the pain away, eye contact for support and strength, an embrace until grief had lessened. Some told the story only to each other, not to me. These were couples that had dealt with so much heartache that they had few inhibitions, tears were only ever a breath away. How did they cope? Although they were "never going to be okay with it," it was clear that they leant on each other and on their relationship to get through.

Divorce is eight times more likely after child bereavement.[55] Divorce and mental illness in parents with a child with severe impairment is even more common.[56] The interviewed couples used various coping mechanisms: mutual support, teamwork, respecting individual grieving, re-introducing humour, relying on faith, sharing emotions, and even dancing. There was, however, always hope: "A curve ball can do what it did to us: it glued us" (Rob and Jo, 47 yrs).

Threat 2: an affair

I had no idea that Wayne had a lady. I was in total shock: and what I found really hard was the fact that he didn't love me anymore. My friendship had been broken. I wasn't good as a woman to him. *Crying*. He betrayed our values of honesty and integrity by not telling me. He did eventually tell me. I admire him for doing that. . . . And you see things on Facebook all the time: 'It's not going to work.' I didn't have to take him back. But 42 years is worth fighting for. It's only as hard as you're prepared to put the effort in. You have to find again what held it together in the first place. (Veronne and Wayne, 32 years)

LAURE Philippe wanted to see what the world was and what the other women were. For him it was just a play with other women. I had to say again and again that I was not happy about it and it was getting worse and at one point he realized he had gone too far so, maybe not too far but just at the edge. So either he stayed with me only, or I go. We saw one or two [therapists] actually. My friends said, "Oh my god, why are you staying?" People are more selfish so they think of themselves, but not of the family. His father was a good counter-example for him because he got married four times but that did not make him happy. In the end he committed suicide.

PHILIPPE We survived because Laure was very strong in her willingness to keep our marriage together. At the time you say: no, my marriage is the most important thing, we've built something irreplaceable. (47 yrs)

> I had a crazy midlife crisis which lasted a very short time. After the hiccup I got my head together and have been working on that ever since. I try to compensate and make up for that stumble along the way. I believe I'm a better person now. I reflected on it fairly and I've put everything into a commitment to my wife and family ever since, for obvious reasons. "Keep it going. Don't walk away. Do no walk away." I got forgiveness and compassion, and I speak from my heart there. (Lyle and Heather, 69 yrs)

It was very difficult for couples to disclose affairs. Seven couples divulged affairs and four strongly alluded to it. Some were likely left undisclosed.[57] Affairs often lead to divorce, but some marriages can withstand the hurt and conflict:[58]

> When you've been married for quite a long time you have a history and memories that nobody else has and if you throw that away, what was the point of all that? You have to fight for it and build it again. It comes back to values and you realize and appreciate what you do have. There was a glitch, it was stupid, and now we're stronger. (Liz and Kevin, 51 yrs)

Others were clear that the threat was there, but there was no affair:

> In retrospect, it is easier to see what made both of us turn away from each other and seek love elsewhere. In each case seeking the missing TLC from someone else. . . . There was a bishop I was confessing to: "I'm planning to leave, there's somebody else that I am falling in love with and we're so similar, blah, blah, blah." And he said, "You made your vows and you can't just walk out. Besides, you think the

grass might be greener on the other side, it frequently works out not to be so." After a serious discussion of the reality of our potential marriage failure, the effects on the children, and the break up of everything we worked for, we began to see things in a different light. We decided to stay together. And gradually, the feelings began to come back. It doesn't happen overnight. You've got to work on it. (Alex and Alexandra, 58 yrs)

Observations: At moments of disclosure, couples became very emotional as feelings of betrayal, hurt, compassion and forgiveness competed for dominance. One affair was not too long ago and many tears were shed in the interview. Sometimes silences hung heavily in air. Some gave me defensive looks. One couple used humour, another held hands in support. I was awed by the trust. With consent, couples painfully opened their hearts for others to know: "[We] wanted to help as many people as we can." (Veronne and Wayne, 42 yrs)

Threat 3: major physical issue

David fell off the roof. He nearly died. He was on life support, in hospital three months. He broke 38 bones: his spine in 15 places, 17 ribs and his pelvis in five places. And he still has a brain injury. He had to re-learn how to swallow, eat, write, talk. It was a dreadful time, it was a battle minute to minute. (Debby and David, 48 yrs)

GRAHAM Eve had cancer . . . *Crying* . . . she was 40.
EVE Stomach cancer. I had my stomach removed. They said I'd only live for about 18 months. I'm [still] here.[59] (Eve and Graham, 65 yrs)

I was injured at work as a seaman. Hurt my spine. Because of the drugs they gave me I lost two thirds of my gut. We nearly lost the house because Sharon had to nurse me, had to give up work. We got through it with just sheer determination and dedication to each other. (Peter and Sharon, 57 yrs)

I had a serious accident. I was a papermaker, so couldn't use my hand. That's when Heather came to the fore. She took a job alongside her mothering role [of eight children]. She went out and became a salesman because our budget dropped. I was off work. That was the incentive also for me to get myself rehabilitated and back to work earning a full wage. And that happened through sheer pig headedness. (Lyle and Heather, 69 yrs)

No-one left the relationship, but these were identified as threats.

Observations: I saw the discomfort of their injury through people's difficulty getting out of chairs, limping, not being able to shake my hand. Couples negotiated the pain together, or with a little assistance: twice in the interview when Eve and Graham broke down, their little dog popped out from under the table to comfort them. Cancer was prominent among couples. Other medial issues included heart attacks, Crohn's disease, hyperthyroidism, stroke, and Parkinson's disease. One person was in a wheelchair. "In sickness and health" is a formidable commitment: "[Doctors told] me that most partners leave. They just can't cope with [serious] illness" (Anjelika and Graeme, 46 yrs).

Threat 4: in-law issues

As discussed in Chapter 3, family and friends can help or hinder a relationship; their influence is much greater than appreciated. Some couples had in-laws living with them up to 22 years with little conflict and lots of support: "It was our joy and our privilege" (Malcolm and Jeanette, 64 yrs). At other times, however, in-laws had values "which clashed" with the values of couples when they were young (Linden and Hermann, 54 yrs). Insights were proffered: "It is a whole family that you are getting married into, for life. You've got to know them" (Gennaro and Maria, 65 yrs).

In-law disapproval of spouses lead to rumours, doubts, conflict, and rejection:

> Everything was on his parent's side, Patrick just didn't know how to stand up for me. (Shirley and Patrick, 48 yrs)
>
> [Our decision to adopt children] was not agreeable to our families which we found extremely hurtful. (Beti and Clive, 60 yrs)

Gary and Ruth planned to live overseas: "Ruth's dad was saying things like, 'I'm going to lay down on the runway in front of the plane'" (54 yrs). "Raul's whole entire family didn't want us to get married. 150 people were invited to the wedding, only 20 showed up." Some are "still waiting for us to get divorced" (Olga and Raul, 45 yrs).

Threat 5: living away from home

Although up to ten percent of couples in affluent countries may live apart together,[60] surprisingly few interviewed couples spent any time living apart. When they did, it was generally problematic: "I was alone all the time. He was gone almost all the time. I had a nervous breakdown. . . . [There were a] lot of threats about leaving the relationship" (Mary and Brian, 50 yrs).

Candy was on the road, Gregg was a commanding officer: "we were just so busy. We were being pulled apart." They found something "to do together; one thing that takes time that you have to do every single week, setting apart time to do it together" (49 yrs).

Gunter and Lee had separate interests. Gunter liked "mountain climbing, paragliding, swimming with sharks, and jumping off cliffs. Crazy things." He was gone six months at a time. Lee wanted to be "the stay-at-home mom. One time I remember, it came to a point, we really got into it and got it out. . . . After that we thought our relationship was wonderful . . . a unique relationship" (Germany/USA, 52 yrs). Similarly, Harry volunteers in China each year. Wendy stays in New Zealand. They balance their separate times with active sporting involvement together, and lots of humour (50 yrs).

Threat 6: mental illness

JIM I have serious PTSD from Vietnam. How she put up with me after I came back from Vietnam, I don't know.

PAT And nor do I.

JIM A lot of guys went to drugs, alcohol or something; I went to work 50, 60, 70 hours a week. I found it very difficult to maintain close relationships because I learned in combat you don't do that; people die, you lose them. It was really tough for me to get close to family.

PAT In our household the Vietnam War has never ended and that's been hard for me . . . *crying*

JIM It's okay to cry if you want to. For me it's been very, very tough because I believe we're both very intelligent individuals. I'm smart enough to fix things and I can't fix this one. If you lose cabin pressure, put your mask on first so you're capable of helping the other person. If you're not totally satisfied with self you can never be satisfied with anything else. I never expected her to be perfect. But I *knew* I wasn't. (54 yrs)

WENDY I had a lot of depression through the last 20 years. I've had about 300 ECTs and my memory is shot, and I was in and out of hospital all the time and David had to cope. I would say "I'm in a dark, a very dark place at the moment."

DAVID Wendy can go from really on a high to very suicidal in a very short period of time. We had a very long stretch in hospital in 1990, just after our youngest was born. And that was incredibly tough for all of us. And Wendy was blaming herself. We just kept communicating to get through it all. I was saying "it's not your fault. It's the same as if I had a heart attack." We would go home and keep on putting one foot in front of the other. (41 yrs)

CAROL He's got PTSD. There was a lot of abuse when he was at school so he has night terrors.

STEPHEN We've been through the royal commission with the childhood abuse. Yeah. I was one of those people [who] got abused; and Carol got abused. I'm on antidepressants.

CAROL We had horrendous fights. And when all that was going on, my mom often said to me, "your bedroom's always there, you can always come home." And I just had it in my mind, that will never happen, because I'm married now. And I had to make it work, and we did. It was just hard work. . . . And because we both had such emotional trauma, it's worked out for us, that basically we need each other. We've found our level of things that are acceptable, things that aren't. It's not going to get the better of us.

STEPHEN We are both very stubborn and we are not quitters. (40 yrs)

Carol and Stephen have determination, as do Wendy and David and Pat and Jim. All of these couples, and others, were still living with mental health as the uninvited guest.

> *Observations*: while discussing mental health issues, these couples could be brittle with each other but balanced this with humour, touch, or raw admissions of difficult memories and emotions. Vietnam Veteran Jim had to check the room before the interview and sat with his back against the wall throughout. I observed the load these couples were carrying, and I felt their anxious energy, often externalized as they nervously tapped their fingers on the table or scrunched up a tissue. There were, however, no elephants in the room with these couples, only stamina, loyalty, and sacrifice: "one thing I've always known, he would always jump into the fire pit if it was a choice, you or me."(Pat and Jim, 54 yrs)

We can reflect on the resilience displayed by all interviewed thriving couples. Some had much more adversity to overcome than others, but they were not defeated by it. How did they build their resilience? This question will be considered in Chapter 7 based on current scientific understanding, their insights, and years of clinical experience. How resilient were our thriving couples? Did they ever consider divorce?

Divorce

Divorce was not identified as a threat by interviewed couples. It was, however, something we specifically asked about:

> "Have you ever considered divorce?"

Only 9% of the interviewed couples had seriously considered divorce. For another 9% "it's not a been a serious thought. Just an angry thought"

(Sharon and Bob, 46 yrs). 82% had never considered divorce and a third of these adamantly stated or yelled "no" or "never" together. "Why not?" became the next question. Answers included:

It's a forever deal 18%
Why would you? 16%
A vow is a vow 16%
The kids would suffer 13%
The grass is not greener elsewhere 9%
I'm still in love 8%
Because of what was modelled to us 6%
Who wants loneliness? 6%
For religious reasons 5%
Too much bother 3%

Important outlying replies included:

It's too painful
Where else have we to go?
I'd lose my security
Because I'm happy
Divorce would be failure
We are a family
Too much to lose
Couldn't live without him/her
You don't just discard something
Are we supposed to divorce?

For the 9% who had seriously considered divorce, the most frequent reason to consider divorce was not discontentment with the partner, but a feeling of inadequacy in themselves:

> I did think of separation. There are times when I felt I was having such a destructive [emotional] impact on my wife and my children. It may be better if I wasn't there. But there was no real concept of divorce. Maybe it would be easier and more helpful for them if I lived separately. (Richard and Pearl, 42 yrs)

> I thought she would be better off without me. Because, you know, I know that I'm not that outgoing a person. But you know, it's the last thing I want to happen. (Ted and Christine, 50 yrs)

Others felt societal pressure: "It's that voice in your head: the world tells you 'just walk if you're not happy' " (Sharon and Bob, 46 yrs) and "I sometimes feel like running away. But it passes" (Christine and Ted, 50 yrs).

As discussing threats and divorce often evoked negative memories, the last interview question helped re-affirm togetherness. Each person was asked "can you tell me a strength or something you love about your spouse?" Answers to this could fill another book:

> When we look in each other's eyes across a room, we connect. I can see his eyes. I just feel a connection. (Helen and George, 48 yrs)
>
> He's a rock that I can depend on, he's got my back. (Annette and Bernie, 60 yrs)
>
> She's beautiful and she's been the driving force behind me. (Harry and Irene, Aus 55 yrs)
>
> He is very, very, very reliable. I knew that right from the very beginning when I was 19 when we met. My mental illness was in a pretty bad state at the time . . . all over the place. I remember saying to him, if I walk out on you, don't let me go. . . . So he never did let me go, he used to drive the streets looking for me. And he wouldn't let me go. (Frances and Wayne, Aus. 42 yrs)
>
> I love her. Her servant heart. I love her patience with me. Faithfulness. The gift of hospitality. (Gary and Ruth, 54 yrs)
>
> He rescued me. (Irene and Harry, 55 yrs)
>
> His integrity. I trust him 100%. (Marilyn and Gerry, 49 yrs)
>
> I've always loved how he is so steadfast, and patient. And his ego never gets in the way. (Candy and Gregg, 49 yrs)

Findings: answering younger couples' questions

We conclude this chapter by presenting an amalgamation of surveyed and interviewed couples' answers to the five most pressing questions asked by younger couples from the Surviving COVID-19 Survey:

1. What is your secret to staying together?
2. Is the spark still there?
3. How do you stop arguing and get through hard times?
4. How do you keep your marriage fun and not boring?
5. How do you keep connected and communicate well?

QUESTION: WHAT IS YOUR SECRET TO STAYING TOGETHER?

The top glue-secrets of relationship longevity for our 90 thriving couples were commitment, altruism, shared values, good communication and compromise. Some young couples did not only ask "what," they asked "how." Here are some key responses on each:

Commitment

> You have to be fully committed to that person and there'll be some rough times. As you get through adversity you'll be stronger . . . and you will have a strong foundation for your life. (William and Mildred, 40 yrs)
>
> It's a commitment to a partnership and partnership is working together, trusting and loving each other. And if there's a problem then you can always go back to your original reasons and say "Hey okay when I started off that was why I wanted to do it and things haven't really changed." (Tony and Cyndy, 49 yrs)
>
> What's gonna happen when you don't love each other? That's where commitment comes, you have to want to work through this. (Howard and Peggy, 48 yrs)
>
> You've made a commitment; you honour the commitment. And yeah, it's tough. But life is tough. And it isn't any better on the outside. (Mary and Brian, 50 yrs)

Altruism

> We are selfish. And if you acknowledge that from the very start, and then work to combat that, by being self-giving, and self-sacrificing to your partner, that's got to help your relationship every single time. (Gary and Ruth, 54 yrs)
>
> A relationship means being prepared not to get your way all the time. (Tiiu and Inno, 66 yrs)
>
> Don't give in to the passion, or the feeling, or the emotion of the moment in order to either gratify yourself, or satisfy yourself, or console yourself. You have to support each other. (David and Trish, 48 yrs)
>
> The secret of our relationship is that we both try not to take the relationship for granted. We consider each other's feelings. We work at it. (George and Lana, 50 yrs)
>
> I often see selfishness on both sides. People maintain that they love each other, but they resent. . . . A relationship is not a football game. There's no offence and defence. (Lucy and Frank, 55 yrs)

Shared values

> We talked about our values when we started dating. And we always discussed what was important to us in values all through our marriage . . . and that we didn't want to break those values either. (Jeneen and Monte, 45 yrs)

> There have been values that we've shared and others we have been able to talk to each other about, and not let them divide us. We talk them out. If Jeanette wasn't too happy with something that I believed in, then she would tell me, and I would do the same. And then we would sort it out between us. (Malcolm and Jeanette, 64 yrs)

> You form your ideas and values as you grow because we were growing together. I think we've made up our own values . . . as you grow together you lean into the same values. (Bruce and Jan, 57 yrs)

> When you have shared values, you can't beat it. I mean it's so important. You might look at a situation, she comes at it from a little different angle, I might need that angle. I might need to understand a little more from that way. (Monte and Jeneen, 45 yrs)

Communication

> You have to keep talking. Communication is the most important thing . . . if you stop talking, then you [are] setting yourself up to go in different directions. (Peter and Elizabeth, 60 yrs)

> If you sense that there's something not right, don't hide it under the covers. You need to ask about it and talk about it. (Veronne and Wayne, 42 yrs)

> I think you have to say what you need, and not expect somebody to know what you need: clear, concise and direct. (Peggy and Howard, 48 yrs)

> I can't say it enough. Communication is the key. If we had communicated more he wouldn't have had an affair. (Online survey)

> It's not what you say, but how you say it: you don't accuse the person. But if there's something that's annoying you or something that is a deal breaker, you could say "do you think you could change this?" or "I don't like the way you do that." (Carol and Stephen, 40 yrs)

Compromise

> What's really held us together is the ability to compromise. Stopping and thinking "it's not about me always," "what can I do to

be a little more flexible?" . . . Allow yourself to go with the flow rather than have your way. (Keith and Stephen, 30 yrs)

It's compromise. If you don't both like something, well find something else that you both do and go and do that. (David and Wendy, 41 yrs)

There has to be some compromise and even sacrifice. Not a "My way or the Highway" attitude. Compromise, meet in the middle. No one is always right. (Online survey)

We've always come up with a compromise. You know, even if it takes a day or two you need a compromise. And you have to see each other's point of view. Sometimes it might mean that you've got to retreat and consider options. (Arnie and Liz, 51 yrs)

Compromise, you can't be "me, me, me" you must be "us, us, us." (Online survey)

Some younger couples may find these responses very disagreeable. Commitment, altruism, and compromise in particular may seem like archaic concepts. They could, however, become progressive again as society comes to count the cost of relationship loss. They could become shared values for couples in our society.

QUESTION: IS THE SPARK STILL THERE?

With a glimmer in their eyes, 84% of interviewed couples replied "yes." Five couples, heartbeats synchronized, answered in unison. Here are some of their descriptors:

Nice spark all the time now, but when [we were] younger it was a bushfire. (Trevor and Sandra, 43 yrs)

It's got a better light now than before. (Graeme and Anjelika, 46 yrs)

Different sort of spark; more mature. (Allan and Carol, 55 yrs)

It burnt brightly when we were young. (Lyle and Heather, 59 yrs)

It's never been a spark, but a steady flame. (Pearl and Richard, 42 yrs)

Spark is still there. (Ben and Isabella, 56 yrs)

If it's not there, it's sad. Your relationship gets rusty. (Gaetano and Dorothy, 49 yrs)

Still there, but not as sparky as it was 45 years ago. (Trish and David, 48 yrs)

It's getting bigger! (Patty and Jorge, 47 yrs)

You can rekindle it. (Alex and Alexandra, 58 yrs)

Further comments included the following:

> Every once in a while we will embarrass our kids by saying there is sex after 60. (Candy and Gregg, 49 yrs)
>
> At 73 years old . . . we're making more love now than we ever did for God's sake! (Gunter and Lee, 52 yrs)
>
> The passion's still there. We're still lovers. I'm just being very frank. (Jeanette and Malcolm, 64 yrs)
>
> The truth of the matter is after 48 years of marriage, intimacy still exists and it's still important, but not the same. (David and Trish, 48 yrs)
>
> It slows down. (Peter and Sharon, 57 yrs)
>
> The mind's really willing but the body mightn't work. (Bruce and Jan, 57 yrs)

Intimacy and romance developed over decades of knowing and loving have replaced frequency and high passion for most. Embers can burn warmly and deeply in a perpetual glow.

QUESTION: HOW DO YOU STOP ARGUING AND GET THROUGH HARD TIMES?

The primary response from the online survey was to listen:

> Listen attentively and see beyond the problem
> Listen . . . take a step back before responding
> First become a good listener before becoming a good narrator
> Really listen to the emotions behind the words, even if it hurts.

Other suggestions, in order, were:

> Talk it through
> Get space and time to think
> Look at both point of views
> Avoid arguing altogether
> Don't go to sleep angry

Many interviewed couples embraced healthy arguing to "manage" conflict underpinned by commitment:

BETI But you don't change.
CLIVE No. I hate confrontation really. But we still argue. You learn to manage it.
BETI We're still here together anyway.

CLIVE I don't like arguing but we're not afraid of it. (60 yrs)

> Stick it out, try and make it work, make it last. . . . Choose permanence over temporary. Temporary is buying something at Cotton On, wearing it twice, and throwing it out. Permanence is quality and making things last: you wouldn't fling your Prada in the washing machine! Nurture what you have and make it last. (Stella and Fred, 42 yrs)
>
> I think it's been harder for Wayne because I suffer mental illness in depression. And it's the commitment that's helped him get through because we've had some very hard times. Very, very hard times. But he stayed committed all the way. (Frances and Wayne, 42 yrs)
>
> Just stick with it because you had the idea that it was a good idea at the start. (Kevin and Liz, 40 yrs)
>
> If you dump a person for two or three things that you don't like about them, you take on another person who's got six or seven things you don't like. So you dump them and you move on to the next one who's got ten things. Stay. Make it work. (Carol and Stephen, 40 yrs)

One younger couple specifically asked "How did you handle the extreme differences between the two of you?" (6–10 yrs). 27% of the interviewed couples had opposite personalities, "like chocolate and cheese" (Lyle and Heather, 69 yrs), but this became a strength: "Two sharp stones do not grind flour" (Bulgarian proverb; Veselina and Boris, 73 yrs). "What makes it work is our personality types are very different, . . . we bring together our differences . . . I think that's been our secret" (Beverly and Allen, 46 yrs). Having opposing personalities has been considered a relationship risk,[61] but recent studies[62] and our findings challenge this. It seems that thriving couples find a way of making personality differences work for you, not against you.

QUESTION: HOW DO YOU KEEP YOUR MARRIAGE FUN AND NOT BORING?

Fun for Couples Thriving 40+ years together differs from what younger couples may consider fun:

> Playing tricks on each other in restaurants: hiding around the corner like a kid. (Kevin and Liz, 40 yrs)
>
> He's a bit cheeky, he likes throwing a glass of cold water on me in the shower, pinching me on the backside. (Rhonda and Peter, 53 yrs)
>
> When we first got married we used to read the newspaper and cut out cartoons that we thought were particularly funny and place them in a booklet. (Michael and Jennifer, 43 yrs)

> We'll run into each other and bump bellies. We just laugh at ourselves. We find a lot of joy with ourselves. (Stephen and Keith, 30 yrs)

> Speleology. Finding caves that have never been found. You just don't walk into them. You've got to slide down in usually backwards. (Margaret and Merv, 59 yrs)

> Chasing her with a hose through the house: ah the things you do for fun! (Peter and Sharon, 57 yrs)

> Board games are a cheap way of having fun. (Carol and Allan, 55 yrs)

> That's one of the reasons I married her. I loved the fact that we can have fun together. Yesterday we played Uno, the card game. I wish we could have recorded that, we had so much fun. We laughed at each other so much that if anybody had been on the outside looking in they would have said "Man I'd like to have some of that." (Jim and Pat, 54 yrs)

> Our son and his wife would never want the relationship we have. Theirs is based on fun love: going out and having a good time. We would never want to do that. It's got to be something else. (Beverly and Allen, 46 yrs)

Irene and Harry had numerous fun adventures together travelling around to the country shows "selling junk jewellery and living in a caravan" (55 yrs).

The word 'bored' was not used once in the entire 450,147 word transcription of the interviews, or in the 40+ online surveys. "Comfort," mentioned 66 times, is (as couples told us) highly underrated: "[we like] being comfortable and happy in our knowledge of each other" (Ken and Ruth, 54 yrs). Sitting together for hours in "comfortable silence" (Keith and Kay, 52 yrs) was highly prized as it "All just feels very comfortable and loving" (Peggy and Howard, 48 yrs) like a "comfortable slipper" (Marge and Ted, 56 yrs). Because "[we] know each other so well" (Samantha and Timothy, 51 yrs), "living, growing old together is so much fun!" (Stephen and Keith, 30 yrs).

QUESTION: HOW DO YOU KEEP CONNECTED AND COMMUNICATE?

To many interviewed couples this question was almost an insult; they *were* connected. After 40+ years none of the couples felt they had any problems keeping connected. They described it this way:

> Through the years, you become almost one because you've shared all these things. (Dorothy and Gaetano, 49 yrs)

> The bond is closer and it's like we are one now. (Lana and George, 50 yrs)

> You're a union of two people. (Gennaro and Maria, 65 yrs)
>
> We've got one brain, it's just how we are. Sometimes you've just got to think together as one to get through it. (Jo and Rob, 47 yrs)
>
> Because we're one, divorce is like saying "no, you're not one, we're gonna rip you apart." (Gary and Ruth, 54 yrs)
>
> If you can say, what *we* want together, let's discuss it. Let's try and live that life. When you step out into marriage, then you forget "I" and you concentrate on "we" because you're no longer an individual, you're a unit comprised of two people. (Jeanette and Malcolm, 64 yrs)
>
> One and one makes one. (Graham and Lynette, 46 yrs)
>
> We've got two things going together, but when they come together, there's a big force. (Arnie and Liz, 51 yrs)

Communication helps achieve this:

> If you're dating someone, if you try to understand and you talk it out, it will go past the next stage, it will work. (Steven and Chuck, 30 yrs)
>
> You communicate silently in a lot of cases. (Peter and Rhonda, 53 yrs)
>
> Talk out every possible scenario before you get married. . . . "I want to go to parties dah, dah, dah." "Your parents were too controlling of you, I don't like that." Get every little possible conflict that may arise in your future out on the table. (Gunter and Lee, 52 yrs)

Relationship happiness

As previously stated, thriving couples did not speak in terms of satisfaction, but of happiness or contentment in their subjective evaluations of their relationship. Although we did not ask a specific question about happiness, the couples volunteered many ideas on the topic when talking about the glue-secrets and the aspects. Without touching on the vast philosophical and psychological literature on the topic of happiness, we include some thriving couples' perspectives on the pursuit of this elusive quality in a relationship.

For many thriving couples, it seems, happiness is being in a relationship and having someone with whom to share life:

> Happy things. We've experienced lots of happy things. (Alexandra and Alex, 58 yrs)
>
> We have been happy with each other so the question of divorce never arose. In fact we would be lost without each other's company. (Vinay and Ramila, Uganda 49 yrs)

> I love the fact that you can sleep well at night knowing you've done the right thing. And you've got a partner and everything's happy. (Steve and Carol, 53 yrs)

> We're together. We're happy. We're comfortable. We don't have to worry about too much. So life's good. (Lyle and Heather, 69 yrs)

> I think also we know each other's strengths and weaknesses. I wouldn't push him to do something if I thought it was going to make him unhappy. If he wasn't going to get anything out of it, what would be the point of it? And I'm gonna have an unhappy husband. (Samantha and Timothy, 51 yrs)

> My whole life has been spent being happy with Lana. (George and Lana, 50 yrs)

> Your heart sings when your family's happy. (Sharon and Bob, 46 yrs)

> We're happy in our own skins. (Fred and Stella, 42 yrs)

> I want him to be happy. He wants me to be happy. (Chuck and Steven, 30 yrs)

> I've never thought of divorce. And I'm sure that comes also from the fact that I'm very happy. (Anjelika and Graeme, 46 yrs)

> You don't have to look for fantastic things to be happy or to find that happiness . . . we've been alone, the two of us for since the end of November so there's no friends. And it's okay. (Philippe and Laure, 47 yrs)

Some thriving couples suggested that relationship happiness may be related to values, altruism, and commitment.

> You got to find your happy . . . you got to work out what your values are. (Frances and Wayne, 42 yrs)

> I live with the word "joyful" in my life. Joy, what brings you joy? What brings somebody else joy that you can do for them? That will make them happy. (Kathy and Jim, 43 yrs)

> We are comfortable and happy in our knowledge of each other and remain fully committed. (Ken and Ruth, 54 yrs)

Relationship happiness, as couples suggest, takes effort and managing expectations:

> The problem [message is] . . . if you're not happy, walk, not work on it. And I think [in] every relationship, you have to work on it constantly. (Sharon and Peter, 57 yrs)

> I would hate to be starting out now to maintain a relationship long term. Because when we started out we weren't well off. And we'd have a great time. Yes, happy with that. We didn't expect to have everything now. (Wayne and Frances, 42 yrs)

Table 5.2 Respondents answer the question "Regarding contentment, please tick all that apply"

	Number of respondents that selected this response
Even through tough times we've stayed content with each other	423
We have grown closer over the years	420
We have been content for the whole of our marriage	417
At first, we were very happy	184
Some things have been great in our relationship, others have been awful	178
The early years of having children were difficult on our relationship	169
We had an issue which threatened our relationship but we are now closer	149
Things got better in our relationship when the children left	106
We grew apart at one stage, but we're back on track	92
We have drifted apart over the years	74
When children left home it was difficult on our relationship	58
We had an issue which threatened our relationship and things will never be the same	47
We've had a rough time but stayed together for the kids	46
We had an issue which threatened our relationship, we're still working through it	39
I have been disappointed with marriage altogether	34

In the online survey, 931 respondents rated our descriptors of relationship contentment (Table 5.2).

Of interest is the top three in Table 5.2. These clearly indicated growing happiness over years. According to Table 5.2, relatively few couples have drifted apart. More than three times as many couples are closer after a threatening issue than things never being the same. Although our information does not encompass couples who have separated, Table 5.2 suggests that things have generally improved for these couples in spite of adversity. Few stayed together for the children and even fewer are disappointed with their marriage. Divorce is always an option, yet these couples still choose to stay together.

Each couple's experience is unique. The subjective nature of happiness, contentment or satisfaction aside, our findings indicate a positive happiness trajectory for long-term relationships in couples choosing to be together. This supports recent evidence.[63] Effort is, however, still required. Happiness in relationships is, we posit, dependant on underlying commitment and attachment and built over years of forging pro-relational values together. These ideals become the subject of Chapters 6 and 7.

Conclusion

A thriving long-term relationship is being committed to make it work even when, at times, you do not feel the love. It is a comfortable slipper, a long quiet drive where you can almost hear each other's thoughts, or it can entail daily arguments. Adversity may threaten to tear a relationship apart, but teamwork can help overcome the despair of the death of a child, major physical and mental health issues, meddling in-laws, and even affairs. It is tough, hard work that leads to happiness and contentment. "The spark" may still be a steady flame in later years. Arguments may sometimes throw cups and yell hurtful words, yet even these can be accepted and managed. Laughing and talking both help and, even in opposing personalities, all is held together by committing to the long haul.

A long-term relationship is *abielu:* help and life. It is putting your needs on the backburner sometimes to balance selfishness and altruism in relational give and take. It reaches for individual and together-actualization:

> Building a lifetime relationship is the most worthwhile thing because you feel as though you've achieved something really good because the relationship is always growing. It's good for your self-esteem to know that you are achieving something that's really good and that it's really good for society. Not just for the couple, but for society as a whole. (Margaret and Ian, 57 years)

Notes

1 A full description of the methodology including recruitment, exclusion factors, limitations is given in the Introduction.
2 Heim, Caroline. *Audience as performer: The changing role of theatre audiences in the twenty-first century*. Routledge, 2016, 21, 22.
3 While the couple is credited collectively for the comments in this chapter, the name of the person who made the comment is always given first. The country born is also noted. The years the couples have been together is taken from the year of the interview.
4 Terman, Lewis Madison, Paul Buttenwieser, Leonard W. Ferguson, Winifred Bent Johnson, and Donald Powell Wilson. *Psychological factors in marital happiness*. McGraw-Hill Book Company, 1938.
5 Stinnett, Nick, Linda Mittelstet Carter, and James E. Montgomery. "Older persons' perceptions of their marriages." *Journal of Marriage and the Family* (1972): 665–670.
6 Lauer, Robert H., and Jeanette C. Lauer. "Factors in long-term marriages." *Journal of Family Issues* 7, no. 4 (1986): 382–390.
7 Roberts, William L. "Significant elements in the relationship of long-married couples." *The International Journal of Aging and Human Development* 10, no. 3 (1980): 265–272.

8 Rowe, G. P., and W. H. Meredith. "Quality in marital relationships after twenty-five years." *Family Perspective* 16, no. 4 (1982): 149–155.
9 For brevity, we have taken to liberty to re-label the findings. Klagsbrun, Francine. *Married people: Staying together in the age of divorce*. Bantam, 1985.
10 Alford-Cooper, Finnegan. *For keeps: Marriages that last a lifetime*. Routledge, 2016.
11 Lauer, Robert H., Jeanette C. Lauer, and Sarah T. Kerr. "The long-term marriage: Perceptions of stability and satisfaction." *The International Journal of Aging and Human Development* 31, no. 3 (1990): 189–195.
12 Fennel, D. L. "Characteristics of long-term first marriages." Paper presented at the *45th Annual American Association for Marriage and Family Therapy Conference*, 1987.
13 Wallerstein, Judith S. "The early psychological tasks of marriage: Part I." *American Journal of Orthopsychiatry* 64, no. 4 (1994): 640–650.
14 Mackey, Richard A., and Bernard A. O'Brien. *Lasting marriages: Men and women growing together*. Greenwood Publishing Group, 1995.
15 Kaslow, Florence, and Shlomo A. Sharlin. *Together through thick and thin: A multinational picture of long-term marriages*. Haworth, 2001.
16 Pillemer, Karl. *30 lessons for living: Tried and true advice from the wisest Americans*. Penguin, 2012.
17 Joel, Samantha, Paul W. Eastwick, Colleen J. Allison, Ximena B. Arriaga, Zachary G. Baker, Eran Bar-Kalifa, Sophie Bergeron et al. "Machine learning uncovers the most robust self-report predictors of relationship quality across 43 longitudinal couples studies." *Proceedings of the National Academy of Sciences* 117, no. 32 (2020): 19061–19071.
18 Mudd, Emily H., and Sara Taubin. "Success in family living – does it last? A twenty-year follow-up." *American Journal of Family Therapy* 10, no. 1 (1982): 59–67.
19 Humbad, Mikhila N., M. Brent Donnellan, William G. Iacono, Matthew McGue, and S. Alexandra Burt. "Is spousal similarity for personality a matter of convergence or selection?." *Personality and Individual Differences* 49, no. 7 (2010): 827–830.
20 Stanley, Scott M., Galena K. Rhoades, and Sarah W. Whitton. "Commitment: Functions, formation, and the securing of romantic attachment." *Journal of Family Theory & Review* 2, no. 4 (2010): 243–257.
21 See Lauer, Robert H., and Jeanette C. Lauer. "Factors in long-term marriages." *Journal of Family Issues* 7, no. 4 (1986): 382–390.
22 Duemmler, Sandra L., and Roger Kobak. "The development of commitment and attachment in dating relationships: Attachment security as relationship construct." *Journal of Adolescence* 24, no. 3 (2001): 401–415.
23 Darling Rasmussen, Pernille, Ole Jakob Storebø, Trine Løkkeholt, Line Gaunø Voss, Yael Shmueli-Goetz, Anders Bo Bojesen, Erik Simonsen, and Niels Bilenberg. "Attachment as a core feature of resilience: A systematic review and meta-analysis." *Psychological Reports* 122, no. 4 (2019): 1259–1296.
24 Stanley, Rhoades, and Whitton. "Commitment."
25 Reis, Harry T., Michael R. Maniaci, and Ronald D. Rogge. "Compassionate acts and everyday emotional well-being among newly-weds." *Relationships, well-being and behaviour*. Routledge, 2018, 207–233.
26 Acevedo, Bianca P., Michael J. Poulin, and Lucy L. Brown. "Beyond romance: Neural and genetic correlates of altruism in pair-bonds." *Behavioral Neuroscience* 133, no. 1 (2019): 18.
27 Wieselquist, Jennifer, Caryl E. Rusbult, Craig A. Foster, and Christopher R. Agnew. "Commitment, pro-relationship behavior, and trust in close relationships." *Journal of Personality and Social Psychology* 77, no. 5 (1999): 942.
28 Stanley, Rhoades, and Whitton. "Commitment."
29 Ibid.

30 Impett, Emily A., Shelly L. Gable, and Letitia Anne Peplau. "Giving up and giving in: The costs and benefits of daily sacrifice in intimate relationships." *Journal of Personality and Social Psychology* 89, no. 3 (2005): 327.
31 See as examples Riggle, Ellen D. B., Esther D. Rothblum, Sharon S. Rostosky, Jennifer B. Clark, and Kimberly F. Balsam. "'The secret of our success': Long-term same-sex couples' perceptions of their relationship longevity." *Journal of GLBT Family Studies* 12, no. 4 (2016): 319–334. Rosen-Grandon, Jane R., Jane E. Myers, and John A. Hattie. "The relationship between marital characteristics, marital interaction processes, and marital satisfaction." *Journal of Counseling & Development* 82, no. 1 (2004): 58–68.
32 Peifer, Corinna, Gina Wolters, László Harmat, Jean Heutte, Jasmine Tan, Teresa Freire, Dionísia Tavares et al. "A scoping review of flow research." *Frontiers in Psychology* 13 (2022).
33 Keeler, Jason R., Edward A. Roth, Brittany L. Neuser, John M. Spitsbergen, Daniel James Maxwell Waters, and John-Mary Vianney. "The neurochemistry and social flow of singing: Bonding and oxytocin." *Frontiers in Human Neuroscience* (2015): 518.
34 Ogolsky, Brian G., Shannon T. Mejia, Alexandra Chronopoulou, Kiersten Dobson, Christopher R. Maniotes, TeKisha M. Rice, Yifan Hu, Jaclyn C. Theisen, and Carolina Carvalho Manhães Leite. "Spatial proximity as a behavioral marker of relationship dynamics in older adult couples." *Journal of Social and Personal Relationships* 39, no. 10 (2021): 3116–3132.
35 Heim, Caroline. *Actors and audiences: Conversations in the electric air*. Routledge, 2020.
36 Girma Shifaw. "Marital communication as moderators of the relationship between marital conflict resolution and marital satisfaction." *The American Journal of Family Therapy*, (2022): 1–12; Stanley, Scott M., Howard J. Markman, and Sarah W. Whitton. "Communication, conflict, and commitment: Insights on the foundations of relationship success from a national survey." *Family Process* 41, no. 4 (2002): 659–675.
37 Karney, Benjamin R., and Thomas N. Bradbury. "Research on marital satisfaction and stability in the 2010s: Challenging conventional wisdom." *Journal of Marriage and Family* 82, no. 1 (2020): 100–116. Wallerstein, Judith. *The good marriage: How and why love lasts*. Plunkett Lake Press, 2019. Gottman, John. *The seven principles for making marriage work*. Hachette, 2018.
38 Grover, Shawn, and John F. Helliwell. "How's life at home? New evidence on marriage and the set point for happiness." *Journal of Happiness Studies* (2014): 1–18.
39 Heim, *Audience as performer*, 137.
40 Johnson, Heather A., Ramon B. Zabriskie, and Brian Hill. "The contribution of couple leisure involvement, leisure time, and leisure satisfaction to marital satisfaction." *Marriage & Family Review* 40, no. 1 (2006): 69–91.
41 Hatch, Laurie Russell, and Kris Bulcroft. "Does long-term marriage bring less frequent disagreements? Five explanatory frameworks." *Journal of Family Issues* 25, no. 4 (2004): 465–495.
42 Kurtz, Laura E., and Sara B. Algoe. "Putting laughter in context: Shared laughter as behavioral indicator of relationship well-being." *Personal Relationships* 22, no. 4 (2015): 573–590.
43 Hall, Jeffrey A. "Humor in romantic relationships: A meta-analysis." *Personal Relationships* 24, no. 2 (2017): 306–322.
44 For a discussion of sex as a measure of health of your relationships and people shamed for not have enough sex in marriage see Finkel, Eli J. "The all-or-nothing marriage." *The New York Times* 14 (2014): 102–103.
45 Heim, *Audience as performer*, 133.

46 Loh, Chin Ee, and Baoqi Sun. ""I'd still prefer to read the hard copy": Adolescents' print and digital reading habits." *Journal of Adolescent & Adult Literacy* 62, no. 6 (2019): 663–672.
47 Brien has since passed away.
48 Mintz, Steven, and Susan Kellogg. *Domestic revolutions: A social history of American family life.* Simon and Schuster, 1989, 203.
49 Yankelovich, Daniel. *New rules: Searching for self-fulfillment in a world turned upside down.* Random House, 1981, 101.
50 Smith, Ralph E. *The subtle revolution: Women at work.* Rowman and Littlefield, 1979.
51 See for example Pfeffer, Carla A. " 'Women's work'? Women partners of transgender men doing housework and emotion work." *Journal of Marriage and Family* 72, no. 1 (2010): 165–183.
52 Blom, Niels, and Belinda Hewitt. "Becoming a female-breadwinner household in Australia: Changes in relationship satisfaction." *Journal of Marriage and Family* 82, no. 4 (2020): 1340–1357.
53 Bianchi, Suzanne M., Melissa A. Milkie, Liana C. Sayer, and John P. Robinson. "Is anyone doing the housework? Trends in the gender division of household labor." *Social Forces* 79, no. 1 (2000): 191–228.
54 Rauer, Amy, Allen K. Sabey, Christine M. Proulx, and Brenda L. Volling. "What are the marital problems of happy couples? A multimethod, two-sample investigation." *Family Process* 59, no. 3 (2020): 1275–1292.
Lehman, Darrin R., Camille B. Wortman, and Allan F. Williams. "Long-term effects of losing a spouse or child in a motor vehicle crash." *Journal of Personality and Social Psychology* 52, no. 1 (1987): 218.
55 Ibid.
56 Namkung, Eun Ha, Jieun Song, Jan S. Greenberg, Marsha R. Mailick, and Frank J. Floyd. "The relative risk of divorce in parents of children with developmental disabilities: Impacts of lifelong parenting." *American Journal on Intellectual and Developmental Disabilities* 120, no. 6 (2015): 514–526.
57 Lebow, Jay, and Douglas K. Snyder, eds. *Clinical handbook of couple therapy*, 6th edn. The Guilford Press, 2022, 412.
58 Cohen, Orna, Yael Geron, and Alva Farchi. "A typology of marital quality of enduring marriages in Israel." *Journal of Family Issues* 31, no. 6 (2010): 727–747.
59 Eve has since passed away.
60 Duncan, Simon, Miranda Phillips, Julia Carter, Sasha Roseneil, and Mariya Stoilova. "Practices and perceptions of living apart together." *Family Science* 5, no. 1 (2014): 1–10.
61 Robins, Richard W., Avshalom Caspi, and Terrie E. Moffitt. "Two personalities, one relationship: Both partners' personality traits shape the quality of their relationship." *Journal of Personality and Social Psychology* 79, no. 2 (2000): 251. Gaunt, Ruth. "Couple similarity and marital satisfaction: Are similar spouses happier?" *Journal of Personality* 74, no. 5 (2006): 1401–1420.
62 Rosowsky, Erlene, Katherine D. King, Frederick L. Coolidge, Camille S. Rhoades, and Daniel L. Segal. "Marital satisfaction and personality traits in long-term marriages: An exploratory study." *Clinical Gerontologist* 35, no. 2 (2012): 77–87. Shiota, Michelle N., and Robert W. Levenson. "Birds of a feather don't always fly farthest: Similarity in Big Five personality predicts more negative marital satisfaction trajectories in long-term marriages." *Psychology and Aging* 22, no. 4 (2007): 666.
63 Karney, Benjamin R., and Thomas N. Bradbury. "Research on marital satisfaction and stability in the 2010s: Challenging conventional wisdom." *Journal of Marriage and Family* 82, no. 1 (2020): 100–116.

Part III

The techniques

Chapter 6

Techniques to build pro-relational values

Thriving Couples, as seen last chapter, value their comfort and peace. Love-relationships striving for comfort and peace is a universal theme of myths, legends, art, music, and research. Societies too value comfort and peace, and finding peace is also a universal theme of myths, legends, history, and research. The World Values Survey[1] is a program "devoted to the scientific and academic study of social, political, economic, religious and cultural values of people in the world."[2] It values peace and fosters it in the world. Couple therapists have the more modest aim of fostering peace within relationships.

The 'glue-secrets' articulated last chapter by thriving couples as contributing to relationship longevity were essentially values by definition. They served each couple "as guiding principles, . . . cognitive representations of basic motivations as goals to be pursued."[3] Couples did not tell us that these were values, yet these glue-secrets were used to guide their priorities, behaviours, and decision-making.

Values are highly relevant to individuals, society, couples, and to self-actualization. As Maslow pointed out,[4] self-actualization is values dependent: "The fully [self-actualized] human being working under the best conditions tends to be motivated by values which transcend [the] self."[5] Each step in Maslow's hierarchy involves values. Self-actualization arguably occurs when something of what is valued is achieved. Likewise, together-actualization occurs when what is valued together is fulfilled together.

This chapter journeys through three major areas: from values in individuals and values in society to values in thriving couples. Along the way we consider values in the brain, how values are chosen and how we, as individuals, as a society, and as couples, deeply value our long-term relationships. It considers values in couple therapy and its growing shift from valuing conflict resolution, communication, and behaviour change, to valuing attachment, acceptance, and shared values. The chapter then presents over 35 techniques to help couples build pro-relational values. These are based on thriving couples' glue-secrets and on clinical experience to help contemporary couples build resilient relationships and escape hyper-individual binds.

DOI: 10.4324/9781003263395-10

Individual values

Values are "goals and ambitions with a moral connotation"[6] and imperatives of what "ought to be."[7] We leave the fingerprints of our values on everything we do.[8] They inform but are distinct from our personality.[9] Our definition is:

> Values are culturally-inherited principles, refined by choice and important to individuals, couples or societies, to guide priorities, goals, behaviours, and decisions.

Values can be ideals (loyalty), legal principles (do not steal), leisure-based (have fun), socio-political (equality), workplace-based (greed is good), relational (be kind to others), and more. We naturally feel that others 'ought' to live by certain values, particular our own, while knowing that values vary from person to person. This leads to clashes and conflict. A list of values is endless. They are instilled into children by parents, teachers, collective history, culture, beliefs, the legal system, societal trends, and more. As we grow, we accept or reject our parents' and others' values while forming our own unique value system.

If we realize it or not, anything we say, do, decide, or prioritize is based on our value system. As an added complexity, at times we can and do transgress our own values. Values shape our opinions and our motivations. To catch a glimpse of how this happens, we peer into the brain.

Individual choice: the orbito-frontal cortex

Our personal value system is refined by choices made in our orbito-frontal cortex (OFC),[10] the brain's decision-making centre.[11] As an over-simplification, the OFC has major inputs from frontal lobe thinking and limbic system feeling centres. It makes decisions after values-based consideration of options, information, feelings, personal values, beliefs, memories, and the environment. After a decision is made in the OFC, complex brain pathways signal the body into action. To this extent, we freely choose.

Our thinking and feeling, however, can be at odds with each other. This can lead to a situation where, driven by strong emotions or sensations (including sexual arousal), we may transgress our own well-thought-through values and rational choices. This is particularly the case when we are under the influence of a substance, another person's attractiveness, peer pressure, or social media ideas enhanced by engaging music and stunning visual effects.

We are not machines. Our values are, in a sense, culturally-inherited, rationally-chosen, emotionally-driven, and socially-influenced. We understandably do things against our own values to go along with a crowd or a person because we are social creatures who want to be accepted, loved, and to belong (Maslow's level 3). To negotiate this part of the human condition, and to help us be authentically ourselves, it helps to understand how easily our values and choices can be influenced and even manipulated. No brain is independent. Our brains 'map' each other in the anterior cingulate cortex so that we become connected.

Individuals valuing relationships

As individuals we value many things, and 'being in a relationship' is only one thing which we can value. As social creatures, we value our food, shelter, and safety (Maslow's levels 1 and 2), as well as sharing love, being part of humanity, belonging to a group and expressing ourselves within that group (level 3). We also value pleasure, health, and a certain amount of personal achievement and recognition (level 4). Amidst the infinite values we can have, we value couple relationships particular highly. This is true of almost all humans across time and place.[12] With exceptions, adults want to be in a relationship, and if that relationship is lost, it is usual to find another (except perhaps later in life). Over 75% of adolescents consider relationships extremely important.[13] The question is not whether we as individuals value long term relationships; we do, but

If we value them so highly, why are they so hard to find and keep?

More questions become relevant as we aim to fulfil competing values:

> Is relationship longevity compatible with sexual novelty?
>
> How can I balance valuing both my relationship and my career advancement?
>
> Can my relationship thrive when my family and friends don't like my partner?
>
> How can I nurture my relationship when there are so many other things I want?

Choices need to be made and a priority of values is needed. These help negotiate the tension between immediate gratification (limbic system pleasure) and long-term gratification (frontal lobe responsibility). It is in this tension that we can be particularly swayed by prevailing societal values looking to influence us.

Societal values

'Society' means 'community' as the sum of us together. Apart from this, it does not really exist as an entity in itself. The society-individual distinction is an ongoing conundrum for social philosophy.[14] To help understand this distinction, the glue-secrets presented last chapter may faithfully represent the 'society' of thriving couples, but they do not represent any one given couple. They are a consensus. Consensus "emphasizes connectedness and shared beliefs,"[15] but this is almost an anathema in hyper-individualism. Due to increased diversity, fewer individuals feel they are represented in society, so values clashes often occur.[16]

Yet something called 'society' exists. Societal values ideally reflect individual values, but the reality depends on power and influence. Previously, the 'church' held much power and influence and so it strongly influenced euro-centric values. Enlightenment societal values were shaped by emerging scientific and philosophical ideas. Victorian moral values were shaped by those in control: the church, the monarchy, and the aristocracy. In hyper-individualism, values are guided less by religious thinkers, philosophers, or scientists, but by more prevailing commercial and corporate interests due to the wonders of economic prosperity since industrialization. The extreme reach of the internet and social media gives much power and influence to marketing and advertising as tools used to influence individuals' decision-making.

Long-term relationships continue to be valued in society. This is according to the evidence of the multitude of individuals and couples still valuing them. Commercial and corporate interests may, however, value them less. Clinical evidence for this is the 'relationship versus career' bind many people find themselves in. I have dealt with this in people I treat many, many times.

Not everyone values hyper-individualism[17] as it erodes collective identities[18] such as couple relationships, even if these identities are dearly valued by individuals. It also excludes and limits trust and attachment.[19] In the light of this, each of us have the opportunity to choose our values regarding couple relationships rather than blindly accept prevailing attitudes. As Buddhist wisdom suggests, "open your arms to change but don't let go of your values."[20] Conservatism balances progressivism,[21] a multiplicity of values exists, and in the contemporary world there is little guidance for choosing among them[22] outside of our own selves. Making choices in today's society is a frightening and confusing responsibility. We are, as Sartre articulated some decades ago, "condemned to be free."[23]

As seen last chapter, many thriving couples emphasize the importance of shared values. Shared values in society, however, exist less and less. The "culture wars"[24] is society grappling with the clashes. How relationships should function, for example, is largely taken for granted,[25] and assumptions are being challenged. In modern mating and dating, for example, shared values and shared expectations can no longer be assumed.[26] Progressives and conservatives rely on different sets of values:[27] conservatives may find each other in places of worship, and progressives may find each other on social media. Between the extremes, a silent, frustrated majority tries to negotiate the misunderstandings.[28] The imperative is to be aware of personal values and prevailing societal values in seeking what is wanted in personal relationships.

Societal values: changing, evolving, and enduring

Some societal values change, others endure. Like genes, they evolve and spread by imitation with permutations; some decline, but most remain constant.[29] In 1970, for example, a meaningful life was highly valued by 85% of surveyed UCLA students, and finances were highly valued by 40%.[30] By 2010, a meaningful life was highly valued by 40% while finances were highly valued by 70%. Raising a family remained a high value for 70%. Society increases in prosperity, students see others valuing finances, and the value is imitated with mutation: 'I want to be rich as long as I don't contribute to climate change.' Some values evolve, some thrive, some survive, some die out. Upheavals in family life often result from changes in cultural values.[31]

These statistics exemplify changing values (finances and meaning) and enduring values (wanting to raise a family). The UCLA survey shows that family values are enduring. This value relates to the idea that we are social creatures. This too may change as more people begin to believe and enact the idea that population growth is a problem, and that the world may no longer be 'good enough' for children. Evidence on this change, however, is currently lacking.

Societal values change through science, culture, shared personal experience, and technology.[32] Darwin's theories, for example, greatly contribute to the decline of religious values.[33] Science evolves its values: pre-Popper theories were valued for certainty, now they are valued for resisting refutation and applicability.[34] Cultural values-changes are seen in fashion and art. That personal experiences change societal values is seen in the tendency for people to grow more conservative as they age.[35] Technology drives increased valuing of materialism, screen pleasure, travel, novelty, and social media opinions.[36] Pro-relational values, those which prioritize relationships, compete with the lure of materialism, pleasure-seeking, and valuing autonomy and immediate self-benefit. Through this, finding and maintaining couple relationships becomes more complex.

Values have evolved in professions working with couples: doctors, social workers, and psychologists among others.[37] The Hippocratic oath was drafted in an age without the ethical challenges of digital information recording, growing diversity, a loud public voice, resource allocation issues, and risk intolerance. Today, Hippocrates would, perhaps, have included some caveats to negotiate these complexities. Social work values have evolved from an early preoccupation with morality, through examining competing values and decision-making, to currently valuing risk management.[38] From its psychoanalytic roots and through a systems approach, family therapy now values diverse gender roles, divorce laws, inclusivity, and self-disclosure.[39] Individual values, however, remain paramount as therapists tend to emphasize their own values in their work.[40] What remains constant over decades, however, is valuing relationships.

Does society value long-term relationships and marriage?

Yes, society still values long-term relationships. Individually and as a whole, we are largely if not fully preoccupied with personal relationships. If society did not value long-term relationships, they would not be the subject of so many movies, series, songs, and more; and, as discussed in Chapter 3, they would not form in the first place, nor would we extend the right to marry to more and more people. In 2001, same-sex marriage was legalized in the Netherlands. By 2010, ten countries had legalized same-sex marriage, the USA in 2015, and by 2022, it was legalized in over 30 countries. This shows how much societies value marriage and relationships. Marriage correlates higher with life satisfaction and well-being[41] than being unmarried,[42] and relationships correlate with happiness.[43] Well-being, happiness, marriage, and relationships are all highly valued in society so access to marriage is rightfully extended.

The many decades of extensive research into couple relationships are further evidence of how highly relationships are valued. It is a huge field of ongoing research branching into more and more diverse areas. The myriad therapy frameworks developed to help couples is further evidence still. Each type of therapy intrinsically values relationship quality and longevity. In this, psychotherapy is fruitful to all society.

Values in psychotherapy

Psychotherapy, as an applied science, assumes values[44] as has long been known.[45] Essentially, therapists value therapy as an agent of change rather than, say, imprisonment. They value mental health, emotional well-being, individual and couple empowerment, personal growth, and skills. A psychotherapist chooses a modality not only according to its evidence-base but also according to their own personal values. They may choose psychodynamic psychotherapy if they value transference and insight, emotional-focussed couple therapy if they value emotions as the agent of change, acceptance and commitment therapy if they value acceptance and commitment, and so forth. Addiction psychologists particularly value freedom from addictions, psychodynamic psychotherapists particularly value personality change, and couple therapists generally value relationships.

Discussing assumed values helps therapeutic alliance:

> Can we agree that we all want what's best?
> Can we agree on some goals before trying to reach them?
> The treatment I will use values . . . are you comfortable with that?

Some couples may be better suited to say a behavioural, a values-based or an attachment-based approach. Ideally, one looks for the best-fit. Cultural, religious, generational, and intersectional diversities underlie the need for therapists to be values-aware[46] and to refer to sub-specialists when indicated.

Couple therapy: a shift in focus

Last century, the focus of couple therapy was on conflict resolution, communication, and behaviour change.[47] This century, the focus has shifted more towards attachment, commitment, and pro-relational values. We trace some of this shift.

From the 1930s, couple therapy was steeped in psychoanalytic conflict resolution.[48] In the 1960s, the focus shifted towards systems analysis. Cognitive and behavioural therapies of the 1970s opened up new possibilities in thinking, communication, and behaviour as empirical evidence was increasingly valued over theoretical frameworks.

A 1993 review article[49] found good evidence for behavioural couple therapy (BCT) and emotion-focussed couple therapy (EFCT), quoting 50% therapy success rates. BCT emphasized behavioural change and communication skills. This arguably led couples in the general public to believe they had a poor relationship if they communicated poorly, could not resolve conflict, or could not change behaviours. More recent evidence, however, shows that couples can thrive in spite of these difficulties.[50] Our findings strongly support this. The question then becomes:

> What are thriving couples doing well despite poor communication, ongoing conflict, and inability to change?

We suggest that thriving couples adapt, accept, and live out shared pro-relational values rather than change. They strengthen their attachment bond through facing adversity together and display commitment on an ongoing basis. In living out shared values, they enhance intimacy while retaining individual autonomy[51] enacted in a choice to remain together.

A 1998 review article[52] re-affirmed the efficacy of BCT and EFCT but discussed changing theoretical frameworks and study limitations: small effect and sample sizes, measurement problems and biases. It reiterated that too many treated couples remain distressed and questioned how much we scientifically understand about relationships. The sheer number of differing modalities is evidence of our lack of understanding: The *Clinical Handbook of Couple Therapy* (2022)[53] gives detailed explications of over 20 established therapies and mentions many more. If one therapy held ‘the answer’ to relationship quality and longevity we would use it alone.

Highlighting the importance of attachment in client-therapist alliance, in 2004 it was suggested[54] that therapy effectiveness depended not on treatment rationale but on client, therapist, and non-specific factors:

Client: learning style, perseverance, and compliance with tasks
Therapist: alliance-building, matching expectations, and emotional connection
Non-specific: emotional experience, cognitive mastery, behavioural regulation

To reflect progress made by 2012,[55] the effectiveness of EFCT was quoted as 75%,[56] a leap from the 50% noted in 1993. In 2020 it was articulated[57] that marital satisfaction does not decline with time, that good communication is not always necessary, and that findings are not generalizable across socio-economic groups due to the effects of accumulated life stressors.[58] A 2022 review article[59] described BCT, EFCT, cognitive-behavioural couple therapy, and integrative behavioural couple therapy as "well-established," while noting that real-world success rates were significantly less than in controlled conditions.[60]

EFCT, strongly underpinned by attachment theory, moves towards acceptance and pro-relational values by reframing conflict in terms of unmet need. A pro-relational values approach, discussed hereafter, is seen in relationship education programs[61] such as PREP.[62] Values are central to acceptance and commitment therapy (ACT). ACT for couples was articulated in 2008[63] and again in 2017[64] after randomized trials confirmed its effectiveness.[65] "Shared Values and Symbols" is one of Gottman's "Four Pillars of Shared Meaning"[66] and he offers a useful Shared Values Questionnaire.[67] Positive psychology couple therapy – emphasizing pro-relational values such as gratitude, love, authenticity, growth, and compassion – is being developed.[68] This reflects the shift in focus towards pro-relational values.

Our research findings are consistent with conceptions noting that behaviour change is difficult, that poor communication does not always lead to distress, and that improvements in these do not always improve outcomes.[69] Thriving couples, we surmise, adapt, accept, or adjust to each other's behaviours and communication limitations. Our findings support evidence showing that relationship satisfaction does not necessarily decline but can increase to a rich maturity.[70]

Interviewed couples clearly went through difficult times. All, however, have grown through their experiences. Attachment as a resilience-building resource in these couples took "time to emerge" and involved "trade-offs"[71] elsewhere in life: altruism in their lives, as shared in Chapter 5, involved forsaking some aspects of self for the relationship. Our findings are further evidence for the importance of pro-relational values in couple relationship education, as an adjunct to couple therapy,[72] and as part of a preventative approach.[73]

Couples tend to seek out therapists because they value their relationship. This choice often puts relationship needs ahead of individual wants.[74] All glue-secret values we articulated involved putting relationship needs ahead of individual wants.

Couples' values

Earlier we discussed how 'being in a relationship' was valued by individuals and that this value is reflected in society. A couple self-evidently values 'being in a relationship.' They are living out their value. They are two people wanting to stay together long-term but need to negotiate their own individual values as well, particularly at times of conflict.

To be in a long-term relationship, you allow another person to influence you and your personal value system. Choosing another person as a partner is consciously allowing and even wanting this. This seemingly limits your autonomy but actually enhances it if this is what you want to happen. When two people say 'I choose you' to each other, they become more of their autonomous selves. To unite further, however, they need to forge something together; a together-story. Together values become increasingly important. The relationship itself needs to be valued by each individual, and together, shared values need to be forged.

Couples married 40+ years stayed together through growing hyper-individual values: growing equality, materialism, social media, and no-fault divorce. They negotiated any resultant tensions with little or no guidance through together valuing their relationship and their glue-secrets values. They

Prioritized 'we' before 'me'
Negotiated shared values
Live out their shared values

Forming and maintaining a long-term relationship is a complex values-based choice made by two independent individuals. By discovering and negotiating shared values, these couples interlock their individual values. This, over time, added to their attachment bond; their together life-story. This is being pro-relational. It balances couple intimacy and individual autonomy[75] to enhance both. Autonomy facilitates couple intimacy[76] and is enhanced when togetherness is freely chosen. Shared values facilitate individual and together growth in two people choosing to be together. Essentially, shared values are pro-relational values.

Pro-relational values

Shared values and pro-relational values are not necessarily the same, but shared values in couples almost always tend to be pro-relational. Pro-relational values "put attachment security ahead of other values . . . [to] ultimately make or break [relationship] stability and satisfaction."[77] Consciously or intuitively, they help navigate relationship threats and values clashes.

Two sets of individual values can be in harmony, dovetail or clash. They can be

Relationship-neutral
Relationship-threatening
Pro-relational

Relationship-neutral values – 'I value fun, money, and sexual satisfaction' – neither enhance nor threaten the relationship. Relationship-threatening values – 'I value my career at all costs, my sexual satisfaction even outside the relationship, my self-fulfilment above the needs of other people' – place the relationship at risk if an individual lives them out. If they are a lower priority than the relationship – 'but I wouldn't do anything to harm our relationship' – the relationship is protected. Pro-relational values – 'I value our fun together, our shared trust, our sex-life, my partner's feelings' – protect the relationship and even nourish it.

The pro-relational glue-secret values of couples we interviewed and surveyed

Half of UK married couples do not make it to forty years and 69% of cohabitating parents break up before their eldest is 17.[78] What values helped our thriving couples stay together?

1. Commitment
2. Altruism
3. Shared values
4. Communication
5. Compromise: give and take
6. Love
7. Never give up
8. Patience/forgiveness/tolerance
9. Teamwork
10. Respect

Many people may baulk at the absence of certain values. Values common in hyper-individualism – fun, sexual novelty, career development, financial success, kudos, and travel – are 'icing-on-the-cake' values and are not excluded. Some of our thriving couples also reach for these, but pursue them with pro-relational values (such as those hitherto listed) firmly in place. This becomes a priority of values: the relationship itself is valued highly so that it cannot be harmed by the pursuit of other values. With pro-relational values in place, all 'icing' values can then happily be pursued. With judgement and choice, a thriving couple can reach for both.

Younger couples, bewildered by a multiplicity of social media opinions and the pitfalls of hyper-individual errors and binds, may need permission to choose pro-relational values if relationship longevity is what they choose:

It's okay to do what you want
If sacrifice and perseverance work for you, that's okay
It's okay to choose to be altruistic
You can both put each other first if you want
Shutting out social media opinions can help improve a relationship
What's 'right' is what works for your relationship
It's okay to prioritize your relationship if you value it

The challenge is for each individual to integrate self-wants and partner needs by choosing pro-relational values as a priority over self-values. Nurturing attachment and keeping autonomy are both enhanced when each individual freely chooses couple togetherness. This shapes a together life-story towards together-actualization to build resilience.

Commitment + altruism + shared values

The top three glue-secrets are especially important to strengthening the attachment bond. Commitment, altruism and shared values directly strengthen the couple-bond. In our research, these three were the strongest glue-secret values by a significant margin.

Commitment

> Because my parents were divorced, commitment meant everything to me. I wasn't going to ruin anything good for any other self-pleasure, or be out there doing something that isn't me just to do it for me. (Judy and Jack, 60 yrs)

Commitment is intention to maintain the relationship. It involves personal desire, dedication to nurturing the relationship and restraint from harming it.[79] It involves "values and beliefs that promote persistence"[80] and is fundamental to attachment.[81] Clinical situations in my office indicate that just believing a partner intends to leave leads to insecurity and compensatory behaviours.

"Commitment readiness"[82] is a useful concept when deciding whether to enter a long-term relationship. People become commitment-ready when they think they are running out of options,[83] so a world of perceived limitless possibilities breeds commitment-phobia.[84] Once committed, however, continued commitment requires altruism: delaying gratification, long-term perseverance, personal sacrifice, and reconciling positive and negative relationship aspects.[85] In this, commitment, altruism and attachment are linked.

Altruism

Altruism leads to positive interactions, deepened trust, relational safety, and attachment.[86] It involves what Bowlby called the "caregiving system"; the willingness to fulfil another's needs, protect and soothe a partner, and foster their personal growth.[87] This requires personal effort for the longer-term gain for two. Abuse situations aside, the most selfish thing two people can do for their long-term selves, is to nurture their partner and their relationship.

'Sacrifice,' a term used by the thriving couples, holds little currency in hyper-individualism. With growing intimacy, the willingness to sacrifice grows,[88] but making sacrifices still comes at a cost. It is easier to put effort into the things we cherish.[89] Cherishing, valuing something dear, was implicit in couples interviewed: "For our vows it was love, honour and cherish" (Debby and David, 48 yrs). Through cherishing, altruism is strongly linked to commitment and attachment.

Shared values

Shared values lead to relationship longevity through increased satisfaction.[90] Sharing values is enjoyable,[91] pro-relational, and is often the glue in bi-cultural couples.[92] Sharing values is more than liking the same things, it involves inhabiting a shared reality[93] while preserving individual autonomy and together intimacy.[94] Selfishness preserves individual identity, altruism preserves relationship identity, while shared values link the two.

Shared values involve "intuition" brain connectivity:[95] "we tend to gravitate to the same values" (Merv and Margaret, 59 yrs), "sharing values is being on the same wavelength" (Helen and George, 48 yrs). As an oversimplification, each of our brains holds a subjective representation of the objective world. Sharing values means sharing more of each other's subjective representations. This engenders trust. Through this, couples share subjective reality: "we formed our values together" (Annette and Bernie, 60 yrs). Living out shared values over decades cements underlying attachment through increasing shared reality. This may be how a relationship becomes a peak[96] life experience.

These three – commitment, altruism, and shared values – are strongly linked to attachment. Commitment and attachment reinforce each other,[97] altruism deepens attachment,[98] and sharing values cements commitment[99] and attachment through brain connectivity. These help couples negotiate hyper-individualism, social isolation, and the mental health crisis through an attachment anchor. More shared reality widens the safe harbour from which to explore the world.

One-off historic commitment, however, does not suffice. Relationships require daily displayed commitment, altruism, and shared values through availability and responsiveness:[100] "relationship longevity becomes prima facie evidence of the partner's availability and commitment."[101] With day-to-day availability and responsiveness, attachment strengthens. After decades of commitment + altruism + shared values, relational security approaches the safe haven provided in carer-infant dyads:[102]

> I'm happy just knowing that I have the safety of that commitment. (Beverly and Alan, 46 yrs)
>
> I just find our relationship is very safe for me, and lovely. (Albert and Clare, 40 yrs)

VALUES-BASED TECHNIQUES FOR RELATIONSHIP LONGEVITY

These techniques enhance pro-relational values based on the Surviving COVID-19 Survey couples' questions (Chapter 4), Thriving Couples Interview insights (Chapter 5), Married 40+ Years Survey, literature evidence, and Dr Christian Heim's clinical experience. Discernment for the appropriateness of any technique for a given couple is always assumed. Each technique can be adapted as a hand-out or written out as needed.

Techniques appear under four headings:

1. Techniques for individual and shared values
2. Techniques based on glue-secret values
3. Therapist values
4. Getting out of hyper-individual binds presented in Chapter 1

1. TECHNIQUES FOR INDIVIDUAL AND SHARED VALUES

These techniques are for awareness of individual and shared values and for fostering pro-relational values and handling values clashes.

Armed with my values

Knowing our most important values helps guide priorities, goals, behaviour and decision-making. The acronym, ARMED with my values, helps uncover them.

Admire. What do I most Admire in myself and others?
Right thing. What do I believe is the Right thing for me to do?
Motivation and Meaning. What Motivates me and fills my life with Meaning?
Esteem. When do I feel full of Esteem and self-respect?
Dying. If I knew I would Die soon, what would become important to me?

It is also helpful to know personal values regarding our relationship.

Admire. What do I Admire in our relationship when it works well?
Right thing. What do I believe is the Right thing for us to do?
Motivation and Meaning. What is Motivating and Meaningful about us together?
Esteem. When do I feel full of Esteem about our relationship?
Dying. If I were to Die soon, what would I want in our relationship?

Our shared values

This technique is for awareness of each other's values: "when we don't agree on a value, we talk it through" (David and Wendy, 41 yrs). A couple can work individually first, then discuss values together.

What are my values?
What do I believe are my partner's values?
What values did I bring into the relationship from my family and culture?
What values have I received from my partner?
What values do we share and which have we forged together?
What are our together-values; where do we clash?

Forging pro-relational values #1

Evidence suggests the following values enhance relationship resilience:

Commitment[103]
Honesty[104]

Authenticity[105]
Respect[106]
Trust[107]
Open communication[108]
Mutual emotional support[109]
Gratitude and forgiveness[110]

Do we value these in our relationship?
Can we value some of these more?

Forging pro-relational values #2

When values align, it is easier to move forward: "With our children, we're always a united front. If there's an issue of discipline or whatever else, we definitely work as a team. We don't play one off against the other" (Merilyn and Gregory, 50 yrs). Consider the following areas:

Balancing independence and interdependence
Our work/life balance
Love, sex, and intimacy
Travel and entertainment
Where we feel at home
Interacting with family and friends
Finances
Parenting

What are my values in these areas?
What are my partner's values in these areas?
Where are we together, where do we clash?

Forging pro-relational values #3

Couples married 40+ years told us that these were their top values:

1. Commitment
2. Altruism
3. Shared values
4. Communication
5. Compromise: give and take
6. Love
7. Never give up
8. Patience/forgiveness/tolerance
9. Teamwork
10. Respect

Which of these values are relevant to us?
Could these become more relevant to us in decades to come?
What will we value in decades to come?
Can we work towards some of these values now?

Valuing shared rituals

Resilience is increased in couples valuing small shared interactions to affirm attachment:

> Touch him and kiss him and just tell them how much they mean to you. Yeah, and going to bed, even if we sometimes have words, give each other a hug and kiss and say sorry. And we say "see you in the morning." (Lana and George, 50 yrs)
>
> Touch for no reason at all when you're walking past your partner. Also just turn around and have a hug for no reason at all. (Lynette and Graham, 46 yrs)
>
> Show love during the day not just in bed. Know what your partner likes, communicate, take time. (Online survey)

What small rituals do you share that show you belong together?
Do you share in-jokes, secret touches, or do you have pet names for each other?
What special little things do you do to show your love?

Think from the same side of the fence

In a long-term relationship, you begin to know your partner's point of view:

> You put a different value on things as you mature. And I think we've learned to sort of think from the same side of the fence. (Ted and Marge, 56 yrs)

The fence tends to be values clashes. Ideally, you discuss values before committing to the relationship. Often this does not happen. People change their values, or only discover them later. Clashes need to be managed.

When a clash comes up:
Can you write down the clash?
Do you agree this captures the clash?
Where is this issue on your priority list of values?
Can a compromise be found?
Can someone choose to be altruistic in this?

What will help prevent future resentment?
Can you think from the same side of the fence?

Valuing laughter and play

Laughter and play works; value it. Humour shares happiness, defends against anxiety, and helps forgive.[111] Even after 40 years, couples have fun: "we're very wacky and don't take ourselves too seriously" (Helen and George, 48 yrs). They developed their own together-humour language. Play can be competitive or non-competitive. Positive, affirming humour is helpful.[112]

Ask:

What silliness or humour did you share early in your relationship?
Can you rekindle some of that?
Can you rediscover each other's laughter and play?
What activities leave you laughing and joyful together?
Can you be competitive without power struggles?
Is playfulness part of your love-making?
What is your 'together-humour?'

Handling value clashes, A – G

Value clashes are inevitable in two autonomous individuals:

> I guess we can clash sometimes. But it's not that one of us has to be right or wrong, as long as it works. You know, it can work that way. It can also work this way. It's just looking at it from the two different perspectives. (Nicia and Juanito, 48 yrs)
>
> She's more of a gift purchaser, I'm more frugal. (William and Mildred, 40 yrs)
>
> He wants to climb mountains and paraglide, I want to stay at home. (Lee and Gunter, 52 yrs)
>
> I like dancing, Fred doesn't. (Stella and Fred, 42 yrs)
>
> His communication style is more indirect and mine is more direct. That drives him crazy. (Ruth and Russell, 40 yrs)

Behind each of these comments is a values clash. Negotiating this requires give and take. Acknowledge the clash, blame no-one, and gently discuss and understand it. Handling clashes is summed up from A to G:

Acknowledge and be Aware of the clash
Blame no-one
Calmly Communicate the Clash

Discuss it to understand it
Empathize. Aim for 'me too, I feel that too, I understand.'
Feelings underneath need to be Fine
Generously Give and take to move forward

2. TECHNIQUES BASED ON GLUE-SECRET VALUES

These techniques aim to enhance the top ten glue-secret values as articulated by thriving couples interviewed and surveyed.

Techniques based on glue-value 1: Commitment

These techniques enhance commitment. Without commitment, there is no relationship; the greater the commitment, the greater the relational safety. Commitment has two components:

1. An outer shell that others see: 'we live together,' 'we're a family,' 'we wear rings'
2. An inner shell that cannot be seen: 'we feel attached,' 'we belong,' 'we share intimacies,' 'we consider each other'

Our contract

As discussed last chapter, couples together 40+ years often revisited marriage vows to get through tough times. Every long-term relationship starts with written and/or unwritten contracts: to live together, sexual exclusivity, an assumption to not be abusive, and to add value to each other's lives. A couple can reread vows or articulate underlying assumptions. They may draft up a new commitment contract with or without exclusion clauses and cooling off periods. They may have a re-commitment ceremony and take time away to celebrate:

> On our 50th we renewed our vows. The first [time] was really a business transaction. It's terrible, isn't it? But love is more important: we've been together all these years. (Irene and Harry, 55 yrs)

Commit to the person you fell in love with

It may be difficult for two people in conflict to commit to each other now, but once upon a time, they fell in love: "Sometimes you think people change so much, they can't see that person they married in the other one anymore. I can still see that person in Allen" (Beverly and Allen, 46 yrs).

> The person you fell in love with is right in front of you, perhaps under layers of anger and resentment. Can you commit to that person inside while working on things now?

Valuing my investments

Couples together 40+ years stuck through hard times. This increased the value of the relationship until it became their greatest asset.

How much have you already invested in this relationship?
Do you recall good times you enjoyed and hard times you've survived?
What led you to value the relationship so much?
How has your relationship increased in emotional and monetary value?
What would it take for you to value the relationship more?

The wedding cake

"To put icing on the cake, after all these disagreements we went on our first two-week cruise in the Pacific" (Alex and Alexandra, 58 yrs). Commitment in a long-term relationship is like a wedding cake:

The icing is the fun, sex, travel, and novelty
The sponge is the cosy comfort of togetherness
The cardboard is the commitment-base to get through "all these disagreements" and problems. It isn't tasty, but without it, the cake could fall
You commit to the whole cake, not just to the icing
This analogy opens up discussion on 'taking the good with the bad'

Techniques based on glue value 2: altruism

"Considering the other person is more important than yourself, that's a basic guiding principle . . . love is giving rather than love is taking" (Gary and Ruth, 54 yrs). Altruism is a response to attachment[113] and balances our selfish genes. Altruism benefits self[114] to be part of self-actualization[115] and together-actualization. The following techniques help to be more giving.

Appreciate your partner

It helps to notice and appreciate your partner for no particular reason: "He will put his hand out to me all the time, and I tell him how much I appreciate it. It is just a lovely thing" (Kay and Keith, 52 yrs) and "I told him as we walked out of the lecture: you're my precious treasure" (Marilyn and Gerry, 49 yrs).

Generously appreciate your partner. Honestly compliment them for their mind, personality, emotions, aspirations, and body. Be grateful for how they enrich you. Tell them positive things you may think but not share. Say 'thank you' to them often.

Don't kick the cat

"Maybe they had a hard day at work, the stress . . . things that are going on that might be driving your partner's behaviour . . . try to understand things or see things through their eyes" (Mildred and William, 40 yrs). In stress, we are able to give to others less. Stress, however, needs to be discharged to keep you free to give to others rather than take things out on them. That is what this technique is about.

Pressure at work builds up, so your boss yells at your colleague, who then yells at you, you come home and yell at your partner, who yells at your eldest child, who yells at your youngest child, who kicks the cat. This is an anger chain. It would have been less painful if your boss came home with you to kick your cat.

Between work and home is an important transition time, an opportunity to discharge frustrations so you can be more giving to others. Here are some suggestions:

Workout at the gym before coming home
Walk in a park and talk out the day's frustrations
Dance-along to loud music in the car on the way home
Swim, jog, shower, or take the dog for a walk as soon as you get home
When working from home, at finish time, do any of the above
Don't dampen frustrations with alcohol or cannabis
Don't let anyone kick your cat

THANKS morning and night

This acronym is a reminder to use gratitude in a relationship: "If ever I felt unhappy about something Russ had said or was doing, I would pause and make a list of all the things that I appreciate in him. Then I would often forget to be upset" (Laura and Russell, 50 yrs). Brain imaging shows that gratitude is linked to altruism to benefit self and others.[116] The acronym is 'THANKS morning and night.'

THINK about how precious your relationship is
HELP your partner
APPRECIATE them
NOTICE their beauty and fine points
KEEP perspective; see the bigger picture
SAY 'thank you' to them often
Morning, say 'thanks' for a new day in relationship
Night, say 'thanks' for a day experienced together

Try not to hurt

"To show Helen I love her, sometimes it's just an improvement in my behaviour. Yeah, you really have to work at it" (George and Helen, 48 yrs). This technique requires monitoring words and actions: "Yeah. And I know I'm a self-opinionated, egotistical bastard. But I have mellowed a lot" (Peter and Sharon, 57 yrs). This is difficult to do.

1 Aim not to intentionally hurt your partner:

   Try not to manipulate or control, criticize or blame, be mean or cynical, withholding or distant, vindictive or resentful. Try not to stomp around in anger or gaslight. Be aware of the impact of your words and actions. Mellow. Try it just for one day first

2 For couples in a better space, aim not to hurt unintentionally:

   Try not to be too direct or indirect, too controlling or too lenient, too energetic or too quiet. Try to be less of whatever it is that your partner finds difficult in you or more of what they need. Try it for one day

Techniques based on glue value 3: shared values

This has been covered in the techniques for individual and shared values.

Techniques based on glue value 4: communication

Say it with style

"I used to push him after five minutes and say, 'why aren't you responding?' And then I got to the point of saying, 'Okay, I'm not gonna push.' I finally decided that's his nature. . . . I have accepted that" (Yin-Len and Mike, 48 yrs). Yin-Len shifted to acceptance. This technique shifts away from trying to communicate well to accepting communication styles (while trying for small, helpful adjustments):

1 Know your communication styles.

What's my communication style, what's my partners?
What do I say through words, innuendo, gestures, tone of voice, looks, or behaviours?
Am I a direct communicator or more indirect?
How is my style influenced by my culture and family background?
Am I stuck in any unhelpful communication patterns?

2 Accept each other's communication styles. Can I accept that . . .

. . . my style is okay?

. . . my partner's style is okay?
. . . our styles can get in the way of love?
. . . even if things don't change, we can still have a good relationship?

3 Try to adjust for my partner.

Can I try to adjust something in my communication style for my partner? As suggestions:

Put negatives into words, not actions (say "I'm angry" rather than slam doors)

Put positives into actions (say 'I love you' and do something to show it)

Lighten up when things go wrong

Say 'oh well, that's just our different styles' (or choose a helpful phrase)

Use humour and touch

Say what you mean and mean what you say

Be more direct when you tend not to be

Be more circumspect when you tend to be too direct

Be kind rather than use truth as a weapon

Speak more truth rather than say things just to be nice

Notice and respond when your partner does things that say 'I love you'

In any of these, you may fail, but the love is in the trying

4 Value adjustments made by your partner. Making adjustments takes real effort. Notice and appreciate their effort: 'Thanks, I really appreciate it'

Learn to listen

Every therapist learns listening skills. Couples could benefit from them too, but it takes a lot of effort.

> With all the therapy and things, I've learnt how to listen, and now, I find it much more important to listen to what means something to him, rather than trying to find it out in an argument. (Frances and Wayne, 42 yrs)
>
> Listening wasn't quite so easy at home because I just wanted to solve problems. I wanted to fix it. So I had to learn. And Helen will allude to the fact that I may not have been overly successful. (George and Helen, 48 yrs)

Here are six basic principles of listening.

1 The EARS roadmap: Establish an Environment to talk and listen
   Ask questions so they talk 80% of the time
   Reflect their responses in their words
   Summarize the situation and say 'have I got it?'
2 Listening is "being there" for the other person
3 Listening is not a two-way conversation; it is a one-way street
4 Listening means shelving your beliefs and judgments
5 Listening is not problem-solving
6 Listening takes trust

Accept conflict

LANA I'm still listening to the same old repetitive stuff. It still goes on. I'm still listening . . . still.
KEITH Those things never go away. (49 yrs)

It may surprise younger couples, but thriving couples can still argue about 40 year old issues. Much conflict is never resolved, it needs to be accepted, listened to, and carried by two.

What are some of your unresolved issues?
Can you adapt, accept, or adjust rather than solve?
What would it take to see unresolved conflict simply as part of a together-story?

Techniques based on glue value 5: compromise: give and take

These techniques help compromise:

> If I want an orange wall and he wants a brown wall, you stop and think. You can't just dig your heels in demand: "I want orange and I'm having orange." Because it's just going to make him miserable. So you say, "okay, well, then green, I can live with that." So we compromise. (Carol and Stephen, 40 yrs)

A long-term relationship makes demands: not sleeping with others, not being overly controlling, and not being abusive. These demands limit freedom just like the law limits your freedom to drive on the wrong side, shop while naked, or to steal. In a close, personal relationship, both people make demands, so give and take and compromise become norms.

I prioritize you

You do not have to be there every minute for your partner, you just have to let them feel that, above anything else, you would be there for them if that is what they need: "If anything comes up where there's either a desire or need to be together, we drop everything and do it" (Don and Paula, 57 yrs).

Ideally, in a long-term love-relationship, it's your job to love them the way they want to be loved and it's their job to do the same for you.

> Is your partner your number one priority?
> How can you make sure they know and feel that they are?

More give, less take

"It's give and take, but you have to be more prepared to give" (Gaetano and Dorothy, 49 yrs). Giving is difficult. Sometimes, some things are never given and a partner gives up asking. Aim not to give up on each other. At any time, you can decide to give more and take less:

> Share more thoughts and feelings (or keep things more contained)
>
> Be more enthusiastic about sex (or less demanding)
>
> Be more direct in communication (or less)
>
> Find more solutions to problems (or offer less solutions to listen more)
>
> Each person's task in a relationship is to love the other person the way they need and want to be loved. In the best relationships, two people aim to fulfil each other.
>
> Could you each find a relationship area where you could give a little more and take a little less?

Techniques based on glue value 6: love

No romance pressure

As seen last chapter, romance does not have to be a part of every relationship in narrow, clichéd, commercialized terms. It may be more important to be kind, thoughtful, or considerate. Forcing romance is counter-productive:

> I always wanted the whole romance, I wanted the movies. And Howard was from a different family, different feelings, and that wasn't important to him. And that bothered me at first. . . . I think I've really had to relearn what's really important, because I understood that he still loves me very

> much; and I might not have gotten flowers on a certain day, but then one day he surprises me with something big. (Peggy and Howard, 48 yrs)

> We do things together and we focus on each other's best points. And that, to us, is most important for romance. (Monte and Jeneen, 45 yrs)

> We think of each other a lot, try and help, because I think we're always trying to think how we know how the other one feels. That's our romance. (Bruce and Susan, 49 yrs)

ALLEN I guess I've never been that romantic . . . she doesn't like it. Wouldn't want me to bring home flowers. But on the other hand, it is something that I kind of wish I did more.

BEVERLY I'm not romantic. I don't think I required that, no, *he cries* sweetheart, . . . just as long as I have the commitment. (46 yrs)

Thriving couples found alternatives for clichéd romance. Some watch sunsets, give each other massages, or go to concerts together. Others spend time together, do favours for each other, walk together, compliment each other, travel together, or talk intensely:

> We used to go out, gaze in each other's eyes, and sit in a dark bar somewhere and dance. It's basically the same: we get together, we look at each other, we hold hands. I can't dance anymore. When you're 80 years old, your romance changes. (Tony and Pat, 54 yrs)

How important is romance to each of you, really?
What do you already do as a couple that says 'I love you'?
What could you do for romance without forcing it?

More love languages

Chapman's *The Five Love Languages*[117] shows that we express love in different ways: time, words, acts of service, gifts, and touch. Some other love languages expressed by our thriving couples include:

Forgiving your partner (Maria and Gennaro, 65 yrs)

Finding a middle ground (Anne and Ergun, 41 yrs)

Being grateful (Richard and Pearl, 42 yrs)

Deferring to your partner (Gary and Ruth, 54 yrs)

Laughing with your partner (Lucy and Frank, 55 yrs)

Doing large, unexpected favours (Yin-Leng and Mike, 48 yrs)

Learning to listen (Jack and Judy, 60 yrs)

Letting your partner shine when socializing (Heather and Lyle, 69 yrs)

Working together towards a goal or charity (Merv and Margaret, 59 yrs)

Knowing your partner well (Sharon and Peter, 57 yrs)

Fulfilling your partner's needs even more (Harry and Irene, 55 yrs)

What do you already do as a couple that says 'I love you'?
Do any of these love languages have meaning to you?

Techniques based on glue value 6: keeping the sex spark alive

Under the rubric of 'love' we have included techniques for approaching sexual intimacy. This was a pressing question from the Surviving COVID-19 Survey, and insights from the Married 40+ Years Survey on this topic were enlightening. Sex is highly valued. It did not rate as a glue-secret but is, perhaps, an 'icing' activity needing the support of pro-relational 'cardboard' values underneath.

Pro-relational values do not kill the sex spark: sex, romance, and commitment run together,[118] and consistent with evidence,[119] most thriving couples were sexually active. Frequent sex was important for some, but not for the majority. Many accepted diminished sexual activity due to medical conditions. To others, sex was a secret garden.

Talk about it

The number one tip regarding sex from the 40+ Years Married Survey was to talk about sexual wants and needs:

Don't always "expect" one knows what the other needs or wants.

Don't be embarrassed: this is the person you are going to be together with for the rest of your life.

Talk about your needs and be playful. Always consider the other first.

Talk . . . about what you want and what [they] want, and meet in the middle. (Online survey)

Do you know each other's sexual and emotional wants and needs?
Do you feel you fulfil each other sexually and emotionally?
Can you accept things the way they are or do things need adjusting?

Sexual give and take

Sex becomes a battleground if someone demands or withholds. It flows more easily with give and take. Love-making is protective, caring, sharing, and pro-relational. Thriving couples bring their values into their love-making: commitment, altruism, shared values, communication, compromise, patience and forgiveness:

> You have to sort of compromise if one wants it, and the other doesn't. (David and Wendy, 41 yrs)
>
> You do need to work on what the other needs because it's often quite opposite to what your needs are. (Sharon and Bob, 46 years)
>
> Love your partner unconditionally. (Online Survey)
>
> Sex is the most important part of life. So, for full intimacy, try to see her with full romanticism and sink with her into full fun and wildness. (Online survey)

When does sex work for both of you? Can you do more of that?
Can you be more giving in sex? What does that mean to you both?
Can you be more patient and forgiving in sex?
Can you be more altruistic, communicative, and loving?

Kitchen foreplay

Foreplay can start during the day, in the kitchen, with a spark in your eyes, or with words to build connection:

> Sexual intimacy is not just intercourse. Take time to touch, stroke, pat, and cuddle throughout the day, even for a few seconds. (Online survey)
>
> I'll be in the kitchen and Graham will turn up the music and we'll dance to the music in the kitchen, just us two. Then we move and dance around the dining room. (Lynette and Graham, 46 yrs)

Can I tenderly prepare my partner for a romantic night?
Do I convey my love as well as my desire?
Can we fulfil both in each other?

Just keep having sex

Things had slowed down greatly for many thriving couples, but a few told us they "just keep having sex" (Online survey) or they "do it at least occasionally" (David and Wendy, 41 yrs) or "always have some sort of sex" (Online survey). Others described the attraction:

> Life is still very romantic for us . . . I make him very happy in bed. (Laura and Russell, 50 yrs)
>
> I still find Jo very attractive . . . I'd like to jump her all the time" (Rob and Jo, 47 yrs).
>
> He's quite a romantic. Very good in bed. (Frances and Wayne, 42 yrs)

Here are some suggestions:

> Dissolve the day's problems to focus on each other. Make the time. (Online survey)
>
> Make love when you don't feel like it. (Online survey)
>
> At our age it's still good, we still explore each other's bodies, keep the romance. (Online survey)

Vaseline for the doors

Creating time and space for love-making is a challenge with children around; however, it's worth protecting intimate moments. Here's what some couples remember:

> We took a packet of [treats], and threw them on the floor. And put Vaseline on the door handle so the kids couldn't open it. (Sharon and Peter, 57 yrs)
>
> Make time for love, romance and sex. Get away together or send the kids away. (Online survey)

Naughty dreams

Sex is an activity and "a place you go"[120] together. As Alex explained with a grin: "I discuss anything. Even the naughty dreams I might have" and Alexandra smiles (58 yrs). Through imagination, telling stories, sharing secrets, and rekindling earlier memories, a couple can go places together no matter their age. Some exciting embellishment helps. During love-making, you can

Retell the story of an adventurous shared encounter
Embellish it
Narrate a story based on your partner's desires
Share your naughty dreams and fantasies

Our secret garden

As we saw last chapter, many couples keep their sex lives a secret. It may be problematic for some, but others prefer to keep things private. A few surveyed couples told us they use role-play, explicit material, and sex toys. Being in a long-term relationship has not killed the spark for many couples:

> Now that we're into each other a lot more, we're "sexual partners" again. (Veronne and Wayne, 42 yrs)
>
> It's changed of course. Nobody can keep that up. We'd be dead. (Mary and Brian, 50 yrs)

> It doesn't have to be the physical full-on penetration. You can have sex six million different ways and still satisfy one another. (Jo and Rob, 47 yrs)
>
> We wear ourselves out early. . . . All you guys burn out because you're so rabid when you're younger . . . it's still very nice and it's still there. . . . I think we all need to encourage intimacy as it's an important part of marriage no matter what age. (Gregory and Merilyn, 50 yrs)

Techniques based on glue value 7: never give up

These are covered next chapter.

Techniques based on glue value 8: patience/forgiveness/tolerance

Patience, tolerance, and forgiveness are closely related to altruism but are more specific in practice: it takes altruism to not hurry someone or not be demanding, it takes altruism to allow things in your partner you find disagreeable, it takes altruism to let go of strong negative emotions to forgive. Many couples saw these as essential to relationship longevity:

> Her patience is amazing. Her patience to put up with me. I wouldn't put up with a bloke like me. (Jorge and Patty, 47 yrs)
>
> *Avec patience tu vas passer au travers.* (with patience you will get through) (Online survey)
>
> Well you have to be tolerant of each other's individual aspects. If one person likes something that you don't like, either learn to like it or tolerate it, don't fight over it. (Jack and Carole, 54 yrs)
>
> Forgiveness of the other and then being able to forgive yourself. (Online survey)
>
> Being able to forgive each other, I think that's one of the biggest things. It's very hard, you have to really work at it. (Anjelika and Graeme, 46 yrs)
>
> I think you do need to learn to forgive quickly, not hold on to things. . . . Don't let things fester. (Sharon and Bob, 46 yrs)

Forgiveness repairs relationships[121] and has health[122] and well-being benefits.[123] It is not just a decision; it is a process. After much research and clinical work, I developed a forgiveness technique involving a journey of seven steps.[124] Depending on the hurt, moving through these steps can take many months. Forgiveness can be the focus of therapy, particularly in working through an affair.

Can I forgive?

There is growing evidence that forgiveness is an effective way of moving forward. But it is not just a decision, it is a process of seven steps involving the will, thoughts and emotions. It starts with a decision, but then it moves forward through these questions. Can I . . .

1 Decide to forgive?
2 Accept the reality of what happened?
3 Understand why this may have happened?
4 Pardon from a position of power, like a judge or queen?
5 Give a sacrificial gift of forgiving?
6 Let go of anger, resentment, and bitterness?
7 Overlook this to focus on life's bigger picture?

The love is in the trying

This technique is a catch-phrase to help patience and tolerance.

> You don't need to get everything right in your relationship, but you do need to genuinely try. This shows you care: 'The love is in the trying.' Say this whenever your partner tries and especially when they fail. Say this at times you feel yourself needing to be patient and tolerant with your partner. If you fail yourself, remember: 'the love is in the trying.'

Techniques based on glue value 9: Teamwork

These are covered next chapter.

Techniques based on glue value 10: Respect

Strangers again

A relationship begins as two strangers, then familiarity grows. After years, however, someone may become a stranger again: reveal a deep secret, share a repressed hope, behave hurtfully, reveal an affair. A couple in conflict can feel like strangers: 'do I even know this person?' Respect allows a partner their otherness; it is a form of *xenia*, hospitality love. Respect can be difficult to extend to someone very familiar. In conflict, however, it is needed:

> We each respect if one of us doesn't agree with the other. (Kathy and Jim, 43 yrs)
>
> If you really do love someone, they get respect from you, and you give respect to them. I think it comes back to respect. (Samantha and Timothy, 51 yrs)

We respect each other: allowing each of us that space to do our own thing. Not be controlling of each other. Yeah. That's the main thing. (Pauline and Denis, 44 yrs)

What does respect mean to you?
How did you respect each other when you first met?
How do you respect each other now?
Can you respect differences of opinion, taste, style, and manner?
How did you handle discovering new or difficult things about each other?
During conflict, do you feel like strangers again?
Can you allow separateness until you're familiar again?

Tolstoy's respect

Leo Tolstoy had much psychological insight. In his novel *Anna Karenina*, he wrote that "Respect fills a void in a marriage where passion should be."[125]

Respect, by its nature, keeps boundaries:

I won't touch you unless you want me to
I won't impose my opinions on you
I will let you be yourself even if I do not like it
Tonight, if you agree, we could make love

Passion, by its nature, crosses boundaries:

I want to hold you and kiss you right now
I'll tell you all my thoughts and feelings, tell me yours
I don't want to leave you alone, I feel for you deeply
I want us to make love right here and now

It feels wonderful to have someone respect the full, separate person you are; it also feels wonderful to have someone love you passionately: "Respect is the nuts and bolts, . . . and then as you grow with the respect, then you allow yourself a little bit more freedom" (Chuck and Marion, 44 yrs). Both are desirable, but this becomes a balance: respect for independence and passion in inter-dependence. Some people are very respectful, others more passionate. Both work within a relationship. With flexibility and insight, more of both is achievable.

Are you happy with the respect-passion balance in your relationship?
At what times are you passionate, when are you respectful?
If you are not very passionate, can you feel okay about that?
Would you like more respect or more passion?
Can you add flexibility to increase both?

3. THERAPIST'S VALUES

These techniques examine therapist values and how they impact therapy. The aim is to be values-aware.

What do I value?

What are my personal and professional values?
How do I show that I value personal relationships?
How much do I value and respect others' relationships?
When do I believe a couple 'should' break-up or stay together?

'Should' invokes an ethical dilemma: who decides what 'should' be done? Couple therapy is bound by the ethics of the couple, the therapist, their professional body, the theoretical basis of modalities used, and the law.

A therapist's work is informed by personal experience.[126] Therapists naturally deal with varying degrees of relationship conflict in their own lives. Leading researchers have been divorced multiple times; others have been in the same relationship for more than forty years. One life experience always negates another. With awareness, any experience can inform practice to serve a couple's needs.[127] Self-awareness, supervision, and regular review of evidence help avoid biases.

How do my personal experiences cloud my objectivity?
Where are my personal experiences useful?
How do I keep perspective in a complex world?
Can I remain therapeutic no matter what my personal experience?

Applying my skills to myself

Therapists naturally apply their knowledge and skills to their own lives. Each modality adds insight, yet each falls short of human need. The aim is to keep perspective.

How much do I practice what I learn?
How difficult is it for me to apply my knowledge and skills in my own life?
How does this enhance my compassion for the people I serve?
What does this tell me about the limits of the work I do?

My work with diverse values

Beliefs and worldviews inform our values. Therapists need to negotiate others' beliefs, worldviews, and values as well as their own. Each relationship is unique and is informed by two people's worldviews, values, cultures, belief-systems, and more. Cultural, religious, and diversity groups have distinct approaches to relationships, and a relationship can cross two or more diverse groups.

> Do my values clash with those of the couple? With one partner?
> Can I shelve my values to serve the couple and their values?
> Do suggestions I make enhance, challenge, or affront their values?
> Can I begin to understand the world and their situation from their world-view?
> Is it appropriate for me to ask about cultural, faith, or diversity issues?
> Is referral to a faith, culture, or diversity-group specific therapist indicated?

4. GETTING OUT OF HYPER-INDIVIDUAL RELATIONSHIP BINDS

Here we consider the eight hyper-individual relationship binds articulated in Chapter 1. These insights are needed when a relationship seems pitted against self-wants or societal expectations. In each, the value principle is to choose to prioritize the relationship.

Bind 1

Can two individuals keep their individuality and values but stay together as a couple?

This pits self against partner in a false dichotomy. Relational contentment is part of individual contentment not contrary to it. When you make a conscious choice for togetherness, you enhance rather than diminish your own autonomy. These two ideas are explored.

Firstly, aside from hermits and solo explorers, few people are content to remain alone. For self-benefit, we choose a relationship. If the relationship thrives, we thrive as individuals. A relationship, however, needs effort to balance self-wants and partner-needs, give and take, and independence and inter-dependence. It takes forsaking immediate self-pleasure for long-term together-gain rather than forsaking your partner for yourself. In most cases, you either both win or you both lose.

Secondly, individual autonomy is enhanced if the togetherness is freely chosen.[128] 'I choose you' means that the 'I' doing the choosing is enhancing its autonomy, not diminishing it. Nurturing a secure, chosen, long-term relationship is one of the most worthwhile things two people can do to benefit and enhance themselves and each other:

> Building a satisfying relationship will give you more fulfilment than anything you might pursue individually. (Don and Paula, 57 yrs)

In practice, however, self-wants often *are* pitted against relationship-needs: a career move, doing something for yourself, values clashes, or prolonged self-indulgence. At these times, consider:

> What are the deal-breakers in our relationship?
> How do I expect my partner to react to this?
> Will this harm our relationship?
> How much do I value our relationship; am I devoted to it?
> Can I talk about this with my partner to get a 'we' perspective?
> Do I value being hurt, betrayed, manipulated, or railroaded?

Thriving couples often had to consider these things:

> I said "this Bed and Breakfast is causing too many disagreements with us. Either one of us buys the other one out, or we break up. But I will not stay with you under these conditions, I am too unhappy. I'm getting angry." He said, "I don't want the relationship to end." . . . So we sold it. (Steven and Chuck, 30 yrs)

The venture was causing harm; it became a deal-breaker. Options were considered and a hard decision was made. The relationship was valued.

Value clashes are inevitable in two autonomous individuals and cannot always be reconciled. With a higher priority value, valuing the relationship itself, a way forward may be found. Self-values often need to take a backseat to pro-relational values. This is hyper-individual judgment and choice shaping a together life-story reaching for together-actualization *and* self-actualization.

Bind 2

To pursue Maslow's self-esteem and self-actualization, I have less time for my love and belonging needs. Which do I choose?

Self-esteem and self-actualization are not set *against* love and belonging; both are desired. Getting love and belonging needs met and fulfilling them for someone else helps facilitate self-esteem and self-actualization. Impeding love and belonging needs leads to mental illness.[129] This is clearly an error. Many people, Maslow explains, are unaware that fulfilling love needs is part of reaching for higher needs.[130]

Bind 3

In hyper-individualism, can people freely choose for their partner to make decisions for them?

It may seem archaic, but in a long-term relationship, it is natural to flow with your partner and let them influence you and for you to influence them. This is how shared values are negotiated, and strengths are dovetailed: 'you budget, I'll take care of the social schedule.' You trust your partner with some things while they trust you with others. This strengthens attachment. Choosing to trust, however, can be difficult in practice:

JACK She likes to make decisions and I'm kind of "okay whatever you want."
CAROLE But you're very quick to say "let's talk about this" if you don't like it. (54 yrs)

In abuse and dependence, autonomy is progressively lost, whereas in interdependence, autonomy is enhanced. In hyper-individualism, you can do what you want with your autonomy, even share it with another person.

Bind 4

How can a couple strengthen their relationship-identity by challenging societal norms when the norm is 'anything goes'?

'Anything goes' as a societal norm may not exist. No matter what you do, there is always someone to criticize you: parents, jealous siblings, apparent friends, workplace gossipers, and others. Your individuation will always challenge someone. In the spirit of hyper-individualism, you can challenge others and even challenge hyper-individualism itself. One ideal is that, over time, your partner's opinion of you becomes more important than what others think of you. When your partner respects your decisions, you individuate and strengthen your identity in their eyes and in your own. This is in line with hyper-individualism if that is what you choose. It strengthens your attachment bond and your individuality.

Bind 5

How can the pitfalls of the psychology of affluence be avoided?

The main pitfall in the psychology of affluence is putting self-gratification first to such an extent that excessive choice and unrealistic expectations drive you towards depression, anxiety, loneliness, narcissism, nihilism, or lost relationships. These are errors. To protect against these, it helps to delay gratification and balance selfishness and altruism through pro-relational values. These maximize the relationship and the self. As couples explain:

> Don't count on material things making you happy because that's not the thing in life that counts. Have a loving relationship with your family, have a loving relationship with your friends. (Jim and Pat, 54 yrs)
>
> Relationships are a hell of a lot more important than how big our home is. (Chuck and Marion, 44 yrs)

Bind 6

In hyper-individualism, can people freely choose to put their partner's needs above their own?

In hyper-individualism, you can choose to do what you want with your autonomy. It is best to not blindly follow anything, not even hyper-individualism itself. Our evidence and Maslow and Bowlby show that being in a relationship brings self-fulfilment. It takes altruism to fulfil partner's needs above self-needs. Outside of enabling abuse, this is a sound choice to make. In thriving relationships, two people often put each other's needs above their own. In hyper-individualism, this choice can be freely made as it is self-serving in the long-term.

Bind 7

How can a couple choose to be we-focussed in me-focussed hyper-individualism?

Self-actualizing, as Maslow explained, almost always involves being in a good relationship. We-focussed couples are secretly living the dream: wanting the best for someone who wants the best for you. This gives life meaning, purpose, and vitality:

> If the two of us don't stick together like glue, life could be incredibly dreary, and sad. Every day, I wake up with the view of a positive thing and having fun. (Merilyn and Gregory, 50 yrs)
>
> She is the love, the beauty underneath everything I do. (Graham and Lynette, 46 yrs)

Bind 8

Why balance selfishness and altruism when hyper-individualism is all about me?

This question hits at the core of the me-versus-the-relationship dilemma. As evidenced by the pitfalls of hyper-individualism, unrelentingly putting yourself first is actually harmful to yourself. You are free to judiciously choose to harm yourself, but we do not recommend it. To benefit yourself long-term, delaying gratification works in your best self-interests.

A blind pursuit of immediate self-pleasure often results in error, harm and long-term pain. Taking amphetamines or heroin, for example, leads to immediate pleasure. but often, long-term misery. I have seen heroic recoveries in previously substance-dependent people who bravely focussed on worthwhile values: self-respect, creative self-expression, regaining family trust, or, in many cases, wanting to save a long-term relationship. Achieving this takes much delayed gratification.

A couple relationship involves continuous delayed gratification. Our thriving couples worked through mental illness, physical hardship, having children with severe impairment, the death of children, families trying to tear them apart, affairs, and more. Through adversity, they achieved gratification and climbed towards together-actualization and self-actualization. In this, a relationship uncovers the gold of working on something worthwhile:

> The relationship is more important than the satisfaction of perceived pleasures. (Don and Paula, 57 yrs)
>
> Why dig in a tin mine, when you own a gold mine? (Ted and Christine, 50 yrs)

Summary of values

The approach in this chapter is based on the premise that "you pull in different directions if you have different values" (Gary and Ruth, 54 yrs). In hyper-individualism, long-term relationships are still valued; being in a thriving long-term relationship is of great benefit to each individual. If, with judgment and choice, a couple forges pro-relational values and lives by them, both individuals grow toward together-actualization. The techniques presented here aim to enhance pro-relational values to build resilience. Couples thriving 40+ years exemplified this. How resilience was built in their lives is the subject of our final chapter.

Notes

1 https://europeanvaluesstudy.eu/ Retrieved 8 May 2022.
2 www.worldvaluessurvey.org/WVSContents.jsp Retrieved 8 May 2022.
3 Sagiv, Lilach, and Shalom H. Schwartz. "Personal values across cultures." *Annual Review of Psychology* 73 (2022): 517–546.
4 Maslow, Abraham Harold. "A theory of human motivation." *Psychological Review* 50, no. 4 (1943): 370–396.
5 Maslow, Abraham Harold. *The farther reaches of human nature*, vol. 19711. Viking Press, 1971.
6 Schroeder, Doris, Kate Chatfield, Michelle Singh, Roger Chennells, and Peter Herissone-Kelly. "The four values framework: Fairness, respect, care and honesty." *Equitable Research Partnerships*. Springer, 2019, 13–26.
7 Tsirogianni, Stavroula, and George Gaskell. "The role of plurality and context in social values." *Journal for the Theory of Social Behaviour* 41, no. 4 (2011): 441–465.
8 Attributed to Elvis Presley.
9 See Allport, Gordon W., Philip E. Vernon, and Gardner Lindzey. *Study of values*, 3rd edn. 1960. First published in 1931.
10 Brass, Marcel, Margaret T. Lynn, Jelle Demanet, and Davide Rigoni. "Imaging volition: What the brain can tell us about the will." *Experimental Brain Research* 229, no. 3 (2013): 301–312.
11 Hilgard, Ernest R. "The trilogy of mind: Cognition, affection, and conation." *Journal of the History of the Behavioral Sciences* 16, no. 2 (1980): 107–117.

12 Fisher, Helen. *Why we love: The nature and chemistry of romantic love*. Macmillan, 2004, 3.
13 Finkel, Eli J., Chin Ming Hui, Kathleen L. Carswell, and Grace M. Larson. "The suffocation of marriage: Climbing Mount Maslow without enough oxygen." *Psychological Inquiry* 25, no. 1 (2014): 1–41.
14 Hossain, F. M. Anayet, and Md Korban Ali. "Relation between individual and society." *Open Journal of Social Sciences* 2, no. 8 (2014): 130.
15 Stover, Sue, and Harriet Brown. "Consensus: In theory and practice." *Early Education* 53 (2013): 27–28.
16 See Baker, Wayne E. "America's crisis of values." *America's Crisis of Values*. Princeton University Press, 2013.
17 Throop, Elizabeth A. "Psychotherapy and hyperindividualism." *Psychotherapy, American culture, and social policy*. Palgrave Macmillan, 2009, 25–40.
18 Pakulski, Jan. "Postmodern social theory." *The New Blackwell Companion to Social Theory* (2009): 251–280, p. 277.
19 Liddell, Belinda J., and Bronte S. Courtney. "Attachment buffers the physiological impact of social exclusion." *PLoS One* 13, no. 9 (2018): e0203287.
20 Gill, Roger. "Change management–or change leadership?" *Journal of Change Management* 3, no. 4 (2002): 307–318.
21 Chae, Haesook, and Steven Kim. "Conservatives and progressives in South Korea." *Washington Quarterly* 31, no. 4 (2008): 77–95.
22 van der Walt, Johannes Hannes L. "The search for a moral compass and a new social contract in the context of citizenship education." *HTS Teologiese Studies/ Theological Studies* 75, no. 4 (2019).
23 Sartre, Jean-Paul, and Philip Mairet. *Existentialism and humanism*. Methuen, 1960, 6.
24 Duffy, Bobby, et al. "Culture wars in the UK: How the public understand the debate." 2021. https://www.kcl.ac.uk/policy-institute/assets/culture-wars-in-the-uk-how-the-public-understand-the-debate.pdf Retrieved 27 December 2022.
25 Yodanis, Carrie, and Sean Lauer. "Is marriage individualized? What couples actually do." *Journal of Family Theory & Review* 6, no. 2 (2014): 184–197.
26 Thielmann, Isabel, Benjamin E. Hilbig, and Ingo Zettler. "Seeing me, seeing you: Testing competing accounts of assumed similarity in personality judgments." *Journal of Personality and Social Psychology* 118, no. 1 (2020): 172.
27 Graham, Jesse, Jonathan Haidt, and Brian A. Nosek. "Liberals and conservatives rely on different sets of moral foundations." *Journal of Personality and Social Psychology* 96, no. 5 (2009): 1029.
28 Private clinical communications.
29 Blackmore, Susan. "Evolution and memes: The human brain as a selective imitation device." *Cybernetics & Systems* 32, no. 1–2 (2001): 225–255.
30 Pryor, John H., Sylvia Hurtado, Victor B. Saenz, Jose Luis Santos, and William S. Korn. "The American freshman: Forty year trends." *Los Angeles: Higher Education Research Institute* 3 (2007).
31 Mintz, Steven, and Susan Kellogg. *Domestic revolutions: A social history of American family life*. Simon and Schuster, 1989, 205.
32 Calman, Kenneth C. "Evolutionary ethics: Can values change." *Journal of Medical Ethics* 30, no. 4 (2004): 366–370.
33 Downie, J. R., and N. J. Barron. "Evolution and religion: Attitudes of Scottish first year biology and medical students to the teaching of evolutionary biology." *Journal of Biological Education* 34, no. 3 (2000): 139–146.
34 Maxwell, Nicholas. "A critique of Popper's views on scientific method." *Philosophy of Science* 39, no. 2 (1972): 131–152.

35 Peterson, Johnathan C., Kevin B. Smith, and John R. Hibbing. "Do people really become more conservative as they age?" *The Journal of Politics* 82, no. 2 (2020): 600–611.
36 See, for example, Hanks, Craig, ed. *Technology and values: Essential readings.* John Wiley & Sons, 2009.
37 Calman, Kenneth C. "Evolutionary ethics."
38 Reamer, Frederic G. "The evolution of social work ethics." *Social Work* 43, no. 6 (1998): 488–500.
39 Doherty, William J. "Values and ethics in family therapy." *Counseling and Values* 30, no. 1 (1985): 3–8.
40 Ibid.
41 Dush, Claire M. Kamp, and Paul R. Amato. "Consequences of relationship status and quality for subjective well-being." *Journal of Social and Personal Relationships* 22, no. 5 (2005): 607–627.
42 Eckermann, Elizabeth. "Living alone and living together – Their significance for wellbeing." *Global handbook of quality of life.* Springer, 2015, 435–444.
43 Saphire-Bernstein, Shimon, and Shelley E. Taylor. "Close relationships and happiness." Susan A. David, Ilona Boniwell, and Amanda Conley, eds. *Oxford handbook of happiness.* Oxford University Press, 2013.
44 Wilholt, Torsten. "Bias and values in scientific research." *Studies in History and Philosophy of Science Part A* 40, no. 1 (2009): 92–101.
45 Strupp, Hans H. "Humanism and psychotherapy: A personal statement of the therapist's essential values." *Psychotherapy* 17, no. 4 (1980).
46 Redding, Richard E. "Sociopolitical values: The neglected factor in culturally-competent psychotherapy." *Prejudice, stigma, privilege, and oppression.* Springer, 2020, 427–445.
47 Lebow, Jay L., and Rachel M. Diamond. "Brief history of couple and family therapy." Fiese, Celano, Deater-Deckard, Jouriles, and Whisman, eds. *APA handbook of contemporary family psychology: Family therapy and training.* American Psychological Association, 2019, 3–18.
48 Gurman, Alan S., and Peter Fraenkel. "The history of couple therapy: A millennial review." *Family Process* 41, no. 2 (2002): 199–260.
49 Jacobson, Neil S., and Michael E. Addis. "Research on couples and couple therapy: What do we know? Where are we going?" *Journal of Consulting and Clinical Psychology* 61, no. 1 (1993): 85.
50 Karney, Benjamin R., and Thomas N. Bradbury. "Research on marital satisfaction and stability in the 2010s: Challenging conventional wisdom." *Journal of Marriage and Family* 82, no. 1 (2020): 100–116.
51 Kluwer, Esther S., Johan C. Karremans, Larisa Riedijk, and C. Raymond Knee. "Autonomy in relatedness: How need fulfillment interacts in close relationships." *Personality and Social Psychology Bulletin* 46, no. 4 (2020): 603–616.
52 Baucom, Donald H., et al. "Empirically supported couple and family interventions for marital distress and adult mental health problems." *Journal of Consulting and Clinical Psychology* 66, no. 1 (1998): 53.
53 Lebow, Jay, and Douglas K. Snyder, eds. *Clinical handbook of couple therapy,* 6th edn. The Guilford Press, 2022.
54 Sprenkle, Douglas H., and Adrian J. Blow. "Common factors and our sacred models." *Journal of Marital and Family Therapy* 30, no. 2 (2004): 113–129.
55 McMahon, James, and Candice Siu Woo. "Introduction to counseling couples." *Cognitive and rational-emotive behavior therapy with couples.* Springer, 2012, 1–15.
56 Johnson, Sue. *Hold me tight: Your guide to the most successful approach to building loving relationships.* Hachette, 2011, 3.
57 Karney and Bradbury. "Research on marital satisfaction."

58 Hogendoorn, Bram, Matthijs Kalmijn, and Thomas Leopold. "Why do lower educated people separate more often? Life strains and the gradient in union dissolution." *European Sociological Review* 38, no. 1 (2022): 88–102.
59 Doss, Brian D., McKenzie K. Roddy, Stephanie A. Wiebe, and Susan M. Johnson. "A review of the research during 2010–2019 on evidence-based treatments for couple relationship distress." *Journal of Marital and Family Therapy* 48, no. 1 (2022): 283–306.
60 Bradbury, Thomas N., and Guy Bodenmann. "Interventions for couples." *Annual Review of Clinical Psychology* 16, no. 1 (2020): 99–123.
61 Markman, Howard J., Alan J. Hawkins, Scott M. Stanley, W. Kim Halford, and Galena Rhoades. "Helping couples achieve relationship success: A decade of progress in couple relationship education research and practice, 2010–2019." *Journal of Marital and Family Therapy* 48, no. 1 (2022): 251–282.
62 Markman, Stanley, and Blumberg. *Fighting for your marriage*, 294–317.
63 Harris, Russ. *ACT with love: Stop struggling, reconcile differences, and strengthen your relationship with acceptance and commitment.* New Harbinger Publications, 2009.
64 Lev, Avigail, and Matthew McKay. *Acceptance and commitment therapy for couples: A clinician's guide to using mindfulness, values, and schema awareness to rebuild relationships.* New Harbinger Publications, 2017.
65 Morshedi, M., R. Davarniya, K. Zahrakar, M. J. Mahmudi, and M. Shakarami. "The effectiveness of acceptance and commitment therapy (ACT) on reducing couple burnout of couples." *Iranian Journal of Nursing Research* 10, no. 4 (2016): 76–87.
66 Gottman, John M. and Nan Silver. *The seven principles for making marriage work.* Seven Dials, 2015, 263.
67 Ibid, 271–272.
68 Genç, Emel. "Transforming stress to happiness: Positive couple therapy with distressed couples." *Journal of Happiness and Health* 1, no. 1 (2021): 4–15.
69 Karney and Bradbury. "Research on marital satisfaction."
70 Proulx, Christine M., Ashley E. Ermer, and Jeremy B. Kanter. "Group-based trajectory modeling of marital quality: A critical review." *Journal of Family Theory & Review* 9, no. 3 (2017): 307–327. Williamson, Hannah C., and Justin A. Lavner. "Trajectories of marital satisfaction in diverse newlywed couples." *Social Psychological and Personality Science* 11, no. 5 (2020): 597–604.
71 Eastwick, Paul W., Eli J. Finkel, and Jeffry A. Simpson. "Relationship trajectories: A meta-theoretical framework and theoretical applications." *Psychological Inquiry* 30, no. 1 (2019): 1–28.
72 Halford, W. Kim, and Douglas K. Snyder. "Universal processes and common factors in couple therapy and relationship education: Guest editors: W. Kim Halford and Douglas K. Snyder." *Behavior Therapy* 43, no. 1 (2012): 1–12.
73 Mortazavi, Mahnaz, Roya Rasooli, Simin Hoseinian, and Hassan Zareei. "Effectiveness of the prevention and relationship enhancement program based on Gottman & Glaser's integrated approach to love, respect, and marital intimacy." *Journal of Applied Psychological Research* 11, no. 1 (2020): 137–149.
74 Solomon, Marion F., and Stan Tatkin. *Love and war in intimate relationships: Connection, disconnection, and mutual regulation in couple therapy (Norton series on interpersonal neurobiology).* W. W. Norton & Company, 2011, 46–47.
75 Goodman, Catherine. "Intimacy and autonomy in long term marriage." *Journal of Gerontological Social Work* 32, no. 1 (1999): 83–97.
76 Hadden, Benjamin W., Zachary G. Baker, and C. Raymond Knee. "Let it go: Relationship autonomy predicts pro-relationship responses to partner transgressions." *Journal of Personality* 86, no. 5 (2018): 868–887.

77 Solomon and Tatkin. *Love and war*, 46.
78 https://marriagefoundation.org.uk/half-of-todays-newlyweds-will-celebrate-their-ruby-anniversary-together/ Retrieved 5 May 2022.
79 Stanley, Scott M., and Howard J. Markman. "Assessing commitment in personal relationships." *Journal of Marriage and the Family* (1992): 595–608.
80 Stanley, Scott M., Galena K. Rhoades, and Sarah W. Whitton. "Commitment: Functions, formation, and the securing of romantic attachment." *Journal of Family Theory & Review* 2, no. 4 (2010): 243–257.
81 Duemmler, Sandra L., and Roger Kobak. "The development of commitment and attachment in dating relationships: Attachment security as relationship construct." *Journal of Adolescence* 24, no. 3 (2001): 401–415.
82 Hadden, Benjamin W., and Christopher R. Agnew. "Commitment readiness: Timing, the self, and close relationships." *Interpersonal relationships and the self-concept*. Springer, 2020, 53–67.
83 Brady, Ashlyn, Levi R. Baker, Christopher R. Agnew, and Benjamin W. Hadden. "Playing the field or locking down a partner?: Perceptions of available romantic partners and commitment readiness." *Journal of Experimental Social Psychology* 101 (2022): 104334.
84 Stanley, Rhoades, and Whitton. "Commitment: Functions, formation."
85 Bergeron, Sabryna, Audrey Brassard, Josianne Mondor, and Katherine Péloquin. "Under, over, or optimal commitment? Attachment insecurities and commitment issues in relationally distressed couples." *Journal of Sex & Marital Therapy* 46, no. 3 (2020): 246–259.
86 Bayraktaroglu, Deniz, Gul Gunaydin, Emre Selcuk, Miri Besken, and Zahide Karakitapoglu-Aygun. "The role of positive relationship events in romantic attachment avoidance." *Journal of Personality and Social Psychology* (2022).
87 Mikulincer, Mario, and Philip R. Shaver. "An attachment perspective on compassion and altruism." Gilber, Paul, ed. *Compassion: Concept, research and application*. Routledge, 2017, 187–202.
88 Righetti, Francesca, John K. Sakaluk, Ruddy Faure, and Emily A. Impett. "The link between sacrifice and relational and personal well-being: A meta-analysis." *Psychological Bulletin* 146, no. 10 (2020): 900.
89 Bhattacharyya, Pratishtha, and Rabindra Kumar Pradhan. "Exploring cherishing: A qualitative approach." *The Qualitative Report* 24, no. 7 (2019): 1511–1536.
90 See Parry, Travis G. *The association between shared values and well-being among married couples*. Utah State University, 2016.
91 Gabb, Jacqui, Martina Klett-Davies, Janet Fink, and Manuela Thomae. "Enduring love? Couple relationships in the 21st century." *Survey Findings Report*. The Open University, 2013.
92 Brahic, Bénédicte. "The politics of bi-nationality in couple relationships: A case study of European bi-national couples in Manchester." *Journal of Comparative Family Studies* 44, no. 6 (2013): 699–714.
93 Rossignac-Milon, Maya, Niall Bolger, Katherine S. Zee, Erica J. Boothby, and E. Tory Higgins. "Merged minds: Generalized shared reality in dyadic relationships." *Journal of Personality and Social Psychology* 120, no. 4 (2021): 882.
94 Kluwer, Karremans, Riedijk, and Knee. "Autonomy in relatedness."
95 Hyon, Ryan, Yoosik Youm, Junsol Kim, Jeanyung Chey, Seyul Kwak, and Carolyn Parkinson. "Similarity in functional brain connectivity at rest predicts interpersonal closeness in the social network of an entire village." *Proceedings of the National Academy of Sciences* 117, no. 52 (2020).
96 Woodward, Anne J., Bruce M. Findlay, and Susan M. Moore. "Peak and mystical experiences in intimate relationships." *Journal of Social and Personal Relationships* 26, no. 4 (2009): 429–442.

97 Duemmler, Sandra L., and Roger Kobak. "The development of commitment and attachment in dating relationships: Attachment security as relationship construct." *Journal of Adolescence* 24, no. 3 (2001): 401–415.
98 Bayraktaroglu, Deniz, Gul Gunaydin, Emre Selcuk, Miri Besken, and Zahide Karakitapoglu-Aygun. "The role of positive relationship events in romantic attachment avoidance." *Journal of Personality and Social Psychology* (2022).
99 Stanley, Rhoades, and Whitton. "Commitment: Functions, formation."
100 Gunaydin, Gul, Emre Selcuk, Betul Urganci, and Sumeyra Yalcintas. "Today you care, tomorrow you don't: Differential roles of responsiveness variability and average responsiveness in romantic attachment." *Social Psychological and Personality Science* 12, no. 5 (2021): 839–849.
101 Fraley, R. Chris. "Attachment in adulthood: Recent developments, emerging debates, and future directions." *Annual Review of Psychology* 70, no. 1 (2019): 401–422.
102 Hazan, Cindy, and Phillip R. Shaver. "Attachment as an organizational framework for research on close relationships." *Psychological Inquiry* 5, no. 1 (1994): 1–22.
103 Farrell, Jennifer E., Joshua N. Hook, Marciana Ramos, Don E. Davis, Daryl R. Van Tongeren, and John M. Ruiz. "Humility and relationship outcomes in couples: The mediating role of commitment." *Couple and Family Psychology: Research and Practice* 4, no. 1 (2015): 14.
104 Chaney, Cassandra. " 'No matter what, good or bad, love is still there': Motivations for romantic commitment among black cohabiting couples." *Marriage & Family Review* 50, no. 3 (2014): 216–245.
105 Wickham, Robert E. "Perceived authenticity in romantic partners." *Journal of Experimental Social Psychology* 49, no. 5 (2013): 878–887.
106 Eckstein, Donna, Sarah Eckstein, and Daniel Eckstein. "Creating respect in couples: The couple's respect questionnaire (CRQ)." *The Family Journal* 22, no. 1 (2014): 98–104.
107 See Gottman, John M. *The science of trust: Emotional attunement for couples*. W. W. Norton & Company, 2011.
108 Schmidt, Christopher D., Wade Luquet, and Nathan C. Gehlert. "Evaluating the impact of the "Getting the love you want" couples workshop on relational satisfaction and communication patterns." *Journal of Couple & Relationship Therapy* 15, no. 1 (2016): 1–18.
109 Molden, Daniel C., Gale M. Lucas, Eli J. Finkel, Madoka Kumashiro, and Caryl Rusbult. "Perceived support for promotion-focused and prevention-focused goals: Associations with well-being in unmarried and married couples." *Psychological Science* 20, no. 7 (2009): 787–793.
110 Wu, Qinglu, Peilian Chi, Xiuyun Lin, Hongfei Du, Nan Zhou, Hongjian Cao, and Yue Liang. "Gratitude and satisfaction in romantic relationships: Roles of decisional forgiveness and emotional forgiveness." *Current Psychology* (2020): 1–9.
111 Turliuc, Maria Nicoleta, Octav Sorin Candel, and Lorena Antonovici. "Humour in romantic relationships." *The Palgrave Handbook of Humour Research* (2021): 325–340.
112 Martin, Rod A., Patricia Puhlik-Doris, Gwen Larsen, Jeanette Gray, and Kelly Weir. "Individual differences in uses of humor and their relation to psychological well-being: Development of the humor styles questionnaire." *Journal of Research in Personality* 37, no. 1 (2003): 48–75.
113 Wolfe, Alan. 'What is altruism?." Ott, J. Steven, and Lisa Dicke, eds. *The nature of the nonprofit sector*. Routledge, 2021, 381–392.

114 Aknin, Lara B., and Ashley V. Whillans. "Helping and happiness: A review and guide for public policy." *Social Issues and Policy Review* 15, no. 1 (2021): 3–34.
115 Maslow, Abraham. "Self-actualization and beyond." (1965).
116 Karns, Christina M., William E. Moore III, and Ulrich Mayr. "The cultivation of pure altruism via gratitude: A functional MRI study of change with gratitude practice." *Frontiers in Human Neuroscience* (2017): 599.
117 Gary, Chapman. *The five love languages: How to express heartfelt commitment to your mate*. Moody Publishers, 2009.
118 Campbell, Lorne, and Timothy J. Loving. "Love and commitment in romantic relationships." D. M. Buss, ed. *The handbook of evolutionary psychology: Foundations*. John Wiley & Sons, Inc., 2016, 482–498.
119 Sinković, Matija, and Lauren Towler. "Sexual aging: A systematic review of qualitative research on the sexuality and sexual health of older adults." *Qualitative Health Research* 29, no. 9 (2019): 1239–1254. Banerjee, Debanjan, and T. S. Sathyanarayana Rao. "'Love in the later years . . .': Perceptions of sex and sexuality in older Indian adults – a qualitative exploration." *Consortium Psychiatricum* 3, no. 1 (2022): 62–75.
120 Esther Perel. "The secret to desire in long-term relationship." *Ted Talk*. 15 February 2013. www.youtube.com/watch?v=sa0RUmGTCYY video.
121 Karremans, Johan C., and Paul A. M. Van Lange. "Back to caring after being hurt: The role of forgiveness." *European Journal of Social Psychology* 34, no. 2 (2004): 207–227.
122 Harris, Alex H. S., and Carl E. Thoresen. "Forgiveness, unforgiveness, health, and disease." Worthington Jr, Everett L., ed. *Handbook of forgiveness*. Routledge, 2007, 345–358.
123 Wade, Nathaniel G., William T. Hoyt, Julia E. M. Kidwell, and Everett L. Worthington Jr. "Efficacy of psychotherapeutic interventions to promote forgiveness: A meta-analysis." *Journal of Consulting and Clinical Psychology* 82, no. 1 (2014): 154.
124 See Heim, Christian. *7 steps to forgiveness (using neuroplasticity)*. Vivid Publishing, 2021.
125 Part Seven, Chapter Twenty-four.
126 See, as examples, Valente, Sharon M. "Psychotherapist reactions to the suicide of a patient." *American Journal of Orthopsychiatry* 64, no. 4 (1994): 614–621. Vamos, Marina. "The bereaved therapist and her patients." *American Journal of Psychotherapy* 47, no. 2 (1993): 296–305.
127 Lebow and Snyder. *Clinical Handbook of Couple Therapy*, 475.
128 Kluwer, Karremans, Riedijk, and Knee. "Autonomy in relatedness."
129 Maslow, Abraham Harold. "A theory of human motivation."
130 Ibid.

Chapter 7

Techniques to build resilient relationships

'How do I cope with pressure? Will our relationship last? Can you deal with the consequences?' These questions relate to resilience: a treasured commodity which cannot be bought, sold, stolen nor given away. It can, in a sense, be shared. For all our interest in more resilience for children, adults, and relationships, resilience is not fully understood. Some people who have a little more of it have their insights:

> The world is full of suffering but also full of overcoming – Helen Keller[1]
>
> She stood in the storm and when the wind did not blow her way, she adjusted her sails – Justice Elizabeth Edwards[2]

For survival, building resilience is a prerequisite, yet in prosperous thriving, we may be losing it. This paradox is explored after a maritime metaphor.

Seas off the east coast of Northern England are stormy and treacherous. In 1850 alone, 784 lives were lost from 681 shipwrecks.[3] The very next year, the Duke of Northumberland held a competition for a lifeboat design to withstand the tempests. The winning design, by James Beecher, had the inherent tendency to 'self-right' after being tossed about. This design principle has saved many lives.

Do people have a tendency to 'self-right' after life's tempests? Self-righting has been appropriated by writers in psychology and psychoanalysis to describe resilience,[4] the "inherent ability to rebound."[5] We all possess this tendency to some degree, but arguably, the climate has intensified. Can more resilience be cultivated in adults, children, and couple relationships to withstand today's tempests? To build more resilience, we look beyond mere stoic enduring for real resilience.

This is our last chapter. Readers have put in effort to digest previous chapters and now have had a small but significant experience of resilience. We invite each reader to examine the incentives which helped them reach this point. Our brain is wired to build resilience through two joint incentives: gaining pleasure and overcoming pain. Resilience seeks for longer-term

DOI: 10.4324/9781003263395-11

contentment while some social forces focus us more on shorter-term pleasures.

What contributes to relationship resilience? Our thriving couples' insights support the idea that "relationship resilience is founded upon the couple's mutual self-sense or 'we-ness.' "[6]

> A relationship is like an elastic band. You have to know how much it can stretch. You can't pull at it all the time and then be surprised at the consequences. You have to know how far to go. We now know each other so well. (Gaetano and Dorothy, 49 yrs)

This chapter gives an overview of the extensive yet inconclusive research into resilience, including psychological, social, biological, and evolutionary viewpoints. Resilience is strongly connected to attachment.[7] Childhood attachment helps build adult attachment[8] and resilience,[9] but deficits can be overcome. No life story is set in stone, and learning skills and overcoming obstacles is always possible. We present techniques to help build relationship resilience before closing with a consideration of together-actualization.

Resilience definitions

To some, resilience means to stoically "suck it up"[10] leading to victim-blaming. In the first year of the pandemic, for example, many health-care workers were caught in this misunderstanding: they heroically saved lives, yet felt guilty over their personal burnout[11] leading to tragic outcomes.[12] Resilience has become a "dirty word"[13] as young people in particular feel judged and called upon to 'just be more resilient.' Building resilience, however, is complex:

> Little adversity decreases resilience
> Mild to moderate adversity increases it
> Severe adversity may reduce or shatter it[14]

Myriad diverse factors impact this principle; generalizations are inadequate. One person's mild adversity may be someone else's severe adversity and individual exceptions abound. Yet this general principle is reliable enough to help explain how, in affluence, resilience can decrease.[15]

Resilience (Latin *re* + *salient*: "back" + "leaping") is not a personality or character trait. It is a "dynamic process encompassing positive adaptation within the context of significant adversity."[16] How much resilience an individual may or may not have can only be inferred from their functioning and how they withstand stress.[17]

Mental[18] and physical illnesses[19] are adverse consequences of stress; resilience is withstanding stress. As such, illnesses indicate a general lack of resilience.[20] Yet physical health and mental health do not necessarily indicate resilience but may indicate a level of untested resilience. Under enough stress, we would all fail. We each possess resilience to varying and limited degrees.

Our interviewed couples have bounced back from the death of a child, mental and physical illness, wartime displacement, financial ruin, an affair, significant cultural difference, in-law problems, and more. With individual variation, they overcame adversity by helping each other "adapt and maintain well-being during stressful life situations"[21] to enhance their togetherness and relationship stability.[22] Much of their self-righting resilience, however, may have been rooted in their early life experience.

Resilience in young children

In children, building resilience requires minimizing factors hindering development[23] and maximizing protective factors.[24] This already highlights the primacy of attachment, which becomes wired into developing brain networks.[25] Positive childhood experiences ameliorate adverse childhood experiences to build resilience.[26] They include a child having:

A family who acknowledges their feelings
A family who stands by them in difficult times
Community traditions in which they participate
A sense of belonging at school
Supportive friends
Genuine interest from two or more non-parent adults
Safety and protection provided by adults

These are attachment factors. If a child lacks resilience, the problem is not with the child, it is in the parental and societal factors failing to meet attachment needs. These positive childhood experiences make for resilient adult relationships.[27] Attachment failure, on the other hand, has devastating consequences:[28] 65–82% of children with a depressed mother, for example, develop a psychiatric disorder during childhood[29] and all remain at higher risk throughout adulthood.

In my clinical work, I invariably ask about someone's early life. The quality of their life and attachments at that time impact their whole lives. Clinical experience validates the evidence. Protective factors for childhood resilience include:[30]

Parental: being close, setting limits, able to soothe,[31] family cohesion[32]
Individual: intelligence, internal locus of control, easy-going, adaptable[33]
Social: close extended family, peer group, and after-school activities[34]

Involvement in religious and community groups is protective.[35] Chronic social disadvantage is problematic.[36] Early life experiences and role modelling set strong life tendencies, but these are not set in stone; resilience can always be built. Human resilience will continue to flourish while children's attachment needs continue to be met.

Childhood mental illness indicates a lack of resilience in children, but they are blameless.[37] One seminal study found that US children at home in the 1980s were more anxious than those taken to see psychiatrists in the 1950s.[38] This was due to "low social connectedness"[39] demonstrating "the singular importance of social bonds and attachment"[40] to resilience and illustrates how children in affluent societies may become less resilient. Because the change is over decades, however, we may eventually notice but feel powerless to change it. In this a subtle loss in resilience, as suggested in this study, mirrors the insidious nature of growing social isolation.

Children cannot be taught to be resilient as part of their education.[41] A lack of resilience is not due to ignorance, uneducated choices, or character weakness,[42] but due to accumulated risk factors or a lack of protective factors. Attachment and healthy families[43] protect brain development and resilience so much so that resilience and secure attachment walk hand-in-hand to affect the rest of a child's life.[44]

The effects of childhood attachment and modelling were seen in our thriving couples:

> I would say that the example of my parents helped, yes. And of Ian's parents, with their lifelong commitment to each other. (Margaret and Ian, 57 yrs)
>
> I was raised up in a family where my parents were very honest . . . and I told Ergun honesty is very important for me, I don't mind what the truth is but it has to be the truth. (Anne and Ergun, 41 yrs)
>
> I find most of my relationship issues go back to childhood fear. Because I came from a dysfunctional family, there was a lot of fear: being out of control, and not feeling like I had a voice. You can get lost. (Sharon and Bob, 46 yrs)

Adolescent resilience

Adolescence, the transition from childhood to adulthood,[45] is a time to develop skills to fulfilling others' needs while continuing to get one's own needs met. This is crucial to adult relationship success. Some brain circuits are pruned (amygdala-striatum) to decrease impulsivity, while others are strengthened (amygdala-prefrontal cortex) to increase self-regulation of complex emotions. These changes prepare for adult reasoning[46] and adult resilience, but make for emotional complications. To help cope, adolescents rely on their early childhood attachment experiences. Protective in adolescence are a sense of proficiency, family support, positive peer interactions, and having positive role models. Risks include low self-esteem, low parental support, and underdeveloped social skills.[47]

Societal changes such as lowered age for voting, drinking, and independent medical consent place more of an adult burden on adolescents. This is not, however, matched by a growth in meeting their immediate attachment needs, as evidenced by the loss of family cohesion through shared meals mentioned in Chapter 3. This makes the adolescent task as a transition to adult reasoning and resilience that much harder.

Finding romantic attachment in late adolescence or early adulthood is a marker of resilience. Success in this depends on secure childhood attachment.[48] Not finding a love relationship in early adulthood is a predictor of anxiety and depression[49] and poor attachment predicts life-long singleness.[50] Society must, however, provide structures and opportunities to find genuine attachment.

Resilience for humans, adolescents included, is the norm.[51] In a tendency to look for problems, we overlook that child holocaust survivors can thrive in adulthood without mental illness,[52] people with disabilities can obtain actualization, and children can become adults forging relationships lasting more than 40 years. Up to 70% of children growing up with significant adversity develop social competency,[53] and at-risk children become more not-at-risk.[54] The safe harbour of attachment as a shelter from adversity facilitates self-righting.[55]

Parenting impacts on resilience

Protecting children too much from adversity does not build resilience.[56] 'Cotton wool' parenting may seem to benefit an infant or toddler but does not build resilience for the future adult.[57] For resilience, a Goldilocks approach is just right: not too much and not too little adversity.[58] Mild adversity prepares for severe adversity as small failures build resilience for larger ones. Parents need not plan adversity for their children, however; life usually presents enough of it. When a 'good enough' parent provides secure attachment safety rather than an impenetrable protective shield, a child will encounter adversity and withstand it as well as possible.

Children of divorced parents are at increased risk of problems,[59] but most children of divorced parents do well.[60] As children grow to adulthood and choose their own values, individual choice and values become more important:

> My parents split up. So I never want to go through that trauma. So yeah, commitment is the glue for us. (Keith and Lana, 49 yrs)

> My parents were divorced. But I wasn't going to let that happen because I knew what it was like to grow up without a father present, even though my father was a good father. I wasn't going to let that happen, so I worked hard on that. (Judy and Jack, 60 yrs)

Resilience in adulthood

Adult resilience stems from childhood and adolescent resilience. Skills learnt and choices made, however, become more important.[61] Protective to adults are all previously discussed factors, and individual competence in these.[62]

Certain physical illnesses can be directly linked to childhood attachment trauma (particularly abuse and neglect).[63] Depression, obesity, diabetes, hypertension, and heart disease *may* have their genesis in childhood attachment trauma in the following way[64]

> Childhood abuse or neglect leads to
> Feeling anxious, worthless, and hopeless leads to
> Overeating, smoking, alcohol or drug misuse leads to
> Mental and physical illness and relationship difficulties

'Don't smoke, don't take drugs and don't overeat' may be sage advice, but the pertinent question is: 'how do I stop feeling bad after what happened to me as a child?' This merits emphasis: knowing the 'right thing to do' is not enough, the real obstacles have to be discovered, understood, and overcome. In this, secure attachment in adulthood can be powerfully ameliorating:

> As a child, I suffered rape, neglect and homelessness under Pinochet's regime but I've never seen a psychiatrist. I'm surrounded by the love of my husband, children and grandchildren. Their love is a healing bath I take every day. (54 year-old Isidora is a university professor)

Childhood vulnerability is ameliorated by secure adult attachment.[65] Professor Isidora is remarkably resilient and science does not fully understand this. Yet attachment now, in her present, compensates for previous trauma. Children, adults, all of us are adaptive. Everyone can build resilience through strengthening our close relationship ties. This may alleviate some of the need for excessive unhealthy coping mechanisms.

The continued use of unhealthy coping mechanisms is reflected in binge drinking. As several young adults have told me in my office: "at 30 I stopped binge drinking because I thought 'it's time to grow up.' " This may represent an extended time of transition to responsible adulthood, to make up for attachment losses in adolescence. This may also give insight into the tendency to commit later to a long-term relationship.

Overcoming adversity builds resilience

Adapting to or overcoming adversity is the very mechanism of survival. Our brains can remarkably rewire to learn new skills and adapt. Children who experience trauma, for example, can become exceptionally resilient through learnt attention, perception, memory, and problem-solving skills.[66] People who grew up in chaotic environments, for instance, may have adapted their thinking to be able to shift topics effortlessly.[67] This becomes a worthwhile skill. Rather than stigmatize, we can discover the "hidden talents"[68] and strengths of anyone who grew up in adversity, and likewise the "hidden strengths" of any particular couple who have gone through adversity.

Learning from experience builds resilience. What is unknown is how personal choice and experience interact to determine who learns to move forward and who does not or which couples thrive when others break-up (see Jo and Rob, 47 yrs in Chapters 1 and 5). What is certain, however, is that avoiding adversity means avoiding an opportunity to increase resilience. Couples working through thorny issues are, by definition, more resilient than previously: "adversity drives the commitment" (Graeme and Anjelika, 46 yrs). Facing fears, then, holds promise not only for treating and overcoming anxiety and PTSD but for building resilience in the brain.[69]

Nietzsche's maxim "what doesn't kill me makes me stronger"[70] reflects reality but needs qualifying. Perseverance after failure predicts future success[71] but people suffering severe adversity are rarely physically stronger, though they may become mentally and emotionally stronger. Adversity effects each of us uniquely and generalizations are inadequate. The presence or not of resilience is not a value judgment (although it feels like it) but is a reflection of risk and protective factors, particularly attachment. Nietzsche, then, is partially right: 'in moderate adversity, what doesn't kill us may make us stronger, if we can overcome it:'[72]

> We battled through. (Heather and Lyle, 69 yrs)
>
> We toughed it out. (Patrick and Shirley, 48 yrs)
>
> That nearly broke us. (Carol and Stephen, 40 yrs)
>
> We were shattered. (David and Debby, 48 yrs)

Biological perspectives on resilience

Resilience has genetic hereditability[73] impacted by attachment-related epigenetics.[74] Earlier trauma is worse,[75] but secure attachment with a carer is a shock-absorber[76] with measurable biological effects into teenage years.[77] Through oxytocin, attachment catalyzes specific biological processes to build resilience. These were discussed in Chapter 2, *how close relationships protect against mental illness*. Oxytocin biologically links present attachment with future resilience and ameliorates the effects of past trauma in people like Professor Isidora. Oxytocin can do this for all of us when we take care of people who are close and they take care of us.

Secure couple attachment biologically protects individuals against physical and emotional pain[78] and depression and suicide.[79] Adversity, however, happens. Loss, abuse, witnessing violence, separation, or carer impairment are attachment traumas for infants.[80] Attachment trauma is not what happens externally but the internal consequences: brain changes affecting future relationships.[81] In adults, attachment traumas include divorce, separation, abuse, control, and infidelity.[82] These too cause brain changes to adversely impact future relationships. Adversity can, however, be overcome.

In summary, diverse factors lead to resilience: biological (oxytocin-induced changes), psychological (learning skills), attachment (relationships), and the intensity of the adversity and our unique responses to it.[83] Attachment is the most protective factor[84] and underlies other protective factors. It may impart the courage needed for individuals to face and overcome adversity to further increase resilience.

There is still something science does not understand: individual variation in people like Professor Isidora. Science cannot make strong generalizations about the role of individual and societal factors. With this in mind, I believe that the best current equation for enhancing resilience is

Secure attachment + overcoming adversity + learning skills = increased resilience.

Enhancing resilience together

Resilience is enhanced through attachment.[85] Yet we each cope differently.[86] Through social supports, we cope together.[87] In adversity, we naturally seek out our close attachment figures. Close people must, however, be accessible to us and in our growing social isolation; this cannot be taken for granted.[88]

Resilience is enhanced in all of us through the processes of learning information and skills, and through people contact. Through learning skills, IPT,[89] CBT,[90] behavioural activation therapy,[91] problem-solving,[92] psycho-education,[93] and social skills training[94] all enhance resilience. Gratitude, forgiveness and compassion,[95] increased sociability,[96] ACT,[97] prosocial behaviour,[98] guided imagery,[99] and mindfulness[100] have also been shown to enhance resilience not only through learning information and skills but through people contact and oxytocin release. Positive psychology increases resilience[101] through an emphasis on people connection, wellness, healthy thinking, and meaning.

Adversity is part of the human condition and close supportive relationship is always protective. A mountain-climber who breaks a leg at 8000 feet, for example, is in danger of death if climbing alone; as part of a group, however, there is hope. We depend on each other, and mountain-climbers will always learn from each other for future climbs. This is how resilience works in individual-group interactions: in mountain-climbing or in relationships, we can learn from each other's experiences. Younger couples can learn from the insights and experiences of thriving couples to help them face their future.

Resilience is the norm for human beings and the brain can rewire to learn, adapt, and increase in resilience.[102] The mechanism of this change is neuroplasticity. All psychotherapy modalities, and our learning and developing of skills, make use of its principles. We do not yet know for certain what accounts for individual differences,[103] but attachment[104] and family cohesion[105] enhance resilience for everyone. The biological mechanisms of this effect are becoming clearer.

Relationship resilience

A long-term relationship protects individual resilience,[106] emotional wellbeing,[107] physical health,[108] and protects against loneliness,[109] unhappiness,[110] drug addiction,[111] anxiety, bipolar and depression,[112] and suicide.[113] It fosters resilience through continued attachment, opportunity for self-righting in a safe-haven of trust, and continued overcoming of adversity.[114] This evidence underlines the parallels between the infant-carer dyad and the couple dyad in adulthood, particularly in the light of the biological importance of both.

To build resilience as individuals requires attachment. As inviting and optimistic as this reality sounds, it still takes a lot of effort. Conscious judgment and choice are needed to prioritize the relationship above immediate self-pleasures to enhance individual and relationship resilience.

Relationship resilience can be enhanced through couple therapy, gratitude, and forgiveness[115] to increase satisfaction, commitment, and harmony.[116] "There are few stronger predictors of happiness than a close, nurturing, equitable, intimate, lifelong companionship."[117] Following adversity, a relationship may be more resilient or more fragile.[118] Knowledge, skills, therapy, values, and individual choices may make the difference.

Relationship longevity remains the "engine that provides so much of the power for resilience,"[119] and couple stability is fundamental to individual resilience.[120] Forty years of thriving is a marker of a resilient relationship. What follows are techniques, based on insights from thriving couples to help improve couple resilience.

TECHNIQUES TO IMPROVE RELATIONSHIP RESILIENCE

A couple in therapy gain knowledge and skills. Therapy increases these to increase resilience. The techniques presented here are based on our research findings from thriving couples, existing evidence, and clinical experience. Discernment for the appropriateness of any technique is always assumed. Each technique can be adapted as needed, a couple can be encouraged to write down techniques and undertake suggestions as fitting.

Techniques to enhance couple resilience are considered under six headings:

1 Encouraging teamwork
2 Techniques for couples facing external adversity
3 Handling conflict within a relationship
4 Techniques for constructive arguing
5 Techniques for therapist resilience and effectiveness
6 Insights for therapists

1. TECHNIQUES ENCOURAGING TEAMWORK

These techniques help unite two people who may currently feel separate. A couple may overlook the gold they once saw in each other. Our thriving couples spoke often about effort and teamwork:

> We ran a dance performance troupe for 14 years. We both had to work together to do it. As a team, you make it work. (Barbara and Lance, 52 yrs)
>
> We've learned between us that we've got the opportunity to rely on each other for a big input so that we're not both absolutely, individually overwhelmed. (Carol and Brien, 50 yrs)
>
> We share all house chores, cooking. We are a team. (Online survey)
>
> We worked as a team: I was a carpenter and she was a nurse and we worked very hard. (Harry and Wendy, 50 yrs)

BECALM

This technique helps a couple gently face difficult realities.

Teamwork comes when you can BECALM. It is an acronym to help discuss things fruitfully:

Be a team, be accepting, be gentle

Choose a **C**omfortable **C**onversation time: private, undisturbed, with coffee

Ask useful questions:

> What's going right and can we do more of that?
> What's not going right and can we do less of that?
> What have we learnt and how can we apply it?

Listen. Really listen to hear another's point of view before sharing yours.

Move forward. Turn new information into an action plan. Small adjustments may yield big results. Recognize that some things, however, will need to be accepted.

Our relationship is our greatest asset

This technique blames problems on anything but the relationship.

> Dealing with a pandemic has really stressed me out. My husband has been more understanding and will help me by just letting me vent without trying to solve my problems. We have started focussing more on each of our strengths and weaknesses. . . . If things get super crazy we blame it on "Covidness." (11–15 yrs)
>
> Name your problems as 'our finances,' 'my drinking,' 'your parents,' 'our sex life,' 'my sister,' anything but your relationship. With this attitude you can team up against anything. Then, as a reminder you can say: "Our relationship is our greatest asset."

Call it 'our relationship'

"But it's we, it's always we" (Malcolm and Jeanette, 64 yrs). 'Our relationship' is an entity of 'we-ness.' Family systems theory, closely connected to attachment theory,[121] shows that a relationship has meaning to children, parents, friends and society.

> Can you talk in terms of 'our relationship'?
> What does your relationship mean to you?
> What does your relationship mean to your children, parents, and friends?
> How much effort have you put into your relationship?
> How does your relationship serve society?

Relationship sculpture

People in therapy often come feeling like broken failures:

> Because I came from a broken family I had a very minor, but quite poignant sensitivity, about commitment. I went through three periods where I was unsure about commitment. . . . [My] mother, she left, she left home when I was four years old, and I never saw her for another 20 odd years. So difficult to handle. (Keith and Lana, 49 yrs)

Their very brokenness, however, can lead to something beautiful. This metaphor can motivate people to put in effort together to draw out their gold together. Have pictures of Kintsugi sculpture at hand. *Kin-tsugi* means "gold-repair:"

> A relationship sculpts you. A sculptor can gently polish and refine but also harshly chisel and cut. One feels good, the other hurts. The result is still beauty. A Kintsugi artist takes a shattered vase or bowl

and puts it back together with gold. The brokenness becomes part of the beauty.

As one couple shared:

> You need time to rub the corners off each other. You've come from two different backgrounds, two different people, two different attitudes. And all of a sudden, you're supposed to be one. It doesn't work like that. There will be abrasion points. You have to rub up on one another, you know, to smooth the points and you need patience for that, it doesn't happen overnight. (Ben and Isabella, 56 yrs)

How do the two of you polish each other to expose more beauty?
How has past pain strengthened you?
Do you feel beauty in your partner's vulnerability?
Could past pain lead to future beauty in your relationship?
What would that look like for you?

I need to be heard

"We both suffer from not listening at times" (George and Franky, 44 yrs). If a partner keeps bringing up a past hurt, perhaps the reason is that their partner has not fully heard the pain. A quick, easy apology is ineffective. Being heard, understood, and accepted can bring back teamwork.

Has your partner really heard your pain?
What do you need to feel heard?
(Your partner may also want to hear about things you enjoy.)

Apologies and thanks

This technique is about deep emotional connection for couples comfortable with it, through listening, understanding, accepting and forgiving. It presupposes that the couple are still committed to going forward, otherwise it can bring up more hurt.

> Listen to how you have helped each other over the years. Thank each other. Then gently listen to some of the hurt over the years, and apologize. Resilience grows through help and hurt, listening and thanks. You grow together through shared emotions and understanding.

PERSON 1 How have I hurt you?
PERSON 2 . . . .
PERSON 1 I'm sorry
PERSON 2 Thank you for listening

PERSON 1 How have I helped you?
PERSON 2 . . . . Thank you
PERSON 1 Thank you for telling me

Carry a reminder

This technique is a metaphor reminding a couple of each other's strengths. Gemstones are the reminder; it helps to have some to hand out.

> He'll always be the rock. (Lana and Keith, 49 yrs)
>
> She's the rock that holds it all together. (Ben and Isabella, 56 yrs)
>
> I made a conscious decision: why don't I treasure him rather than harbour things against him? (Annette and Bernie, 60 yrs)
>
> She's solid, the cement that holds it all together. (Timothy and Samantha, 51 yrs; Timothy just happens to be an engineer)
>
> If you want, you can carry a gemstone to remind you that you carry someone's hopes and dreams, and that you can be their rock. Look at it, feel it, and ask
>
> > How could our relationship be as solid as this stone?
> > What goes smoothly like its surface?
> > What hard edges need to be polished off?
> > What makes this person precious to me?
> > How am I precious to them?
> > My partner, like this stone, is more beautiful than I realize.
> > So am I to them

Congratulations

As a therapist, you can congratulate a couple for seeking help and for their continued effort. Couples can congratulate themselves. Help-seeking is adaptive to help improve a valued relationship. At times you may ask if they feel like a team, or you may use the word 'teamwork' judiciously to test the waters of growing allegiance.

Change the meaning of the past

Changing the past is impossible, yet the meaning of the past can change depending on choices made now. Timing this technique is essential: asking these questions too early will back-fire, but as therapy progresses so will the idea that the meaning of the past can change.

You can't change the past but you can change the meaning of the past, depending on the outcome of the work you are doing now. What would you like to see happen?
Will that event mean the end of your relationship, or can you grow closer through it?
How can you choose what that event means to your relationship now?
What do you need to grow through the event rather than be defeated by it?

The strengths of our relationship

Relationships already have resilience. Early on, when someone said to some of our thriving couples, "you're making a big mistake," wild horses could not tear them apart. To help bring back forgotten strength, ask a couple to consider some of these questions, slowly over weekly catch-ups:

What first attracted you to your partner?
Any particular reason you chose this person?
Did you have to fight for this relationship at all?
What was the reason you fought for it?
When did you feel most together as a couple?
What helped you stay together?
What was going on then that isn't going on now?
What adversity have you overcome in the past? How did you do that?

Weekly catch-ups

Sitting and talking shows teamwork. In weekly (or more) catch-ups, without distractions, a couple can discuss the following:

What's going right in our relationship? How can we do more of that?
What's going wrong in our relationship? How can we do less of that?
What's helping in therapy? What's not?
What have we learnt? How can we apply it?
How can we keep these skills going for the long-term?
Why is our therapist such a jerk? (This question is a good sign of teamwork)

2. TECHNIQUES FOR COUPLES FACING EXTERNAL ADVERSITY

You and me against the world

Fighting the world makes it easier to forgive[122] and be resilient[123] within the relationship. Many of our thriving couples did this. Maddy and Bryce played 'you and me against the world' rather than let consumer values rule their lives:

> Maddy's a busy lawyer, Bryce runs a business. There was no time for affection, sex, or meals together. Bryce had an affair but didn't want to lose his family. Maddy too had an affair. This was not the life they wanted, so they changed. Bryce cut back his business, Maddy cut back her workload. They downsized their house, and now spend more time together. Affection has increased, sex is better, the kids are happier, and the family's emotional account is thriving, even if the bank account isn't.[124]

Here are some suggestions to play "you-and-me-against-the-world."

Technology:

Have boundaries towards technology

Turn off mobile phones to enjoy meals together

Forsake screens and movies for conversations and love-making

Know the difference between healthy privacy and unhealthy secrecy

Use 'we' language in public:

'We're going on a holiday'

'We're visiting family'

'I'll check with my partner'

If people say you're 'lucky' in your relationship, say:

Lucky we sit down every week to discuss things

Lucky we don't leave things to chance

Well, it seems the more we work on 'us,' the luckier we get

Lucky she loves me the way I need her to and I do the same for her

When outsiders interfere, say something like this to your partner:

I love you and it's their fault if they can't see how amazing you are

I'm sick of them. Let's just get out there and kick some ass

Stuff them. I'm sticking with you

It's not a relationship problem

Relationship resilience is staying united against all problems. To do this, the problem needs to be clearly identified. Your relationship is your greatest asset, so it is never the relationship. It is time to find the real source.

"He keeps looking at other women"
He has a wandering-eyes problem. Together you can fight it

"She never listens, she badgers and harasses me"
She has a listening problem. Together you can work on it

"He takes his work stress out on me"
The problem is managing stress. Together you can make it better

"Our sex-life isn't great"
This may be a sex, health, managing stress, intimacy, or prioritizing problem. Together you can work it out

"She's so selfish"
Her selfishness may be the problem, but together you can team up against it

"He's a workaholic, I come last"
This is a problem with priorities. Together you can manage it

Problems come from many sources: parenting, extended family, finances, sexual expectations, differing cultures, personalities, differing values and priorities, political and religious differences, drug and alcohol issues, work, friends, ill health, misfortune, broken dreams, technology, busyness, societal values, the weather, and more.

Your relationship is not on the list
Your relationship is your greatest asset

Our ability to cope

For every problem, the brain wants to find a solution: problem – the brain finds a solution – the body moves forward. A couple have developed specialized skills to overcome past adversity: hidden gems of adaptive strengths. This technique taps into these.

When did the two of you overcome a large problem?
As a couple, what did you learn through that experience?

What did you learn about yourselves?
Did you develop any skills to cope with that situation?
How have you grown together in problem-solving skills?
How has previous adversity strengthened you?
Can these abilities help you in your current situation?

The dirty rag

When one person in the relationship has a mental illness or a problem (selfishness, being controlling, anything) a narrative technique is to separate the problem from the person by naming it: Blame *dirty depression*, or *annie anxiety*, *contolling connie*, or *billy bipolar*. A partner can then ask,

> Was that you talking or *dirty depression*?
> Is that your idea or is it from *controlling connie?*

Taking this further, an old laundry rag or a toy crocodile can sit in for *dirty depression* or *narkie nick*. A frustrated partner can then get angry with it rather than the person they love:

> *(with emotion)* Listen, *narkie nick*, I've had just about enough of you, you flea-bitten filthy crocodile-rag entitlement. Now you listen to me . . . !!

It is very helpful if the partner with the problem joins the rant. The couple then become a team again.

Let's go for gold

"Young couples are being short-changed, . . . they're missing out the best things in life when they're told, 'if it doesn't feel good, don't do it' because they're not going through the hard bits" (Frances and Wayne, Aus. 42 yrs).

To explain this to a couple:

> It's like being synchronized divers in the Olympic Games. Your problem means you're doing a more difficult dive right now. It's rated higher so you score more points if you do well. You can go for gold.
>
> Whatever life deals out – cancer, a problem child, financial ruin, anything – the two of you can face it together knowing that some gold awaits you: closeness, understanding, wisdom, and living deeper together.

3. HANDLING PROBLEMS WITHIN A RELATIONSHIP

'Your relationship is your greatest asset' is difficult to remember when problems seem to be within the relationship: selfishness, sexual desire mismatch, not getting needs met, thoughtlessness, a temper, criticism, and more. This section is for times needing extra reminders to maintain the idea that your relationship *is* your greatest asset.

Carry our baggage

This technique helps a couple accept 'baggage' in their relationship: past hurts, childhood trauma, mental illness, unresolved conflict, and more. For Pat and Jim (54 years), it was combat-related PTSD:

JIM But the baggage is still there, we carry it.
PAT I loved that statement. If I remember anything from what you or Christian said [in your seminar] I think that's the one thing I'm probably going to remember forever; it's that "you always carry that baggage with you." And I want to get rid of it, and I realize now that it's always going to be there.

The technique is to get a heavy bag – as we used in our seminars – or a pile of books, and get one person to carry their baggage around. Then show how much easier it is when their partner shares the load. It is just as heavy and it does not go away, but two people manage better than one. The learning is in the experience rather than the explanation.

Our loyalty tapestry

Couples we interviewed were loyal to each other. Minor habits, quirks, cultural differences, emotional jerkiness were kept 'under wraps' as part of their relationship tapestry. A tapestry is beautiful, but it can also hide stains on floors or walls or floors. Many thriving couples showed their loyalty by refusing to talk negatively about each other:

> You've sort of got to accept how they are. There might be things you don't like, that you can sort of work around. I mean, that's who you fell in love with. And you shouldn't try and change them. And you know if it's just something that you can talk about: if they're picking their teeth you say 'don't do that in public." (Margaret and Merv, 59 yrs)

Rather than complain about each other, thriving couples remain loyal to each other by keeping flaws and secrets safe: a loyalty tapestry covers them. These questions help a couple grow loyalty.

Do you know each other's flaws and secrets?
Can you accept these as part of the tapestry of your relationship?
Can you trust each other with these?
What does loyalty mean to you?
What would help keep you loyal to each other?

Adapt, adjust, or accept

Many problems must be accepted rather than solved. Build resilience by adapting, adjusting, or accepting challenges.

You tell me you have very different personalities; they clash:

How have you adapted to these clashes?
What adjustments have you made to relate to each other?
Can you accept these clashes and each other a little more?

You tell me you have different sex drives:

How have you adapted to this?
Have frustration and hurt strengthened you in any way?
Have adjustments made by you helped the situation?
What has worked? What hasn't?
Can you manage or even accept this?
What other habits, quirks, or personality issues have you already adapted to?
What little adjustments would help?
Can you accept these more?
How can you adapt, adjust, and accept to strengthen your relationship?

Take a break-up holiday

Taking a holiday is an obvious circuit breaker, but few couples think of a holiday when they are on the verge of breaking-up. Our optimism bias[125] over-estimates the benefits of breaking-up and underestimates the cost. Problems go, but so do good times and familiarity. A holiday often helps to let go of the bad and remember the good:

> If we broke up I would lose a lot. Because I have literally invested a lifetime in her. What a waste of life: just logically. (Bruce and Susan, 49 yrs)

> If we divorced we'd be totally alone in the world, without a best friend. (Veronne and Wayne, 42 yrs)

> Before breaking up, please take a long, expensive holiday together. This will remind you of the good things you'll miss and may rekindle working together well.

4. TECHNIQUES FOR CONSTRUCTIVE ARGUING

In conflict, it is difficult to remember that your relationship is your greatest asset. This is where arguing helps. Arguing couples are ten times more likely to report being happy[126] than couples who avoid arguing. Our findings are consistent with this: 87% of couples we interviewed regularly argued. It is not enjoyable, but most saw it as a necessary form of honest communication.

In my practice, I articulate that arguing is one of seven types of relationship dialogues:

1 On the fly dialogue (happens anywhere, anytime)
2 Conversation (focussed, two-way interchanges of talk and listen)
3 Listening (one person talks, the other needs to 'be there')
4 Problem solving (dialogue looking for a solution)
5 Romance and flirting fun (private)
6 Arguing (respectful, emotionally-charged confrontation)
7 Not-talking (silent arguing)

The following techniques aim for more fruitful arguing.

Permission to be normal

Often, a couple simply need to be given permission to be in conflict and argue:

> I understand that you hate conflict, we all do; but conflict is normal and you're allowed to be normal. Evidence shows that arguing couples are happier.

Go with the flow, talk, or agree to disagree

One couple developed a comprehensive approach to handling conflict:

> Go with the flow whenever you can. If you can't, you try not to let your emotions take control and you try and talk things out. . . . Reach an agreement, even though it may well be an agreement to disagree. (Fred and Stella, 42 yrs)

This is a three-phase approach:

1 Go with the flow when you can; pick your battles
2 Talk things out without letting emotions take control
3 Agree if you can or agree to disagree, but move on

It can be extremely difficult to talk without letting emotions take control. 'Emotions being in control' almost defines a difficult argument. The aim in this is to connect thoughts with feelings through noticing what you are feeling, labelling what you are feeling with a word, then safely speaking this out:

> 'I am very angry at the moment'
> 'I feel hurt and frustrated'
> 'Give me a moment, what you said just really shook me'

This allows your partner access to your mind and this builds relationship in a difficult situation. Aim to discharge the energy of strong emotions safely.

See their point of view

This technique would suit a couple who tend to retreat into themselves and avoid conflict, or suit one partner who does this. Useful arguing means staying in relationship and seeing each other's point of view, even after days of silent retreat.

> Some arguments start off with silly things, and then you revisit something [from the past], right? But . . . you have to see each other's point of view. Sometimes it might mean that you've got to retreat and consider options and things like that. . . . If you don't argue the worst situation is that you don't have a relationship. (Arnie and Liz, 51 yrs)

> That's been the secret of my success . . . seeing the other person's point of view, and [being] willing to go with it. That's true of our relationship too. (Peter and Elizabeth, 60 yrs)

In a retreat after an argument, it helps to think about your partner's point of view and what you may be overlooking. Even after days, it helps to have a conversation about each other's point of view so that you both really understand.

Dance each other's steps

This technique suits a couple who tend to be more direct with each other. Useful arguing means staying in relationship even if you are stepping on each other's toes. Susan and Bruce met at dancing school, still compete in competitions, and practice 4–5 times a week:

> Do we disagree? We do. We can each do each other's steps.

> She'll say, "you're doing this, but you're doing this wrong."

> I say, "you're not stretching out enough, you need to extend more on beat three."
>
> She'll say, "Yes, I understand that. But if you had your little finger in the right position, then I could do it properly."
>
> We do each other's steps until we can work it out. (Bruce and Susan, 49 yrs)

In conflict or harmony, dancing each other's steps is more than seeing their point of view, it is feeling each other's energy and motivation.

> In the heat of an argument, we tend to be preoccupied with what the other person is doing wrong and what they don't understand about us. At any point, someone can say "Stop! I want you to dance my steps!" At that point, stop and think about what your partner is saying, why they are saying it, and why they are so worked up about it. This will get you to see things from their point of view. They will have to do the same for you.
>
> The ultimate 'dancing each other's steps' is for you to start to argue their point of view while they argue yours. You will need to coach each other to get it right. This can be insightful but even comic for some couples. Through this, you may not only see their point of view but also feel it. Then you can go back to dancing together.

Handle conflict

To avoid avoiding, couples often require reassurance on the benefits of talking or arguing things out: arguing couples do better. The following may help a couple process conflict.

1. Affirm love even in the midst of an argument
2. Develop listening skills
3. Have weekly catch-ups
4. Use assertiveness: 'when you . . . I feel . . . could you please . . .'
5. Put negative emotions into words not actions
6. Put positive emotions into actions as well as words
7. Debrief a day or two after an argument to understand the other's point of view

How do you handle conflict? 'Not talking' or 'the silent treatment' is silent arguing with the same emotions. You do not have to argue, but you do need to process conflict.

Pick your battles

You do not have to argue about everything, but you do not have to back down either. Many couples pick their battles while retaining self-respect:

> If she feels strongly about something, I go with it. That's my perspective, that's not avoidance behaviour. That is because I truly believe that it doesn't matter. . . . But there are things that do matter, and there probably are things that I would put my foot down on. (Don and Paula, 57 yrs)
>
> I pick the hill to die on. . . . There are some things that I won't budge on. And there are the ones that I suppose I would consider an argument. The other things I give away easily. (Peter and Elizabeth, 60 yrs)
>
> There are certain things where we need to stand and I take a stand over it and I won't change my opinion and it's because it's the right stand. (Monte and Jeneen, 45 yrs)
>
> When we were first married, you're always vying for power, understanding, and who's going to be boss. Power struggles. So then you have to learn what's worth fighting over and just forget the rest. (Marge and Ted, 56 yrs)

Ask couples to make a note of the things that:

1. Are worth battling over
2. Are not worth battling over
3. Can be sorted without an argument

Don't sleep on an argument

"Don't let the sun go down on your wrath."[127] 15% of couples mentioned this in interviews and 65 respondents wrote it in the 40+ Years Married Survey:

> Don't ever let the sun go down on an argument. And that was pretty much the way we worked, we very rarely had big debates. (Rhonda and Peter, 53 yrs)

> How could the two of you work things so that an argument doesn't spill into the next day?

Surrender and disarm

The usual dynamic during conflict is 'attack and defend.' 'Surrender and disarm' makes for better communication by dissipating ill feelings. This difficult technique can genuinely stop an argument before it begins to move forward. It is based on good listening.

Surrendering is admitting to wrongs: 'I see what you mean, maybe you're right, I'm sorry and I'll try to get it right next time.' Surrendering is not weakness; it is giving reasonable ground to someone you love. It is encapsulated by

> I see what you mean . . .
> I'm sorry . . .
> I will try to . . .

Disarming is staying understanding and accepting while venom is being thrown at you. Reasonable people will usually only throw things until they have been heard and understood (but you would be surprised). Anger is often a veiled cry for connection. Disarming says 'I see you are hurt/angry . . . I'm beginning to understand your point of view. What do you need from me right now?' These words are difficult to say when fired up; again, it takes listening. This is encapsulated by

> I see you are angry
> I'm beginning to understand that . . .
> What do you need from me right now?

'Surrender and disarm' gives ground to break down walls. This unites two people in conflict to build resilience. To use the technique, a couple will need to learn and prepare the words to mindfully use them during conflict. Experiences can be talked about in sessions.

Break arguments with humour

During an argument, humour breaks tension:

> You think you're not achieving anything and it's not going anywhere, then I'll crack a funny, or say something to stop and I'll start laughing! (Carol and Steven, 40 yrs)

Humour links thinking and feeling to lighten things up, but sarcasm is damaging. The following may sound corny, but convey care to ease tension:

> Will this be a long or a short argument?
> Should I make some tea or should we fight over dinner?
> Do you want make-up sex now or after we finish this argument?
> Sorry, I just never noticed that beautiful freckle on your nose before
> Before we go on, I just want to apologize for the next ten things I'll say
> Can I phone a friend before I answer that one?

If you avoid each other, you can say essentially the same things:

> Will this be a long or a short silence?
> Should I make a cup of tea or should we not talk over dinner?
> Do you want make-up sex before or after we finish not talking?
> Sorry, I just never noticed that beautiful freckle on your nose before
> Before we go on, I just want to apologize for the next ten things I won't say
> Can I phone a friend before I don't talk to you?

If humour falls flat, you can always say 'I'm just trying a technique our dumb therapist taught us.'

Break arguments with affection

Using affection during an argument is disarming:

> If there is a bit of an argument, there might be a bit of quiet. Then we use humour and then . . . I grab her like this and hold her. (Phil and Christine, 49 yrs)

Affection gives the underlying message that we are not going to break up over this. Here are some suggestions to give a couple:

> Give a soft touch, a hug, a gentle kiss or a look of encouragement
>
> In the heat of an argument say 'and that's another thing! I love you very much.'
>
> If you avoid each other, just walk up and say or do the same things.

Why bother arguing?

If you recognize your argument pattern and can articulate it, 'hey, we're heading for an argument,' you may find another way forward:

> I think [arguing] happens without you ever thinking about it . . . there's no point huffing and puffing and blowing the house down. You stop and you think about it and then, generally, a compromise comes out. (Tony and Cyndy, 49 yrs)

To articulate this as a technique:

1. Notice when you're heading for an argument
2. Have a reminder-phrase: 'we need to talk' or 'no point huffing and puffing'
3. Talk: 'well, what I feel is . . . what about you?'
4. The 'BECALM' technique helps to find a compromise

Go straight to making up

Another way of not arguing is to go straight to making up:

> We argue all the time. I think I'm more accepting of the arguing . . . because I've learned that I'm not going to change my wife and maybe I'm not going to change either. . . . It's like all of a sudden, I'll stop and it's like "How important is this?" And I'll just [say] "Let's forget it, let's make up" and we try to make up as soon as we can. (Ruth and Russell, 40 yrs)

Making up after an argument may mean a kiss and a cuddle, love-making, sharing some ice-cream, going for a walk, watching a movie, or just talking about fun stuff.

> What's your way of making up and feeling together again?
> Could you find a way to skip the argument and go straight to that?

Let go of anger and hurt sooner

"Whenever we get upset at each other, we settle it real quick" (Jack and Carole, 54 yrs).

We often hold on to residual anger and hurt out of pride, selfishness, or vengeance. Unfortunately, we can be like that sometimes. Altruism, however, means letting go quicker to get back to kindness and truth.

Monitor your emotions on a scale of 1–10 and tell your partner when it gets less:

> 'I'm still bloody angry. I'm at 8/10'
>
> 'Just want to let you know, my anger is down to 6/10, still not good'
>
> 'Ok I'm getting there; it's now 4/10'

The partner can help by saying 'thanks for letting me know.'

If your partner is not able to let go of anger or hurt, ask:

> 'What can I do to help you let go of the anger?' This encourages them to articulate their needs. Often the answer is 'just give me time.' Then, just give them time.

Can we sit down and discuss it?

> When we were just married we did a lot of arguing, but mostly because of my insecurities and trust issues. He never did anything wrong but I had to understand men in general. And I would go at him about something and he would retreat. And that didn't get anywhere . . . so

> we've learned over the years . . . [to] come at it in a gentle way, communication, and ask questions instead of just attack. . . . I gently have him open up about the situation. . . . More of a "can we sit down and have a discussion." (Jeneen and Monte, 45 yrs)

It takes many years to become proficient in knowing your partner and how to best communicate with them. With time, however, most couples learn that talking is easier than arguing.

Rather than argue, can you sit down and have a discussion?

5. TECHNIQUES FOR THERAPIST RESILIENCE AND EFFECTIVENESS

Avoid burnout

Take care of yourself to take care of others. Burn-out has long been a problem for therapists[128] and even couple therapy trainees.[129] We have developed a specific tool to help prevent it.[130] These questions help:

Am I physically, emotionally, and mentally fit enough to do my work?
Is there something else in my life that needs attention?
Am I optimizing my lifestyle so I can render my best services?
Do I treat myself as well as I treat others?

My approach to this couple

Therapist self-appraisal and awareness optimizes effectiveness.

How can I ensure I do no harm to this relationship?
What does 'well' look like for this couple?
Are there risks, or physical and spiritual issues that require other input?
For this couple, what can be adjusted and what needs to be accepted?
What useful skills and resources does this couple already have?
What skills can be developed in this couple? How much effort is needed?
Are they willing to put in the effort and resources? Am I?
Can I keep my personal biases from interfering with their goals?

What's the problem, really?

A relationship becomes more resilient if a couple overcomes the presenting problem. To facilitate this, a therapist needs to have a grasp of what the underlying problem is. Relevant questions to oneself include:

What is the problem, really?

Why is it surfacing now?
Have they overcome something similar in the past?
What personal, informational, and social resources can they draw on?
Can this problem be solved without introducing a new world-view?
If something new needs to be introduced, what would suit them best?

How does this relationship work?

Discovering 'how this relationship works' helps tailor the therapy to a couple's unique strengths and needs. No-one can actually explain the intricacies of how their relationship works; they can, over time, share insights into this. A couple may hide how their relationship works for fear of judgment. With trust and sensitivity, their strengths can be emphasized and utilized. Ideas to ponder include:

How does this relationship work?
How do they dovetail strengths and personalities?
How do they help and fulfil each other?

6. INSIGHTS FOR THERAPISTS

Insight 1: a relationship is like a tree

This insight is a metaphor to encourage a couple to be gentle with each other.

A tree combines strength and flexibility to be resilient
Problems batter relationships like tempests batter trees
A storm strengthens trees, but sudden gusts or lightning bolts can snap trees
Be careful of sudden insult gusts or big-secret lightning bolts
Aim to share concerns like a gentle breeze rather than a huge storm
Be as gentle as you can

Insight 2: speak truth kindly and be truly kind

'Should I be kind or should I be truthful?' is often seen as a dilemma: facing reality is important, yet being blunt with truth can be wounding. Both are needed.

With people who are close,
Rather than choose between truth and kindness,
Aim to speak truth kindly and to be truly kind.

Insight 3: deal-breakers

A couple need to be aware of the limits to their resilience; their deal-breakers. At some stage in therapy this may need to be discussed.

> If you can survive this, you must be strong
> What are your relationship deal-breakers?

If a couple is already in deal-breaker territory, one option is to wipe the slate clean.

> Now you've discussed the deal-breakers and know them. You can choose not to go there again.

Insight 4: you're the expert

A therapist cannot fathom the many ways two people in a long-term relationship know, care for, and affect each other. Yet what you don't know can still be affirmed.

> You know each other and relate to each other better than anyone. It's a skill learnt over many years. You're the only experts on each other.

Conclusion: together-actualization

After exploring the context of hyper-individualism, the mental health crisis and social isolation, the evidence from younger couples surviving COVID-19 and thriving couples married 40+ years in interviews and surveys, and techniques to develop pro-relational values and resilience, we conclude our book by returning to the idea of together-actualization. Together-actualization is a continuous, long-term, authentic encounter in two people resulting in personal and relational growth and shared meaning-making. All couples we interviewed displayed together-actualization in some way. Together-actualization is not always fun, novelty, pleasure, or contentment. It includes these but also includes hardship, sorrow, pain, and overcoming. Like night and day, pleasure and pain are subsumed and integrated into a bigger picture of deeper meaning, purpose, and life experience. It is a relationship becoming more of what it can be.

Great love is available to any couple willing to accept it and the continuous delayed gratification it entails. It is worthwhile but often difficult effort. In twenty-first century complexities, the challenge is for individuals to sustain the necessary effort, value relationship attachment to build resilience, and reach for together-actualization.

We conclude with one modest, flawed, but beautiful couple. They reached for and attained much together-actualization. This glimpse into their life story was during their interview with Dr Caroline Heim:

> Judy and Gordon sat side by side in their modest home of 60 years. Glittering pillows adorned their sofa reflecting the sparkle that was part of their romance. They have been singing duets together at nursing homes for over 30 years. Underneath Judy's vivacious smile and Gordon's quiet strength lay the burden of two tragic family deaths and the journey of a troubled grandson. An unwelcome guest momentarily broke their peace, an 'outsider' who had threatened to tear their relationship apart. At the end of the interview I asked, "Do you have a special song that is just yours?" Having travelled some difficult terrain during our talk, Gordon gently took Judy's hand in his and the two started singing "Perhaps Love."[131] The words reflected their restless sea of conflict protected by a safe harbour of security and a warm fire of comfort. The memories of their love hung in the air between the two of them as they sang their song of 63 years of individual and together-thriving.

Notes

1 www.tribuneindia.com/news/thoughtfortheday/all-the-world-is-full-of-suffering-it-is-also-full-of-overcoming-%E2%80%94-helen-keller-106343 Retrieved 15 July 2022.

2 www.goodreads.com/author/quotes/6439373.Elizabeth_Edwards Retrieved 15 July 2022.

3 www.hastingsobserver.co.uk/arts-and-culture/books/hastings-and-the-tale-of-the-self-righting-lifeboat-3308684 Retrieved 26 November 2021.

4 See, as examples, Pancheri, Lucia, and Franco Paparo. "Fattori terapeutici specifici e comuni in psicoanalisi: Il self-righting." *Rivista di psichiatria* 38, no. 3 (2003): 105–116. Werner, Emmy E., and Ruth S. Smith. *Overcoming the odds*. Cornell University Press, 2019. Lichtenberg, Joseph D., Frank M. Lachmann, and James L. Fosshage. *Psychoanalysis and motivational systems: A new look*. Routledge, 2011, 217.

5 Schonbar, Rosalea A., and Helena R. Beatus. "The mysterious metamorphoses of Bertha Pappenheim: Anna O. revisited." *Psychoanalytic Psychology* 7, no. 1 (1990): 59.

6 Skerrett, Karen, and Karen Fergus, eds. *Couple resilience: Emerging perspectives*. Springer, 2015, 23.

7 Atwool, Nicola. "Attachment and resilience: Implications for children in care." *Child Care in Practice* 12, no. 4 (2006): 315–330.

8 Pascuzzo, Katherine, Chantal Cyr, and Ellen Moss. "Longitudinal association between adolescent attachment, adult romantic attachment, and emotion regulation strategies." *Attachment & Human Development* 15, no. 1 (2013): 83–103.

9 Darling Rasmussen, Pernille, Ole Jakob Storebø, Trine Løkkeholt, Line Gaunø Voss, Yael Shmueli-Goetz, Anders Bo Bojesen, Erik Simonsen, and Niels Bilenberg. "Attachment as a core feature of resilience: A systematic review and meta-analysis." *Psychological Reports* 122, no. 4 (2019): 1259–1296.

10 Sims-Schouten, Wendy, and Simon Edwards. "'Man up!'bullying and resilience within a neoliberal framework." *Journal of Youth Studies* 19, no. 10 (2016): 1382–1400.
11 Sim, Kang, and Qian Hui Chew. "Understanding resilience: No place to rest on our Laurels – reply to Modesto-Lowe et al." *The Journal of Clinical Psychiatry* 82, no. 5 (2021): 35486.
12 Zangeneh, Masood. "Heroes should not die by suicide: The tragic life of Dr. Lorna Breen." *INYI Journal* (2020): 29.
13 Oliver, David. "David Oliver: When "resilience" becomes a dirty word." *BMJ* 358 (2017).
14 Calabrese, Vittorio, Maria Scuto, and Edward J. Calabrese. "Hormesis, resilience and mental health: Enhancing public health and therapeutic options." *Explaining health across the sciences*. Springer, 2020, 497–520.
15 Luthar, Suniya S., and Samuel H. Barkin. "Are affluent youth truly "at risk"? Vulnerability and resilience across three diverse samples." *Development and Psychopathology* 24, no. 2 (2012): 429–449.
16 Luthar, Suniya S., Dante Cicchetti, and Bronwyn Becker. "The construct of resilience: A critical evaluation and guidelines for future work." *Child Development* 71, no. 3 (2000): 543–562.
17 Ioannidis, Konstantinos, Adrian Dahl Askelund, Rogier A. Kievit, and Anne-Laura Van Harmelen. "The complex neurobiology of resilient functioning after childhood maltreatment." *BMC Medicine* 18, no. 1 (2020): 1–16.
18 Jackson, James S., Katherine M. Knight, and Jane A. Rafferty. "Race and unhealthy behaviors: Chronic stress, the HPA axis, and physical and mental health disparities over the life course." *American Journal of Public Health* 100, no. 5 (2010): 933–939.
19 Stewart-Brown, Sarah. "Emotional wellbeing and its relation to health: Physical disease may well result from emotional distress." (1998): 1608–1609.
20 Hjemdal, Odin. "Measuring protective factors: The development of two resilience scales in Norway." *Child and Adolescent Psychiatric Clinics of North America* 16, no. 2 (2007): 303–321.
21 Haas, Stephen M., and Pamela J. Lannutti. "Relationship maintenance behaviors, resilience, and relational quality in romantic relationships of LGBTQ+ people." *Couple and Family Psychology: Research and Practice* 11, no. 2 (2021): 117–131.
22 Skerrett, Karen. "Resilience in couples: A view of the landscape." *Couple resilience*. Springer, 2015, 3–22.
23 Wolff, Sula, and Sula Wolff. "The concept of resilience." *Australian and New Zealand Journal of Psychiatry* 29, no. 4 (1995): 565–574.
24 Werner, Emmy E. "Risk, resilience, and recovery: Perspectives from the Kauai Longitudinal Study." *Development and Psychopathology* 5, no. 4 (1993): 503–515. Rutter, Michael. "Resilience: Some conceptual considerations." *Journal of Adolescent Health* 14, no. 8 (1993): 626–631.
25 Ulmer-Yaniv, Adi, Shani Waidergoren, Ariel Shaked, Roy Salomon, and Ruth Feldman. "Neural representation of the parent – child attachment from infancy to adulthood." *Social Cognitive and Affective Neuroscience* 17, no. 7 (2022): 609–624.
26 Bethell, Christina, Jennifer Jones, Narangerel Gombojav, Jeff Linkenbach, and Robert Sege. "Positive childhood experiences and adult mental and relational health in a statewide sample: Associations across adverse childhood experiences levels." *JAMA Pediatrics* 173, no. 11 (2019): e193007.
27 Poole, Julia C., Keith S. Dobson, and Dennis Pusch. "Childhood adversity and adult depression: The protective role of psychological resilience." *Child Abuse & Neglect* 64 (2017): 89–100.

28 Beckett, Celia, Diana Bredenkamp, Jenny Castle, Christine Groothues, Thomas G. O'connor, and Michael Rutter. "Behavior patterns associated with institutional deprivation: A study of children adopted from Romania." *Journal of Developmental & Behavioral Pediatrics* 23, no. 5 (2002): 297–303.
29 Hammen, Constance. "Risk and protective factors for children of depressed parents." Luthar, S., ed. *Resilience and vulnerability: Adaptation in the context of childhood adversities*. Cambridge University Press, 2003, 50–75, p. 53.
30 Rutter, Michael. "Psychosocial resilience and protective mechanisms." *American Journal of Orthopsychiatry* 57, no. 3 (1987): 316–331.
31 Freud, Anna, and Dorothy Burlingham. *War and children*. Foster Parents Plan for War Children, 1943. Laor, Nathaniel, Leo Wolmer, and Donald J. Cohen. "Mothers' functioning and children's symptoms 5 years after a SCUD missile attack." *American Journal of Psychiatry* 158, no. 7 (2001): 1020–1026.
32 Daniels, Aubrey D., and Julia Bryan. "Resilience despite complex trauma: Family environment and family cohesion as protective factors." *The Family Journal* 29, no. 3 (2021): 336–345.
33 Masten, Ann S., and L. Powell. "A resilience framework for research, policy." Luthar, S., ed. *Resilience and vulnerability: Adaptation in the context of childhood adversities*. Cambridge University Press, 2003.
34 Ibid.
35 Ibid.
36 Fergusson, D., and L. Horwood. "Resilience to childhood adversity: Results of a 21-year study." Luthar, S., ed. *Resilience and vulnerability: Adaptation in the context of childhood adversities*. Cambridge University Press, 2003, 130–155.
37 Hjemdal, Odin. "Measuring protective factors: The development of two resilience scales in Norway." *Child and Adolescent Psychiatric Clinics of North America* 16, no. 2 (2007): 303–321.
38 Twenge, Jean M. "The age of anxiety? The birth cohort change in anxiety and neuroticism, 1952–1993." *Journal of Personality and Social Psychology* 79, no. 6 (2000): 1007.
39 Ibid.
40 Ibid.
41 Martineau, Sheila. "Rewriting resilience: A critical discourse analysis of childhood resilience and the politics of teaching resilience to 'kids at risk'." Dissertation, University of British Columbia (1999).
42 Bluglass, Kerry. *Hidden from the holocaust: Stories of resilient children who survived and thrived*. Praeger Publishers, 2003.
43 Southwick, Steven M., George A. Bonanno, Ann S. Masten, Catherine Panter-Brick, and Rachel Yehuda. "Resilience definitions, theory, and challenges: Interdisciplinary perspectives." *European Journal of Psychotraumatology* 5, no. 1 (2014): 25338.
44 Darling Rasmussen, Storebø and Løkkeholt. "Attachment as a core feature of resilience."
45 Hopkins, J. Roy. *Adolescence: The transitional years*. Academic Press, 2014, 3.
46 Casey, B. J., Aaron S. Heller, Dylan G. Gee, and Alexandra O. Cohen. "Development of the emotional brain." *Neuroscience Letters* 693 (2019): 29–34.
47 Feder, Adriana, Sharely Fred-Torres, Steven M. Southwick, and Dennis S. Charney. "The biology of human resilience: Opportunities for enhancing resilience across the life span." *Biological Psychiatry* 86, no. 6 (2019): 443–453.
48 Feldman, S. Shirley, L. Kris Gowen, and Lawrence Fisher. "Family relationships and gender as predictors of romantic intimacy in young adults: A longitudinal study." *Journal of Research on Adolescence* 8, no. 2 (1998): 263–286.
49 La Greca, Annette M., and Hannah Moore Harrison. "Adolescent peer relations, friendships, and romantic relationships: Do they predict social anxiety

and depression?." *Journal of Clinical Child and Adolescent Psychology* 34, no. 1 (2005): 49–61.

50 Busby, Dean M., Veronica Hanna-Walker, and Jeremy B. Yorgason. "A closer look at attachment, sexuality, and couple relationships." *Journal of Social and Personal Relationships* 37, no. 4 (2020): 1362–1385.

51 Hetherington, E. Mavis, and Anne Mitchell Elmore. "Risk and resilience in children coping with their parents' divorce and remarriage." Luthar, S., ed. *Resilience and vulnerability: Adaptation in the context of childhood adversities*. Cambridge University Press, 2003, 182–212.

52 Bluglass. *Hidden from the holocaust*.

53 Henderson, Nan, Bonnie Benard, and Nancy Sharp-Light, eds. *Resiliency in action: Practical ideas for overcoming risks and building strengths in youth, families & communities*. Resiliency in Action, 2007, 3.

54 Werner, Emmy E., and Ruth S. Smith. *Journeys from childhood to midlife: Risk, resilience, and recovery*. Cornell University Press, 2001.

55 Vaknin, Orly, and Hadas Wiseman. "Rescue fantasies in the personal and professional relational narratives of psychotherapists." *Counselling and Psychotherapy Research* 21, no. 2 (2021): 442–447.

56 Nikiforidou, Zoi. "The cotton wool child." *Childhood Today* (2017): 11–22.

57 Southwick, Bonanno, Masten, Panter-Brick, and Yehuda. "Resilience definitions."

58 Oliver, David. "David Oliver."

59 Lebow, Jay, and Douglas K. Snyder, eds. *Clinical handbook of couple therapy*, 6th edn. The Guilford Press, 2022, 473–474.

60 Hetherington and Mitchell Elmore. "Risk and resilience in children coping."

61 Bonanno, George A. "Clarifying and extending the construct of adult resilience." *The American Psychologist* 60, no. 3 (2005): 265b.

62 Hjemdal, Odin. "Measuring protective factors: The development of two resilience scales in Norway." *Child and Adolescent Psychiatric Clinics of North America* 16, no. 2 (2007): 303–321.

63 Felitti, Vincent J., Robert F. Anda, Dale Nordenberg, David F. Williamson, Alison M. Spitz, Valerie Edwards, and James S. Marks. "Relationship of childhood abuse and household dysfunction to many of the leading causes of death in adults: The Adverse Childhood Experiences (ACE) Study." *American Journal of Preventive Medicine* 14, no. 4 (1998): 245–258.

64 Felitti, Vincent J. "Reverse alchemy in childhood: Turning gold into lead." *Journal of Preventive Medicine* 14 (2011): 245–258.

65 Cohn, Deborah A., Daniel H. Silver, Carolyn P. Cowan, Philip A. Cowan, and Jane Pearson. "Working models of childhood attachment and couple relationships." *Journal of Family Issues* 13, no. 4 (1992): 432–449.

66 Ellis, Bruce J., JeanMarie Bianchi, Vladas Griskevicius, and Willem E. Frankenhuis. "Beyond risk and protective factors: An adaptation-based approach to resilience." *Perspectives on Psychological Science* 12, no. 4 (2017): 561–587.

67 Mittal, Chiraag, Vladas Griskevicius, Jeffry A. Simpson, Sooyeon Sung, and Ethan S. Young. "Cognitive adaptations to stressful environments: When childhood adversity enhances adult executive function." *Journal of Personality and Social Psychology* 109, no. 4 (2015): 604.

68 Ellis, Bruce J., Laura S. Abrams, Ann S. Masten, Robert J. Sternberg, Nim Tottenham, and Willem E. Frankenhuis. "Hidden talents in harsh environments." *Development and psychopathology* 34, no. 1 (2022): 95–113.

69 Frankland, Paul W., and Sheena A. Josselyn. "Facing your fears." *Science* 360, no. 6394 (2018): 1186–1187.

70 Nietzsche, F. *Twilight of the idols*. Jovian Press, 1889. Quoted in Wang, Yang, Benjamin F. Jones, and Dashun Wang. "Early-career setback and future career impact." *Nature Communications* 10, no. 1 (2019): 1–10.

71 Wang, Jones, and Wang. "Early-career setback and future career impact."
72 Seery, Mark D., E. Alison Holman, and Roxane Cohen Silver. "Whatever does not kill us: Cumulative lifetime adversity, vulnerability, and resilience." *Journal of Personality and Social Psychology* 99, no. 6 (2010): 1025.
73 Amstadter, Ananda B., John M. Myers, and Kenneth S. Kendler. "Psychiatric resilience: Longitudinal twin study." *The British Journal of Psychiatry* 205, no. 4 (2014): 275–280.
74 Burns, S. B., J. K. Szyszkowicz, G. N. Luheshi, P. E. Lutz, and G. Turecki. "Plasticity of the epigenome during early-life stress." *Seminars in Cell & Developmental Biology* 77 (2018): 115–132.
75 van Bodegom, Miranda, Judith R. Homberg, and Marloes J. A. G. Henckens. "Modulation of the hypothalamic-pituitary-adrenal axis by early life stress exposure." *Frontiers in Cellular Neuroscience* 11 (2017): 87.
76 Hostinar, Camelia E. "Recent developments in the study of social relationships, stress responses, and physical health." *Current Opinion in Psychology* 5 (2015): 90–95.
77 Ibid.
78 Failo, Alessandro. "Recent advances in the linkage of attachment and pain: A new review." *Features and Assessments of Pain, Anaesthesia, and Analgesia* (2022): 15–25.
79 Diamond, Guy, Jody Russon, and Suzanne Levy. "Attachment-based family therapy: A review of the empirical support." *Family Process* 55, no. 3 (2016): 595–610.
80 Spinazzola, Joseph, Bessel Van der Kolk, and Julian D. Ford. "Developmental trauma disorder: A legacy of attachment trauma in victimized children." *Journal of Traumatic Stress* 34, no. 4 (2021): 711–720.
81 Ibid.
82 Warach, Benjamin, and Lawrence Josephs. "The aftershocks of infidelity: A review of infidelity-based attachment trauma." *Sexual and Relationship Therapy* 36, no. 1 (2021): 68–90.
83 Feder, Fred-Torres, Southwick, and Charney. "The biology of human resilience."
84 Afifi, Tamara D. "Individual/relational resilience." *Journal of Applied Communication Research* 46, no. 1 (2018): 5–9.
85 Southwick, Bonanno, Masten, Panter-Brick, and Yehuda. "Resilience definitions."
86 Miller-Graff, Laura E. "The multidimensional taxonomy of individual resilience." *Trauma, Violence, & Abuse* 23, no. 2 (2022): 660–675.
87 Pow, Jessica Leanne. "We cope together: Predictors and consequences of social support mobilization." Dissertation, University of British Columbia (2019).
88 Southwick, Bonanno, Masten, Panter-Brick, and Yehuda. "Resilience definitions."
89 Cuijpers, Pim, Blanca S. Pineda, Soledad Quero, Eirini Karyotaki, Sascha Y. Struijs, Caroline A. Figueroa, Jazmin A. Llamas, Toshi A. Furukawa, and Ricardo F. Muñoz. "Psychological interventions to prevent the onset of depressive disorders: A meta-analysis of randomized controlled trials." *Clinical Psychology Review* 83 (2021): 101955.
90 Brunwasser, Steven M., Jane E. Gillham, and Eric S. Kim. "A meta-analytic review of the Penn Resiliency Program's effect on depressive symptoms." *Journal of Consulting and Clinical Psychology* 77, no. 6 (2009): 1042.
91 Madahi, Mohammad Ebrahim, and Mahmoud Godarzi. "The comparison of the effects of choice theory therapy and behavioral activation therapy with and without guided mental imagery on resilience in substance-dependent adolescents." *Scientific Quarterly Research on Addiction* 15, no. 61 (2021): 241–260.
92 Tenhula, Wendy N., Arthur M. Nezu, Christine Maguth Nezu, Michael O. Stewart, Sarah A. Miller, Jennifer Steele, and Bradley E. Karlin. "Moving forward: A problem-solving training program to foster veteran resilience." *Professional Psychology: Research and Practice* 45, no. 6 (2014): 416.

93 Steinhardt, Mary, and Christyn Dolbier. "Evaluation of a resilience intervention to enhance coping strategies and protective factors and decrease symptomatology." *Journal of American College Health* 56, no. 4 (2008): 445–453.
94 Stice, Eric, Heather Shaw, Cara Bohon, C. Nathan Marti, and Paul Rohde. "A meta-analytic review of depression prevention programs for children and adolescents: Factors that predict magnitude of intervention effects." *Journal of Consulting and Clinical Psychology* 77, no. 3 (2009): 486.
95 Chesak, Sherry S., Tejinder K. Khalsa, Anjali Bhagra, Sarah M. Jenkins, Brent A. Bauer, and Amit Sood. "Stress management and resiliency training for public school teachers and staff: A novel intervention to enhance resilience and positively impact student interactions." *Complementary Therapies in Clinical Practice* 37 (2019): 32–38. Van Cuylenburg, Hugh. *The resilience project*. Penguin Random House Australia, 2019.
96 Williams, Lisa A., and Monica Y. Bartlett. "Warm thanks: Gratitude expression facilitates social affiliation in new relationships via perceived warmth." *Emotion* 15, no. 1 (2015): 1.
97 Shahabi, Abbasali, Parvin Ehteshamzadeh, Parviz Asgari, and Behnam Makvandi. "Comparison of the effectiveness of acceptance and commitment therapy and guided imagery on the resilience of cardiac disease patients referring to the heart rehabilitation department." *The Horizon of Medical Sciences* 26, no. 3 (2020): 276–297.
98 Leiberg, Susanne, Olga Klimecki, and Tania Singer. "Short-term compassion training increases prosocial behavior in a newly developed prosocial game." *PLoS One* 6, no. 3 (2011): e17798.
99 Azhari, Rasyidah, and Isti Harkomah. "Progressive muscle relaxation, spiritual guided imagery, music on coping and resilience among cancer patients who undergo chemotherapy." *KnE Life Sciences* (2021): 344–355.
100 Condon, Paul. "Meditation in context: Factors that facilitate prosocial behavior." *Current Opinion in Psychology* 28 (2019): 15–19.
101 Luthar, Suniya S., Emily L. Lyman, and Elizabeth J. Crossman. "Resilience and positive psychology." *Handbook of developmental psychopathology*. Springer, 2014, 125–140.
102 Bonanno, George A. "Loss, trauma, and human resilience: Have we underestimated the human capacity to thrive after extremely aversive events?." *American Psychologist* 59, no. 1 (2004): 20.
103 Southwick, Bonanno, Masten, Panter-Brick, and Yehuda. "Resilience definitions."
104 Perry, Bruce D., Maia Szalavitz, and Corey M. Snow. *Born for love: Why empathy is essential–and endangered*. HarperCollins, 2010.
105 Daniels and Bryan. "Resilience despite complex trauma."
106 Oswald, Ramona Faith. "Resilience within the family networks of lesbians and gay men: Intentionality and redefinition." *Journal of Marriage and Family* 64, no. 2 (2002): 374–383.
107 Waite, Linda J., and Evelyn L. Lehrer. "The benefits from marriage and religion in the United States: A comparative analysis." *Population and Development Review* 29, no. 2 (2003): 255–275.
108 Wilson, Chris M., and Andrew J. Oswald. "How does marriage affect physical and psychological health? A survey of the longitudinal evidence." *IDEAS* Working Paper Series from RePEc (2005).
109 de Jong Gierveld, Jenny, Theo Van Tilburg, and Pearl Dykstra. "Loneliness and social isolation." *The Cambridge handbook of personal relationships*. Cambridge University Press, 2006.
110 Easterlin, Richard A. "Explaining happiness." *Proceedings of the National Academy of Sciences* 100, no. 19 (2003): 11176–11183.

111 Thomas, Nathaniel S., Sally I. Kuo, Fazil Aliev, Vivia V. McCutcheon, Jacquelyn M. Meyers, Grace Chan, Victor Hesselbrock et al. "Alcohol use disorder, psychiatric comorbidities, marriage and divorce in a high-risk sample." *Psychology of Addictive Behaviors* 36, no. 4 (2022): 364.
112 Weissman, Myrna M., Roger C. Bland, Glorisa J. Canino, Carlo Faravelli, Steven Greenwald, Hai-Gwo Hwu, Peter R. Joyce et al. "Cross-national epidemiology of major depression and bipolar disorder." *JAMA* 276, no. 4 (1996): 293–299.
113 Trovato, Frank. "A longitudinal analysis of divorce and suicide in Canada." *Journal of Marriage and the Family* (1987): 193–203.
114 Afifi, Tamara D., Anne F. Merrill, and Sharde Davis. "The theory of resilience and relational load." *Personal Relationships* 23, no. 4 (2016): 663–683.
115 McNulty, James K. "Forgiveness in marriage: Putting the benefits into context." *Journal of Family Psychology* 22, no.1 (2008): 171.
116 Lemay Jr, Edward P., and Rachel B. Venaglia. "Relationship expectations and relationship quality." *Review of General Psychology* 20, no. 1 (2016): 57–70.
117 Myers, David G. *The American paradox: Spiritual hunger in an age of plenty*. Yale University Press, 2001, 43.
118 Thompson, Bryant S., and M. Audrey Korsgaard. "Relational identification and forgiveness: Facilitating relationship resilience." *Journal of Business and Psychology* 34, no. 2 (2019): 153–167.
119 Southwick, Bonanno, Masten, Panter-Brick, and Yehuda. "Resilience definitions."
120 Britto, Pia R., Suna Hanöz-Penney, Liliana Angelica Ponguta, Diane Sunar, Ghassan Issa, Sascha D. Hein, Maria Conceição do Rosário et al. "Pathways to a more peaceful and sustainable world: The transformative power of children in families." *Development and Psychopathology* 33, no. 2 (2021): 409–420.
121 Rothbaum, Fred, Karen Rosen, Tatsuo Ujiie, and Nobuko Uchida. "Family systems theory, attachment theory, and culture." *Family Process* 41, no. 3 (2002): 328–350.
122 Williamson, Hannah C. "Early effects of the COVID-19 pandemic on relationship satisfaction and attributions." *Psychological Science* 31, no. 12 (2020): 1479–1487.
123 Neff, Lisa A., Marci E. J. Gleason, Erin E. Crockett, and Oyku Ciftci. "Blame the pandemic: Buffering the association between stress and relationship quality during the COVID-19 pandemic." *Social Psychological and Personality Science* 13, no. 2 (2022): 522–532.
124 Case study from Dr Christian Heim's clinical practice.
125 Sharot, Tali. "The optimism bias." *Current Biology* 21, no. 23 (2011): R941–R945.
126 Grenny, Joseph, Kerry Patterson, Ron McMillan, Al Switzler, and Emily Gregory. *Crucial conversations*. McGraw Hill, 2022.
127 Based on Ephesians 4:26.
128 Heim, Christian. "Preventing vicarious trauma: A private psychological tool for health care workers." *International Journal of Emergency Mental Health and Human Resilience* 22, no. (2020): 6–10.
129 Glebova, Tatiana, Arpita Lal, Alix Girard, and Jessica Van Ligten. "Burnout in MFT trainees: Impact of demands and resources." *Journal of Marital and Family Therapy* 48, no. 3 (2022): 908–926.
130 www.drchristianheim.com/new-blog/2020/4/18/a-psychological-tool-to-prevent-vicarious-trauma-wash-your-web-introduction
131 Denver Johnny. *Perhaps love*. CBS Masterworks, 1981.

Appendix 1

More couple insights on relationship issues

In this appendix, each couple is represented once by an insight not included in any chapters.

Altruism

Love is giving rather than love is taking. Love is thinking of the other person and helping and promoting the other person and honouring the other person. That just makes you avoid so many of the common pitfalls. (Gary and Ruth, 40 yrs)

I think that you have to put something into the community. Otherwise, what sort of community can you live in? (Harry and Wendy, 50 yrs)

Comfort

Life is more comfortable down the track. (David and Trish, 48 yrs)

Commitment

Marriage is forever. You make a commitment and, irrespective of what happens, you sort it out, argue your case, explain yourself. (Gordon and Judy, 66 yrs)

Marriage does not guarantee you will be together forever, it's only paper. It takes love, respect, trust, understanding, friendship and faith to make it last. (Ramila and Vinay, 49 yrs)

If you're committed then the minute the physical, or emotional, or the attractiveness changes, your commitment changes. But when you have a spiritual basis together, that never changes. That's a solid base to start with. (Monte and Jeneen, 44 yrs)

Commitment to start with. That was an interesting discovery that we thought we'd like to grow old together. That commitment becomes stronger when the children become a focus. When they go their own way, the commitment's there. We don't worry about it. It's just there. (Christine and Phil, 49 yrs)

Chileans have a strong "you're married for life" attitude. If you have a worrying situation you try to work this situation; fix this situation. (Patty and Jorge, 47 yrs)

When you get married, you make a commitment. And you have to make it work. There's no walking away. So if you both put 100% effort, it's gonna work. (Barbara and Lance, 52 yrs)

Communication

I'm not so much a good communicator, but it's true that I'm always trying to find common grounds. (Philippe and Laure, 41 yrs)

Honesty has to be there: speak from the heart. When you speak from the heart you lay yourself out there. (Veronne and Wayne, 42 yrs)

Whenever I'm upset I certainly let him know, which I think is a good thing instead of harbouring it in. (Jack and Carole, 54 yrs)

There has to be trust and openness to be able to have a discussion without it turning into a fight. (George and Helen, 48 yrs)

Okay, one rule we've always adhered to is we never talk about the person being bad. We talk about the behaviour being bad. We don't say "you're an asshole." We say "I don't like what you are doing." (Brian and Mary, 50 yrs)

Never give up talking to each other about problems and be honest. (Ken and Ruth, 54 yrs)

You can't change the other person. You have got to know yourself and know the other person. (Beverly and Allen, 46 yrs)

Compromise

I mean, you really give in actually. Even though you don't want to admit it. (Tiiu and Inno, 66 yrs)

You have to give and take, and once in a while you have to be silent. Listening to each other is important, we continue working on that one, it is a hard one. (Juanito and Nicia, 48 yrs)

You've got to be more considerate. It's not that hard. It's really not that hard, because the benefits are there, you know, having that lifelong partner. I wouldn't have done it with anyone else. (Christine and Ted, 50 yrs)

Conflict

But there's an old Chinese saying that when you have a fight at the head of the bed, very soon, it would have peace at the end of the bed. (Albert and Clare, 40 yrs)

Reach out to each other. Don't hold a grudge. Sort it out immediately, don't hold it in. If you hold a grudge and are resentful about something that's just like a cancer festering. (Wendy and David, 51 yrs)

If one partner wants to blame the other it puts a strain on the marriage. So you have to stick together. (Trevor and Sandra, 43 yrs)

Don't hold grudges. Don't dwell on things. (Eve and Graham, 65 yrs)

Arguing is a part of life, and we get through it. It doesn't determine where we want to go. (Steve and Carol, 53 yrs)

Try and see things through your partner's eyes. (Mildred and William, 40 yrs)

You don't have to keep score. You don't keep score and say "Oh if she won that one I need to win this one." (Michael and Jennifer, 43 yrs)

Division of labour

All our tasks are done in love. They're much more important than just a job being completed. (Hermann and Linden, 54 yrs)

Finances

I never bought anything I didn't need with money I didn't have. (Ben and Isabella, 56 yrs)

Finding a relationship

Know who you marry and know what they're like and what they like. Know their friends, know their family. Know that what you're entering into is not just the wedding, and there's gonna be a long, tough draw, when you return home from the wedding into work. (Tony and Pat, 53 yrs)

There's no such thing as perfection, so don't try to find somebody who's perfect. Try to find somebody who you can live with the imperfections, and they have to live with the imperfections that you have. (Jim and Pat, 54 yrs)

Respect your family, not just the person you marry, but you respect the whole family that you are getting married into. You're marrying for life. (Gennaro and Maria, 65 yrs)

The wedding, it's like a big day, a big party, spending lots of money. Marriage is not about that. It's about all the periods ahead. Not that day, but the future. (Denis and Pauline, 44 yrs)

Trust your gut feelings that this is the right person for you. There is something inside of you that tells you whether it is the right person or not. And trust your partner. (Anne and Ergun, 41 yrs)

Forgiveness

So there are decisions that get made that you don't agree with so there is a lot of tension over many years, and I think that's where the forgiveness has to come in, on both sides, you know. (Sharon and Bob, 46 yrs)

Friendship

Build on the friendship aspect. Because when all else fails, you've got your friend. And friends look after each other. (Liz and Kevin, 40 yrs)

You've got to be friends with your partner. Otherwise, it's only jumping into bed. The lust stops after a while. (Bruce and Jan, 57 yrs)

We believe that marriage is not only for sexual gratification short term, but it's for long term companionship. (Romeo and Lunesa, 48 yrs)

Fun

Have adventures together, do things you're afraid of together. He helps me to do things I'm terrified to do, and once I've done it, I feel this rush of joy. Sharing an adventure where you're scared together creates a bond unlike any other that's so wonderful. (Laura and Russell, 50 yrs)

You can always find a randy man but it's hard to find a handyman. (Irene and Harry, 55 yrs)

Happiness

It's a lot better to go through life with a smile on your face than your head on your chest. (Lyle and Heather, 69 yrs)

Build up some good, good memories. So when the times get difficult, you can look back and think we did that, that's lovely, and then talk about it. (Kay and Keith, 52 yrs)

Humour

Humour is very important in a relationship, because if you try to see the humorous side of things, it'll keep you from becoming overly critical. (Don and Paula, 57 yrs)

We can laugh together, we can do things together, we can also argue together, not always agreeing in the end. (Beti and Clive, 60 yrs)

Individuality

I always say you don't own each other, you're still your own individual person. You have different hobbies and do different things. Trust was a big part of it. (Debby and David, 48 yrs)

You've got to be yourself. You can't be in a relationship and not be yourself otherwise you're fooling the other party all the time. (Rhonda and Peter, 53 yrs)

If you grab a handful of sand and squeeze really tight, it'll try and escape. If you hold it loosely, it'll stay around. It's like that in a relationship. (Marilyn and Gerry, 49 yrs)

He has his own views. And I have my own views. That's not a good enough reason to not stay together. (Avima and Steve, 41 yrs)

Intimacy

Sex is not love. (Stephen and Keith, 30 yrs)

Because you grow into love, it doesn't just happen like that. You know "love at first sight." Lust at first sight is mixed in with love at first sight. Especially for a bloke. (Graham and Lynette, 46 yrs)

In terms of sexual expression, I believe faithfulness starts in the choices I make. In the movies I watch, in the books I read. When you're younger, you expose yourself to things: they stay in your brain . . . they affect your physical response to [your partner]. (Pearl and Richard, 42 yrs)

Listening

You are born with two ears and a mouth. Listen to each other twice as much as you want to speak. (Allan and Carol, 55 yrs)

Longevity in relationship

Take a longer view rather than a short view. (Lana and Keith, 49 yrs)

Hang in there because life is so much better when you've got somebody to share it with. (Carol and Brien, 50 yrs)

A relationship is something that you work out. It's not something that if it works, you stay and if it doesn't work, you don't stay. (Frances and Wayne, 42 yrs)

It's not easy to click straight away. So we had to synchronize. It doesn't happen in one year, two years, three years. It takes a while. (Gaetano and Dorothy, 49 yrs)

Marriage is a long-term thing. And this little problem now is a short-term thing. So understand that and say, well, we can solve this and we can get on with our life. So why don't we do that? (Timothy and Samantha, 51 yrs)

Loyalty

Loyalty is something that's just kind of there in a relationship, that no matter how somebody treats you, you're still loyal. But commitment is a giving of energy to make sure that the relationship is stronger. So commitment makes it better. And that then adds to the loyalty, but it gives the loyalty a lot more texture. (Peggy and Howard, 48 yrs)

Parenting

When you have children, remember that you and he started off together. And you're going to be together at the end. If you've only got your kids keeping you together. What's the point? (Fay and Bill, 57 yrs)

She's always been first, the kids come second. (Jack and Judy, 60 yrs)

The family is critical. And whatever individual decisions you're making, they may benefit a member of the family more than another member. But the aim is to benefit the family unit. (Fred and Stella, 42 yrs)

Personality

I'm never going to change you even though I want you to be a little more outgoing, but that's not going to happen. You are who you are, I am who I am. (Gunter and Lee, 52 yrs)

I realized that because we were so different, we actually complimented or supplemented each other in many different things. (Alex and Alexandra, 58 yrs)

Romance

There are romantic times, and there is the nitty gritty that you have to deal with day by day. It's the pleasure and the pain. You need the balance between the two. (Margaret and Ian, 57 yrs)

Even though he may not be romantic, I know that I am loved. (Marge and Ted, 56 yrs)

Separating

It's very easy to slam the door on somebody, but it's very hard to re-open it. (Carol and Stephen, 40 yrs)

Don't be so quick to give up, it's not worth throwing everything away. Ride it out. (Annette and Bernie, 60 yrs)

No, I wouldn't divorce. Where else have we to go? I can't imagine anybody putting up with me like Peter does: he's faithful and solid, and it's secure. (Elizabeth and Peter, 60 yrs)

Don't be hasty about taking the easy road. Have a good long think about things. There are cases when you have to be hasty like if your marriage is violent: you're out of there. But most things can be worked through. (Merilyn and Gregory, 50 yrs)

We both went through divorces, and they're very, very painful, and they're not good for your ego. Everything seems like a disaster. So when we started dating, we said the most important thing is the relationship. In the end, it's the relationship that makes the difference. And so we've gotten this far. And I think we'll continue till one of us keels over. (Marion and Chuck, 44 yrs)

Don't throw away 80% of something that's good, looking for 20% that's missing. Because you'll end up with only the 20%. Make the 80%, make the 70%, make the 66%, make 53% work, and figure out how to fill in the rest of it. (Chuck and Steven, 30 yrs)

Supporting each other

When you marry, you get couples that are at different levels: the guy gets pulled down or gets pulled up. George feels that he was pulled up. (Franky and George, 44 yrs)

No matter how angry you are at that person for some other reason, you need to take care of each other through thick and thin no matter what. When there is sickness involved stick together. (Lucy and Frank, 55 yrs)

Man is head, woman is neck. Which direction are you going to turn? (Veselina and Boris, 73 yrs)

I'm out there looking at the horizon and she'll stop me from tripping over the curb, it's that kind of understanding. (Arnie and Liz, 51 yrs)

Tolerance

We need to be very compassionate and not get so upset, frustrated or angry with another person because we simply do not know what is going on for them. (Yin-Leng and Mike, 48 yrs)

Don't come with a set of expectations. . . . Your partner will never live up to what you really think is your ideal. (Anjelika and Graeme, 46 yrs)

We all have our moments. But you've got to learn to work around them. (Margaret and Merv, 59 yrs)

Tough times

Marriage is: you go this way, and then that way. You get there, but you don't go straight. (Jim and Kathy, 43 yrs)

It's going the slog and going forward through those really dark hours and finding the sunshine out the other end. (Jo and Rob, 47 yrs)

Don't take the easy way out come thick or hot water. If you find no other way, then work through it. (Patrick and Shirley, 48 yrs)

If you've got rocky times through your life, you don't throw in the towel. (Lana and George, 50 yrs)

So you had to stick at it or you were up the creek. We had to make it work. It was a case of make the decision. I made the decision. I had to fight to get Sharon's parent's permission to marry. (Peter and Sharon, 57 yrs)

We-ness

We think of ourselves as a jigsaw puzzle; if one of us is not there, the puzzle is not complete. (Susan and Bruce, 49 yrs)

It has been a partnership. What he brings to it and what I bring to it come together and it is ours, and it doesn't matter whether he brought more patience or I brought less patience, or my salary was higher than his for the first 20 years: it's ours. (Candy and Gregg, 49 yrs)

We are each other's biggest supporters. (Russell and Ruth, 40 yrs)

But on everything we talk it through first. I call that commitment. Don't do anything without telling the other one. (Jeanette and Malcolm, 64 yrs)

Say "we are a team." Be on the same page: faith, health, parenting, everything. (Olga and Raul, 45 yrs)

It's a commitment to a partnership, and partnership is working together, trusting and loving each other. (Tony and Cyndy, 49 yrs)

Appendix 2

The Surviving COVID-19 Survey

Demographics

There were 290 survey respondents from 21 countries and 37 ethnicities. 63% were female and 36% male and 1% were other. 49% had been together in an on-going relationship for 3–15 years, 41% for 16–40 years and 10% for 40+ years.

Questions

Included here is the list of the Multiple Choice, Likert and open-ended questions. The Surviving COVID-19 Survey results are discussed in Chapter 4.

1. Before Covid, say at the end of 2019, how would you have rated your overall RELATIONSHIP level of happiness?
2. During the Covid crisis and isolation times, how would you rate your overall level of RELATIONSHIP happiness?
3. Before Covid, say at the end of 2019, how would you have rated your partner's level of RELATIONSHIP happiness?
4. During the Covid crisis and isolation times, how would you rate your partner's level of RELATIONSHIP happiness?
5. BEFORE Covid, how much have these contributed to unhappiness in your relationship (rather than in you)?

    - Financial Stress
    - Mental Health Issues
    - Arguing
    - Children's needs
    - Constricted space

6. In comparison, SINCE Covid, how much have these contributed to unhappiness in your relationship (rather than in you)?

    - Financial Stress
    - Mental Health Issues
    - Arguing

- Children's needs
- Constricted space

7. Were their problems for your relationship during Covid Isolation?
8. If there were relationship problems, what were they?
9. If there were relationship problems, what helped?
10. Were your thinking of breaking up during Covid?
11. If you were thinking of breaking up, what contributed to this?
12. If you were thinking of breaking up, how has this been resolved?
13. Were their benefits for your relationship during Covid isolation?
14. If there were benefits, what were they?
15. What did you learn about your relationship during the Covid time?
16. If you could ask someone who has been married for 40+ years a relationship question, what would it be?

Appendix 3

The Married 40+ Years Survey

Demographics

There were 932 survey respondents from 47 countries and 81 ethnicities. 56% were female and 44% male. 68% had been married 40–49 years, 25% for 50–59 years and 7% for 60+ years.

Questions

Included here are the results of the Likert questions and a list of the open-ended and multiple-choice questions. The complete Likert, multiple-choice, and open-ended question answers will be used in future research. Discussing them all in this book is outside the scope of this current research. As discussed in Chapter 5, all the of the answers to the Married 40+ Years Survey broadly support the findings of the Thriving Couples Interviews.

Likert questions

1 How much have each of the following contributed to your relationship contentment?

Question	*None at all*	*A little*	*A moderate amount*	*A lot*	*A great deal*
Financial stability	6.06%	13.97%	38.02%	26.97%	14.95%
Understanding, acceptance, and being known	2.50%	8.70%	26.22%	40.69%	21.87%
Friendship	1.19%	4.88%	18.00%	39.15%	36.76%
Personality compatibility	3.59%	7.50%	25.89%	36.56%	26.76%
A decision for commitment	2.61%	4.46%	18.71%	38.41%	35.79%

Question	None at all	A little	A moderate amount	A lot	A great deal
Fidelity	4.34%	4.88%	18.24%	28.77%	43.64%
Satisfying sexual intimacy	5.18%	9.83%	30.27%	32.10%	22.59%
The ability to solve problems	1.51%	6.17%	21.66%	41.27%	29.36%
Support from parents and siblings	18.41%	17.87%	26.86%	22.96%	13.86%
Forgiveness	2.59%	7.80%	24.24%	37.33%	28.03%
Arguing (and making up) well	5.55%	15.46%	31.15%	32.24%	15.57%
Good communication	3.91%	7.72%	19.36%	38.95%	30.03%
The ability to compromise or sacrifice	1.74%	6.63%	20.02%	40.80%	30.79%
Laughing together and/or having fun	1.51%	8.67%	16.59%	32.86%	40.34%
Sharing values	2.38%	5.74%	15.49%	37.05%	39.32%
Shared activities	4.67%	11.41%	24.34%	33.47%	26.08%
Leaving space for one another	2.27%	6.50%	21.01%	42.68%	27.51%
Respect	1.62%	4.88%	16.50%	32.24%	43.73%
Religious affiliation	30.78%	13.53%	20.85%	17.24%	17.68%
The influence of children	13.52%	11.99%	27.69%	28.68%	17.44%

2 How much have each of the following contributed to your relationship discontentment?

#	Question	None at all	A little	A moderate amount	A lot	A great deal
1	Financial stress	31.20%	36.40%	19.71%	8.12%	4.55%
2	Work pressures	27.59%	34.52%	22.07%	12.44%	3.35%
3	Infidelity	68.11%	13.77%	11.06%	3.79%	3.25%
4	Time spent apart	51.51%	23.70%	15.90%	6.38%	2.48%
5	Poor communication	38.06%	32.97%	16.48%	8.35%	4.22%
6	Cultural clashes	70.91%	15.57%	7.18%	5.33%	0.98%
7	Arguing or "not talking" periods	37.48%	36.61%	14.62%	8.23%	3.03%
8	Inability to forgive or make-up	53.74%	23.99%	12.26%	7.69%	2.28%

#	*Question*	*None at all*	*A little*	*A moderate amount*	*A lot*	*A great deal*
9	Inability to manage problems	52.87%	24.10%	14.00%	7.16%	1.84%
10	High expectations	42.62%	27.54%	17.35%	9.00%	3.27%
11	Control issues	48.26%	22.21%	15.07%	9.00%	4.44%
12	Division of chores	47.60%	23.20%	18.40%	8.38%	2.39%
13	The pressure of child-rearing	46.08%	26.52%	17.71%	7.71%	1.95%
14	Religious affiliation	75.65%	9.89%	7.71%	5.21%	1.95%
15	Pressures from siblings or parents	66.95%	17.17%	10.06%	3.93%	1.85%
16	Dissatisfying sexual intimacy	56.73%	21.63%	12.39%	5.97%	3.26%
17	Personality clashes	47.71%	28.26%	14.45%	6.95%	2.60%

Multiple-choice and open-ended questions

3. What were your main reasons for marrying your partner?
4. What advice would you give your young self about looking for a long-term partner?
5. Looking back, what made this person a good love-partner for you?
6. What little things do you do, even daily, that help keep your relationship together?
7. In your experience, what are the 3 things (in order) of a good relationship?
8. What's your top tip for better arguing or conflict resolution?
9. What's your advice for Satisfying Sexual Intimacy?
10. If you had your time over, what would you change in your marriage?
11. What's your advice to people wanting their relationship to last as long as your relationship has?

Index

Note: Page numbers in *italic* indicate a figure and page numbers in **bold** indicate a table on the corresponding page.

For Product Safety Concerns and Information please contact our
EU representative GPSR@taylorandfrancis.com Taylor & Francis
Verlag GmbH, Kaufingerstraße 24, 80331 München, Germany